Social, Economic, and Political Perspectives on Public Health Policy-Making

Rahmatollah Gholipour
University of Tehran, Iran

Khadijeh Rouzbehani
University of Tehran, Iran

A volume in the Advances in Public Policy and Administration (APPA) Book Series

Medical Information Science Reference
An Imprint of IGI Global

Published in the United States of America by
Medical Information Science Reference (an imprint of IGI Global)
701 E. Chocolate Avenue
Hershey PA 17033
Tel: 717-533-8845
Fax: 717-533-8661
E-mail: cust@igi-global.com
Web site: http://www.igi-global.com

Library of Congress Cataloging-in-Publication Data

Names: Gholipour, Rahmatollah, editor. | Rouzbehani, Khadijeh, editor.
Title: Social, economic, and political perspectives on public health policy-making / Rahmatollah Gholipour and Khadijeh Rouzbehani, editors.
Description: Hersey, PA : Medical Information Science Reference, [2016] | Includes bibliographical references and index.
Identifiers: LCCN 2015046936| ISBN 9781466699441 (hardcover) | ISBN 9781466699458 (ebook)
Subjects: LCSH: Medical policy--United States. | Health care reform--United States.
Classification: LCC RA395.A3 S693 2016 | DDC 362.10973--dc23 LC record available at http://lccn.loc.gov/2015046936

This book is published in the IGI Global book series Advances in Public Policy and Administration (APPA) (ISSN: Pending; eISSN: Pending)

British Cataloguing in Publication Data
A Cataloguing in Publication record for this book is available from the British Library.

Advances in Public Policy and Administration (APPA) Book Series

ISSN: Pending
EISSN: Pending

Mission

Proper management of the public sphere is necessary in order to maintain order in modern society. Research developments in the field of public policy and administration can assist in uncovering the latest tools, practices, and methodologies for governing societies around the world.

The **Advances in Public Policy and Administration (APPA) Book Series** aims to publish scholarly publications focused on topics pertaining to the governance of the public domain. APPA's focus on timely topics relating to government, public funding, politics, public safety, policy, and law enforcement is particularly relevant to academicians, government officials, and upper-level students seeking the most up-to-date research in their field.

Coverage

- Government
- Law enforcement
- Political Economy
- Politics
- Public Administration
- Public Funding
- Public Policy
- Resource allocation
- Urban Planning

IGI Global is currently accepting manuscripts for publication within this series. To submit a proposal for a volume in this series, please contact our Acquisition Editors at Acquisitions@igi-global.com or visit: http://www.igi-global.com/publish/.

The Advances in Public Policy and Administration (APPA) Book Series (ISSN Pending) is published by IGI Global, 701 E. Chocolate Avenue, Hershey, PA 17033-1240, USA, www.igi-global.com. This series is composed of titles available for purchase individually; each title is edited to be contextually exclusive from any other title within the series. For pricing and ordering information please visit http://www.igi-global.com/book-series/advances-public-policy-administration/97862. Postmaster: Send all address changes to above address.

Titles in this Series

For a list of additional titles in this series, please visit: www.igi-global.com

Handbook of Research on Transitional Justice and Peace Building in Turbulent Regions
Fredy Cante (Universidad del Rosario, Colombia) and Hartmut Quehl (Felsberg Institute, Germany)
Information Science Reference • copyright 2016 • 559pp • H/C (ISBN: 9781466696754) • US $295.00 (our price)

Managing Big Data Integration in the Public Sector
Anil Aggarwal (University of Baltimore, USA)
Information Science Reference • copyright 2016 • 337pp • H/C (ISBN: 9781466696495) • US $205.00 (our price)

Management and Participation in the Public Sphere
Mika Markus Merviö (Kibi International University, Japan)
Information Science Reference • copyright 2015 • 399pp • H/C (ISBN: 9781466685536) • US $200.00 (our price)

Teaching Research Methods in Public Administration
Richard W. Schwester (City University of New York, USA)
Information Science Reference • copyright 2015 • 313pp • H/C (ISBN: 9781466681163) • US $185.00 (our price)

Emergency Management and Disaster Response Utilizing Public-Private Partnerships
Marvine Paula Hamner (LeaTech, LLC, USA) S. Shane Stovall (True North Emergency Management, USA) Doaa M. Taha (GMI, Ltd, USA) and Salah C. Brahimi (GMI, Ltd, USA)
Information Science Reference • copyright 2015 • 345pp • H/C (ISBN: 9781466681590) • US $200.00 (our price)

ICT Adoption and Application in the Malaysian Public Sector
Abdul Raufu Ambali (Universiti Teknologi MARA, Malaysia & Kwara State University Malete, Nigeria) and Ahmad Naqiyuddin Bakar (Universiti Teknologi MARA, Malaysia)
Information Science Reference • copyright 2015 • 316pp • H/C (ISBN: 9781466665798) • US $195.00 (our price)

Human Rights and the Impact of ICT in the Public Sphere Participation, Democracy, and Political Autonomy
Christina M. Akrivopoulou (Hellenic Open University, Greece) and N. Garipidis (Aristotle University of Thessaloniki, Greece)
Information Science Reference • copyright 2014 • 371pp • H/C (ISBN: 9781466662483) • US $185.00 (our price)

Table of Contents

Detailed Table of Contents

Policy making is a tool for modern societies to manage an array of public issues including health. At first, the concept and content of policy making will be described in this chapter. In order to do so, first the science of policy making and its history and objectives have been expressed and it is concluded that this science as a branch of political and administrative sciences considers the study of policies and certain functions of government in different fields. Then the concept of policy making and public policy are discussed. Since the current economic, social conditions and political values, government structure and cultural norms affect public policy making, the contexts of public policy making have been reviewed briefly. After that a variety of public policy, qualities of a good policy and the key factors in public policy making and rationality has been reviewed. In this chapter, in fact, the health policy will be studied as one of the crucial issues in this era and its dimensions will be discussed.

Local newspapers spend many square inches each week covering how long the fire department was on the scene of the most recent house fire or how many burglaries the police department had reported. Analysis of this public safety coverage indicated that, as in prior agenda-setting studies, it is correlated with policy change if only minimally yet continues to shed insight into a seldom-examined area of public health policy. Analysis of hundreds of news articles over a 10-year period in dozens of cities revealed that only about 1 percent of community newspaper coverage was devoted to pre-hospital healthcare — EMS. Subsequent qualitative investigation, which included interviews with EMS officials and newspaper reporters in cities identified with both high levels of coverage and low levels of coverage, found five potential reasons for the minimal coverage including that reporters simply were more interested in police/fire coverage and EMS simply was not on the radar screen of the citizens.

The chapter describes policy implementation components of a health system in United States of America and explains how they affect health outcomes (service delivery). It argues that implemented policies affect various components of a health system in terms of service delivery, workforce, information, financing, medical products, technologies, leadership and governance. Using health system as framework of analysis, the paper explains that the outcome of health policy implementation determines the availability, quality and equitability of program service delivery. The chapter goes on to argue that policy implementation barriers, such as demand- and supply-side barriers, market, insufficient resources, cultural barriers, imperfect communication, information, education, coordination, leadership and governance affect the poor and vulnerable groups in developed and developing countries from benefitting from public spending on public health policies and programs.

Annually, many deaths occur in Africa due to infectious diseases. African countries are predominantly low-income. A third of all deaths in low-income countries are caused by lower respiratory infections, HIV/AIDS, diarrheal diseases, malaria and tuberculosis. These preventable diseases continue to kill millions of Africans each year. More recently, Ebola Virus Disease (EVD) has killed thousands in Africa but even with the number of deaths attributable to EVD, it is still a fraction of the deaths caused by any one of the top five causes of deaths in low-income countries. This chapter examined the political economies that have enabled infectious diseases to thrive in Africa. The numerous conflicts, barriers to education, high fertility rates in the poorest countries and the privatization-tied conditions of loans were some of the factors identified. Ecological studies also suggest that changes in climatic conditions around the West African country of Guinea enabled the index case to come from Guinea. The foundational causes of the diseases have made the African nations susceptible. The chapter concludes with recommendations.

Preface

Healthcare is an important industry that touches most, if not all of us at some time in our lives. Healthcare is noted for using leading edge technologies and embracing new scientific discoveries to enable better cures for diseases and better means to enable early detection of most life threatening diseases. However, the healthcare industry globally has been extremely slow to adopt policies which focus on better practice management and administrative needs. Presently, healthcare is grappling with many challenges both nationally and globally, including escalating costs, a move to a preventative care environment and a technology savvy patient with high expectations. Hence, it is useful to think of the major challenges facing today's healthcare organizations in terms of the categories of demographics, technology, and finance. Healthcare organizations can respond to these challenges by focusing on three key solution strategies; namely: 1. Access - caring for anyone, anytime, anywhere; 2. Quality – offering world class care and establishing integrated information repositories; and 3. Value – providing effective and efficient healthcare delivery. These three components are interconnected such that they continually impact on the other and all are necessary to meet the key challenges facing healthcare organizations today.

This book will provide an extensive and rich compilation of various policies i and the role that public policy making plays and will play in the future of healthcare administration, delivery and management. International experts will address one or more of the areas of access quality and value and thereby represent ways in which healthcare delivery can be made superior and the healthcare industry can begin to address the major challenges it faces in the 21st century so that ultimately the most important person in the web of healthcare players, the patient, can be confident of receiving high quality, cost effective healthcare anytime, anywhere.

The purpose of the proposed encyclopedia is to bring together articles by international experts pertaining to critical concepts about the use, adoption, design and diffusion of policy making in healthcare. Ultimately the role of new theories, frameworks and methodologies in healthcare will address the challenges faced by today's healthcare environment. These challenges can be best examined under the categories of access, quality and value and the management of medical technologies and health policies must relate to addressing one or more of these challenges.

There is every reason to expect that this book will be used by all leading healthcare organizations throughout the US and globally as well as be a vital part of any universities' reference collection in the area of policy making, health policies in healthcare sector. Given that we extensively teach, research, and present in the area of management of medical technology and healthcare sector throughout the world, we are in no doubt as to the potential extent of the audience at a global scale.

This book is a compilation of 12 chapters – contributions discussing the approaches and processes for managing healthcare. These 12 chapters are written by 17 authors from all over the world, including many internationally renowned and experienced researchers and specialists in several disciplines and integrate contributions from academe, research institutions, and industry.

Chapter 1, "Policy Making: A New Method to Manage Public Issues" by Rahmatollah Gholipour, introduces the book with an overview of the fact that policy making is a tool for modern societies to manage public issues including health. At the beginning of this chapter, the science of policy making and its history and objectives are expressed and it concludes that this field as a branch of political and administrative sciences considers the study of policies and certain functions of government in different fields. Then the concept of policy making and public policy are discussed. After that a variety of public policy, qualities of a good policy and rationality in policy making is reviewed.

Chapter 2, "EMS Denied 15 Minutes of Fame: Newspaper Coverage of Pre-Hospital Healthcare Related to Policy Change" by Bradley Wilson, deals with analysis of hundreds of news articles over a 10-year period in dozens of cities .This research reveals that only about 1 percent of community newspaper coverage was devoted to pre-hospital healthcare — EMS. Subsequent qualitative investigation, which included interviews with EMS officials and newspaper reporters in cities identified with both high levels of coverage and low levels of coverage, found five potential reasons for the minimal coverage including that reporters simply were more interested in police/fire coverage and EMS simply was not on the radar screen of the citizens.

Chapter 3, "Health Policy Implementation and Its Barriers: The Case Study of US Health System" by Augustine Nduka Eneanya, offers a discussion to the problem of policy implementation components of a health system in United States of America and explains how they affect health outcomes (service delivery). It argues that implemented policies affect various components of a health system in terms of service delivery, workforce, information, financing, medical products, technologies, leadership and governance. Using health system as framework of analysis, the paper explains that the outcome of health policy implementation determines the availability, quality and equitability of program service delivery. The paper goes on to argue that policy implementation barriers, such as demand-and supply-side barriers, market, insufficient resources, cultural barriers, imperfect communication, information, education, coordination, leadership and governance affect the poor and vulnerable groups in developed and developing countries from benefitting from public spending on public health policies and programs.

Chapter 4, "The Political Economy of Infectious Diseases in Africa: Ebola Virus Disease (EVD) as a Case in Point "by Titilola T. Obilade, presents the issue of many deaths which occur in Africa due to infectious diseases. African countries are predominantly low-income. A third of all deaths in low-income countries are caused by lower respiratory infections, HIV/AIDS, diarrheal diseases, malaria and tuberculosis. These preventable diseases continue to kill millions of Africans each year. More recently, Ebola Virus Disease (EVD) has killed thousands in Africa but even with the number of deaths attributable to EVD, it is still a fraction of the deaths caused by any one of the top five causes of deaths in low-income countries. This chapter examines the political economies that have enabled infectious diseases to thrive in Africa. The numerous conflicts, barriers to education, high fertility rates in the poorest countries and the privatization-tied conditions of loans were some of the factors identified.

Chapter 5, "The States as Generators of Incremental Change in American Health Care Policy: 1935 to 1965"by Robert A. Peters and Minerva Cruz, comes to the issue of that literature does not acknowledge the impact of Congressional casework or the initial Social Security (OASI) eligibility criteria. There is, as a result, an inadequate appreciation for (1) the extent to which the initial development of federal policy was a function of Congressional delegations pursuing initiatives that would increase the flow of federal dollars their states could use to expand health services or (2) the way in which the regional cleavages created OASI eligibility criteria combined with the South's control of Congressional leadership positions to yield an expansion of health care for indigent people while intentionally delaying the creation of Medicare. This chapter addresses these gaps and provides a more complete picture of the way in which the incremental, unplanned evolution of federal health care policy was the product of using federal resources to diminish the states' fiscal needs and the south's capacity to temporarily control the health care agenda.

Chapter 6, "The Study of Public Reporting in Healthcare" by Ubaldo Comite exploits that public reporting, intended as the public disclosure of information on healthcare performance, is linked to the improvement of the quality of care through the incentives of selection and change, which are in turn determined by the availability of comparative information that is used by those outside the system (citizens) and those from within (organizations and professionals).The aim of this paper is to highlight how public reporting systems have the potential to not only support healthcare users in making informed choices, but to also foster healthcare structures in the improvement of their services.

Chapter 7, "A Revolutionary Look at Health Policy Analysis in Developing Countries" by Khadijeh Rouzbehani and Goltan Fakhteh Yavari, aims to focus on developing and poor countries. This study begins by looking at the health policy environment, and some of the challenges to researching this highly complex phenomenon. It focuses on research in middle and low income countries. Attention is drawn to the roles of the policy researcher and the importance of reflexivity and researcher's position in the research process and finally ways of advancing the field of health policy analysis is discussed.

Chapter 8, "Stakeholders Engagement and Agenda Setting in a Developing Context: The Case of the Bangladesh Health Policy" by Golam Rabbani, continues the discussion of developing countries. This paper explores this issue in the case of the development of the Bangladesh Health Policy 2011. It has discovered that the policy making process has many well-organized actors with very clear and efficient roles in generating policy outputs. This study indicates that the distinctions between policy making in western and eastern countries, at least in some countries, may be breaking down.

Chapter 9, "A Systematic Approach to Typology of Functions of National Health System" by Mostafa Zamanian and Zohreh Karimmian talks about the attempts which have been made for offering a comprehensive model in describing the functions. The OECD determined principles needed to offer an appropriate typology that should be independent of the names of health programs in different countries. In this chapter, an overview of the proposed models for structures and functions of the health system has been provided in order to propose a comprehensive health model with an emphasis on theoretical aspects of public policy-making and binding functions in any national development system.

Chapter 10, "On-Site Clinics: A New Model of Health Coverage in Local Government" by Robert Yehl, aims at health care costs. With the continued rising cost of health insurance and the fiscal constraints as a result of the 2007-09 economic recession requiring local governments in the U.S. to make cuts in employees, services, and benefits, it appears that on-site health clinics are one method of reducing, or at least, slowing health care costs. This chapter analyzes the use and benefits of such clinics for local government managers which is a new, but potentially effective method of both controlling costs and improving employee health.

Chapter 11, "Bridging the Gaps with Nonprofits: The Intersection of Institutions, Interests, and the Health Policy Process" by Laura Caccioppoli, investigates how nonprofits are both bridging the gaps left behind from health policy, and are at the intersection of institutions, interests, and the policy process. Using cultural competency as a theoretical lens, the chapter will make use of the current literature, demographic trends, and other qualitative and quantitative data to situate three case studies .Finally, the chapter offers an overview and evaluation of these policies as well as an explanation of the role nonprofits have in filling necessary service delivery and advocacy.

Chapter 12, "Redesigning the Organizational Structure to Reach Efficiency: The Case of Ministry of Health and Medical Education of Iran" by Mohammad Arabi, gives insights of the structure of an organization requires partial modification or even total redesigning due to the changes in missions, strategies, policies and objectives once environmental and technological changes take place. This evolutionary redesign and implementation of its plan can have the maximum effectiveness and efficiency when all aspects and components of a coherent structure are considered carefully. This research has considered redesigning the structure of the Ministry and outlines the methodology and undertaken activities in order to evolve the structure of the central department of Ministry to prove how a re-design in organizational structure followed by policy coherence can maximize the output in healthcare sector.

Throughout these 12 chapters, the reader of this book is confronted with the economics of information systems, the players and the market in information systems, and the global information infrastructure.

It presents the various aspects of both theoretical and empirical approaches in economic of information systems, the management of information systems, and digital business/markets. We are grateful to all authors for their efforts as the whole process of writing, reviewing, rewriting, editing, and proofreading needs a lot of time.

Chapter 1
Policy Making:
A New Method to Manage Public Issues

Rahmatollah Gholipour
University of Tehran, Iran

ABSTRACT

Policy making is a tool for modern societies to manage an array of public issues including health. At first, the concept and content of policy making will be described in this chapter. In order to do so, first the science of policy making and its history and objectives have been expressed and it is concluded that this science as a branch of political and administrative sciences considers the study of policies and certain functions of government in different fields. Then the concept of policy making and public policy are discussed. Since the current economic, social conditions and political values, government structure and cultural norms affect public policy making, the contexts of public policy making have been reviewed briefly. After that a variety of public policy, qualities of a good policy and the key factors in public policy making and rationality has been reviewed. In this chapter, in fact, the health policy will be studied as one of the crucial issues in this era and its dimensions will be discussed.

BACKGROUND

In March and in the early days of spring, our friends and I went to the local sports complex to play football. During the match, I had my forearm broken so we went to one of the main public hospitals. At the arrival to emergency ward, I saw many clients, each required special kind of therapy and health service .undoubtedly, chronic

DOI: 10.4018/978-1-4666-9944-1.ch001

health issues, accidents and incidents cause the high volume of visits to health care centers as a result of which these centers are not able to respond to the volume of referrals effectively. Besides that, due to difficulties arising from poor management, including inappropriate structures of health care centers, low-experienced staff, poor management of human resources, and so on that the present article is not seeking to discuss them, health service providers have usually difficulties delivering the right service on time. Having observed this inconvenience and delays in service, I decided to refer to one of the private hospitals in the city. Needless to say that the moment I arrived there the medical staff welcomed me and worked nonstop to treat the injury. During receiving therapy, I was obsessed with this question "who is responsible?" As a scholar in the field of public administration and policymaking, I kept thinking about it while I was resting indoor. A week later, I returned to faculty to have my lecture in policy making class. After greeting, students learned about what happened to me and that was a wonderful opportunity to be exploited to have further class discussions on public policy. My story was a case study to motivate learners to participate in the discussion .After brain storming and sharing various views based on different paradigms, we reached to this very point that there are different topics and issues in each society which need to be managed. Management system, to be more precise, is responsible in each country to manage activities and coordinate them. Usually this management system in each country has three levels: level of political affairs office, level of administrative affairs office and level of private sector management (Danayi fard, 2008).

Those three levels manage the society with close interaction with each other. Political affairs office identify the public issues by different methods and find a solution for them in parliament, public affairs office implements the legislated policies and private affairs office helps public affairs office with implementing policies in the hope of gaining more benefits. Thus the main role of political management is to recognize issues and prioritize them and find solutions for public issues and the main role of governmental management is to find appropriate methods to implement policies. Playing these roles in accepted way whether at political level or implementing level requires rationality and professional knowledge. Therefore, professionalization of these two levels is very important.

SCIENCE OF POLICY MAKING

The science of policy making tries to professionalize mentioned roles. Policymaking is the governance responsibility of governments. These measures are focusing on coordinating role of governments. Governmental management will affect policymaking in its own new role. Governments determine strategies and methods to deal with it, given to available public issues in society and issues that have possibility to be raised in future.Science of policymaking as a branch of political and administrative sciences studies the policies and specific measures of government.

Public policy consists of a series of government functions that are applied directly by the government or their representatives and affect introduced by government formation but it got new order simultaneously with establishing modern governments and got new identity in a scientific form and organized frameworks. From this point of view, experts consider the policy making a new scientific field that has been formed to have new recognition of relations between governments and citizens by efforts of scholars of political sciences, especially after World War II (Howlett & Ramesh, 2003, P. 3) The knowledge of policy making has been evolved based on most of conceptual developments during past 30 years. From late 1960s', the study of politics and its secondary contexts extended to a correct organized subject with courses, curriculums, schools of public policy.

Policymaking is the science of government practically and is a new branch of politics that benefits of sciences including Law, Economics and Sociology or Psychology according to its public scope and multi-dimensional issues that policies are defined to resolve them (Muller, 1998, p.11).

Public policymaking is a phenomenon that appears in a form of state program in one sector or geographic space. This Phenomenon as a process tries to list inappropriate functions that can be seen between one sector and another sector or one sector and the whole system. Three main qualities of knowledge are:

- **Being Multidisciplinary:** Means the science of policy making should go beyond the limited study framework of institutions and political structure and considers the findings and works of other sciences such as Sociology, Economics, Law and Politics.
- **Strongly Normative:** What we meant by quality of normative is that the science of policy making should not be deceived by appearance (scientific objectivity) but it should define the possibility of separation of goals, tools or values and techniques in study of governmental measures.
- **Seeking to Solve Problems:** Solving problems refers to this point that this science should take into account the origin of issues, its goal should be the real world and it should not involve in academic discussions that are mostly based on classic interpretations and sometimes complex and vague political texts. In this regard, the appropriate analysis of context around and community of policy making is very important. President Obama has mentioned social insurance and free health service as the main issue of his presidency

plans in his election mottos but because this policy was not compatible with economic and social realities of US society, there was just relative success in achieving this goal. In this way, the focus of discussion gradually emerges in relation with this title," the context of public policy".

CONTEXTS OF POLICY MAKING

Public policy does not form in a vacuum and it is influenced by social and economic conditions, governing political values, government structure and cultural, local and national norms. These contexts determine which problem is more important? Which alternatives should be considered more and what actions are more practical economically and politically? The context of public policy can be classified as cultural, political, economic and social contexts.

1. **The Social Context:** Social context and conditions affect political decisions in different ways. These conditions are dynamic and non-stationary. Changes in population due to migration, population growth, positive or negative, increasing or decreasing birth rate and other social changes, have changed attitudes and made changes in policies.
2. **Economic Context:** Economy of a government affects its policies and implanting those policies. Economic policies are facing inflation and unemployment. A strong or weak economy will bring various policies inevitably, for example, a strong economy has lower unemployment rates and leads to reduced need for welfare programs.
3. **The Political Context:** It is impossible to understand public policy regardless of the existing political context and politics. Policy context affects policies at every stage of the policymaking process. In order to understand the political context, policy makers and the people should be aware of the power of the major parties, effects of minor and smaller parties, ideological differences among people, especially those who are conservatives, careful and aware and committed Libertarian, and the ability and the power of main groups in order to use pressure. Democrats and Republicans, liberals and conservatives often have different attitudes to the legitimacy of government action and policies are being accepted (Kraft & Furlong, 2012, pp.13-17).
4. **Cultural Context:** One of the much influencing contexts for policy making is cultural context. Order making of a problem is priority and choosing solution and even decision making method influenced by cultural indexes. Hofstede (1980) argues that the continued use of a significant amount of decision-making depends on the cultural characteristics of subordinates, managers and policy

makers. According to Hofstede (1980), for example, managers use more collective decision making in culture of collectivism (Gholipour, 2008, p.53). Also, the fact that what issue should be on the agenda of policy-making and decision-making, and which groups are influencing the policy process, goes back to the cultural context of the organization and society and priorities that policy making groups and authorities consider. Therefore, given the effect of surrounding context on the decision making, decision makers should analyze the contexts in order to solve the problems of society and provide solutions. Policymaking of this context is political in some societies and this rules others. For example, in the case of social insurance in US or in the case of Iranian nuclear issue this is the political context that prevents achieving the optimal model to solve the problems of region with the supremacy of the technical context. Electoral system of US and competition of candidates during last years blocked access to a model for solving the problem of social security and health system.

THREE MAIN AREAS IN POLICY MAKING

Knowledge of policy making covers a wide range of issues because of above characteristics specially being multidisciplinary and many headlines have been considered for it. In one categorization, they can be classified in three main headlines: *Study of theory and conceptual basics of policymaking*, *Implementation and evaluation of public policies Analysis of public policies*

In the first headline, the researcher try to study theories, concepts and patterns of public policy making and different dimensions of a policy and the quality of its development and approvals in a procedural pattern and introduce the scientific methods which are used in policy making community. These sets of activities are called science of policy making.

Science of policy making is the study of who, what, when and how. Classic political science focuses on institutional governments that are combined with philosophical reason. Policy making is nothing more than study of political areas including generalship, elections, polling, legislation and judgment. Political science is the study of state policy making, description and explanation of reason and the effect of government activity. This focus includes the description of content of state policy and its effect on society, economy and political forces on the content of state policy, studying the different effects of institutional systems and political procedures on state policy making and assessing the results of state policies on society. Can one conclude three different motivations in the study of policy making with what has been described?

Scientific Motivation

Understanding effects and consequences of political decisions increases our knowledge toward society. This knowledge helps to develop more appropriate and more realistic analysis of a policy and considers it as basics for defining posterior policies. Scientific investigation based on procedure will keep away managers from managerial myopia and being superficial observers and this leads to consider issues all-encompassing.

Professional Motivation

Perception of causes and consequences of policy let us to use social sciences for solving scientific problems. The study of each policy improves the professional ability of policymakers and helps them to define policies with higher skills.

Political Motivation

Assessing public policies, comparison of predicted goals of policy and its results all are done by governmental or non-governmental authorities.

Carol H. Weiss (1997) believes that paying attention to assessment is for determining the reputation and suitability of programs and public policies. It is what role these programs have in solving public issues and what is their orientation.

The aforementioned motivations over the years have helped policy making to play a role as a series of sciences in policy making atmosphere and attract the attention of policy makers to those who have this knowledge. This knowledge tries to increase the scientific aspect of these policies and prevents policy makers from being politicization in formulating policies. The main pillar of this knowledge is fundamental principle of "rationality in policy making".

RATIONALITY IN POLICY MAKING

According to this principle, it is assumed that when policies have executive ability and can balance the target population and are based on conceptual foundation. It is defined based on the framework of the rationality. Policies which are the developed by governments are affected by various kinds of rationality. There are four types of rationality that affect state policies (Danayifard, 2008,p.38):

1. Economic rationality,
2. Political rationality,

Figure 1. Rationalities influencing policymaking

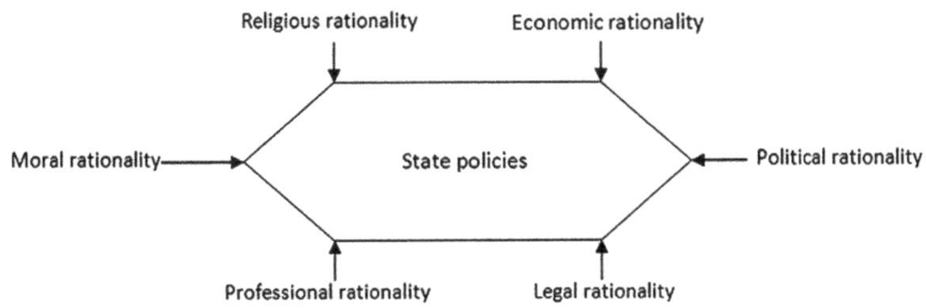

3. Legal rationality,
4. Professional Rationality.

On the other pathway (Danayifard, 2008,p.38), we can also consider two types of rationalities that rule human societies:

5. Moral rationality,
6. Religious rationality.

Therefore government policy is influenced by a variety of rationalities (figure 1).

- **Economic Rationality:** Means the alignment of the policy with limited resources of society. Hence, if economic rationality accomplishes in government policies then policies are implemented in limited resources. Then it is said that this government has put economic rationality in his agenda. Therefore, because the urgent needs of the people are high, which shall be collectively signed and at the same time available resources are limited, economic rationality is necessary.
- **Legal Rationality:** Its main elements are: the right of fair justice, legal security and protection of voluntary measures of citizens." Therefore, It is the policy having legal rationality that is formulated by relying on the Constitution and other laws, and do not distort those elements in formulation, implementation and modification, and termination of policies.
- **Political Rationality:** The government, in which political values are bound in policies in terms of different dimensions, will be government with focus on political rationality and in order to show political wisdom it should make policies as political ones.
- **Professional (Scientific) Rationality:** A wise professional government is the one with scientific policies. Professional rationality will be accomplished when it can develop scientific policies, i.e. they are scientific from the stage

of understanding the problem, formulating the agenda, policy formulation and implementation to evaluation, modification and termination policies based on scientific principles.

- **Moral Rationality:** Policies that are based on ethics and reinforce public morality include a level of moral rationality. Heavy penalty of immoral government in policies is the lack of citizens association by implementing the policies.
- **Religious Rationality:** If government complies with religious values in is various policies, will believe in religious rationality. Therefore policies that are formulated in a political system based on religious values, and reinforce religious values are religiously important. During historical study we can search the amount of institutionalization of rationality in the various processes of policymaking knowledge.

In the analysis of these policies it should be considered a combination of rationalities. In this context, and in the analysis of health policy, for example, the policies of the family doctor, in Iran met many problems while implementing because it was not in framework of economic rationality and not enough resources were determined to implement them and it could not achieve goals. From this point of view we can analyze the mentioned policy as irrational or with low rationality coefficient. Thus it will be opened a new chapter in policymaking literature with this title "policy analysis".

POLICY ANALYSIS

One of main areas in policymaking is policy analysis. Policy analysis is a vast world of concepts, knowledge and dimensions and it is considered as specialty and variable intervening knowledge in improving and developing policies (Gholipour & Faghihi, 2014,p.10). In the words of Harold Lasswell(1971) "policy analysis is to create related and internal knowledge of policymaking". Kraft and Furlong (2012) argue policy analysis can help to clear issues, effectiveness and efficiency of a policy and finally selection and preference of policymakers and public (Kraft & Furlong,2012). Dunn (2007), believes the main aim of policy analysis is improving policymaking (Dunn,2007,p.56). From Dye (1997) point of view, policy analysis includes:

1. First description of target policy (it should not be evaluated at the beginning).
2. Exact search of effects and consequences of policy.
3. Efforts to create and investigate public propositions about effects and consequences of policy.

Also Dye(1997) classified main elements in three items of description, factual basic of information and causes (Dye, 1997).Dunn also extended these items and described policy analysis in five main measures (Dunn,2007, 61): problem structuring, forecasting, recommendation, monitoring and evaluation. So policy analysis is the starting point in order to improve the policy-making process and its consequences. Evaluation based on Dunn's description is one of the policy analysis elements. In Assessment, the amount of achieving goals is considered and to what extent could achieve goals by applying solution. But in policy analysis the whole process of policymaking from problem definition to application and evaluation are investigated. In policy analysis, an organized methodology will be developed in order to solve complex problems that has multi-dimensional variables and because of these it will do quantitative and qualitative analysis and helps policy makers in achieving his rational goal. Thus this area of policy analysis is considered as main headlines of policymaking knowledge.

ORIGINS OF PUBLIC POLICYMAKING

Analysis of policymaking formation is one of the important issues that helps us to study the nature of public policy.

Formation of public policymaking resulted from the different reading of general action that has been developed in an evolutionary process, provides the ability to think about a new relation with people and world. To understand the scientific history of public policymaking we should consider three streams of thought. These are: thinking about bureaucracy, thinking about the idea of organization theory and finally thinking about the management of public affairs(Gholipour,2008,p.109).

1. Idea of bureaucracy that is a product of the nineteenth century and the industrial revolution in the West that focuses on bureaucratic development and development of intelligence in history and government can find insight because of this and by using legal mechanism it will protect public interests(Weber,1994).

Hegel and Wood (1991) believe that this is only government that have public insight and is superior than personal interests and can improve the level of interests. In this stage, government will be developed by using Law and regulations and public policy making will be a necessity. The government here undertakes regulatory activities and public policymaking considers functions and the role of government in civil society. In this regard, the main thought developed is welfare state. The expanding government intervention in civil society and undertaking different roles in society results in maximizing the regulatory role and determining the maximum policies for society. According to Muller(1999), the action scope of bureaucratic system has not been developed and used methods by decision makers of public area became too complex and varied. Opponents argue that the state is used by ruling class and it cannot provide public interests (Marx,2011)

2. Philosophy of organizations and organization theory that were developed after a kind of high dissatisfaction from Taylor organizational impacts has played an important role in public policymaking formation.

Three fundamental concepts in organizational philosophy have showed the policy making a necessity.

The first concept, is the organized concept based on which organization will be considered as an actor that can analyze the action and its relation with context and can determine practical principles for different players despite their preferences.

The second concept, is a concept of power that determines the amount of capacity and people ability in different context in order to maximize their resources and strengthen their position in the organization and in order to institutionalize and control it, requires rules and mechanisms (the policy primarily plays a main role in determining theses rules).

The third concept is the concept of strategy based on which human action is to use and appropriate and non-appropriate operation of relevant rules and regulations, formal and informal regulation of organization. The mobilization of resources that can act assumed to be centered on a strategy which aims to achieve predetermined goals.

3. General management thought as the language of administration in a complex society is a series of logical ways that serve decision makers in public affairs.

The formation of public management along with reinforcing the image of rationality and novelty of bureaucratic system have the same meaning with new reading of government role in society. This will make government to involve effectively in organization affairs and use their power and direct and indirect governmental policies have determining role in organization affairs. Also it makes managers to consider issues out of organization before issues inside the organization and be accountable to certain issues. To value governing values, social priorities and state policies are of issues that managers pay attention to more along with goals of organization. In the idea of public management, organizations have faced changes. One of the main changes is rules of the game in dealing with public issues.

The role of organizations in past was only more production in line with economic mission. Today its role is mostly political-social and political-economic. In line with this role and new mission, issues of organization will be mostly public issues and managers and organizations have collective efforts in order to manage these issues. Based on this view, nowadays issues related to health area are not related to health care organizations but all public organizations are responsible to solve this problem. As private organizations and manufacturing companies play a role in environmental pollutions, they must be responsible the same more and even more.

From this point of view, public policy making resulted from paying attention to public issues that is known as a new dimension in today's management and policy makers and organizational managers try to manage these issues responsively.

POLICY MAKING AND PUBLIC AFFAIRS

Based on the above reasoning, public policymaking is the result of attention to public affairs, issues that are the origin of public policy making and policies are formulated in order to response to them and to solve public problems. In fact the origin of public policymaking is public issues and in order to solve them, applying available strategies by public organizations should be considered in addition to identification of those issues, evaluation of their effects, analysis of issues. Public policy can be defined in context of public problems .Kraft and Furlong (2012) believe that public policy can be defined in different ways but public policy is a set of state measures in order to response to social problems. Social problems are situations that are not acceptable by public and are understood in a wide level and they need an intervention. Issues such as health, work place security, accessing services and serving healthcare services that are required to be solved by government or private sector or combination of both.

In this case, those issues that are required to solve by public organizations, are considered enough serious by policy makers and will be placed in policy making procedures and their results will be a package of policymaking in line with solving their issues. In this regards there is required policymaking in both local and national levels.at local level, health, employment rates and unemployment rates, high rate of inflation and urban fights can attract the attention of mayor or city council to do something about policymaking. At national level, policy makers force to do policy making based the concerns of the lack of access to health care services fairly or the lack of trust on government and similar issues. Thus it can be seen that the main origin of policy making are public issues and social problems that organizations(public or private) and government are responsible for formulating policy and implementing it in order to solve problem.

WHAT IS A PUBLIC ISSUE?

Several definitions of this have been provided some of which are as follows; "Public issue is stress and need that have public aspect and has been created by undermining public interests, therefore it is based on our perception of public interest."(Alvani,1992); "public issue can be considered as a need, shortage, limitation or even an opportunity in society that can be recognized and exploited for betterment"(Dunn,2007); "social issues are social phenomena including structural conditions or interaction patterns that are in a line of social changes, development of status quo and desired status that attract the attention of people and social groups and prevent accomplishment of goals and threaten values. Social issues are considered as not desired issues by elites and people in a way that there will be created a consensus and collective readiness in order to deal with them that make governors to take actions to solve, prevent or modify them"(Abdollahi,2007).

Now according to above definitions we can define public issues: there is a difference between what should be and what it is, people will feel it and are dissatisfied by interests from this phenomena in current situation for all people and they take an action to modify it and find suitable solutions to make the situation desirable in official systems of government.

One of the issues should be considered in above definition is that an issue can cover two subjective and objective dimensions and what makes the need of change is subjective dimension and what is changed is objective dimension of an issue. Of characteristics of public issues differentiate them is its multidimensional. Also a public issue has various aspects and different views govern them. Public issues appear as a set of consistent series and affect each other. Therefore policies should be choose to solve these issues and should have systematic approach. One of the main points in public issues is when it is so obvious that the need of public action will be inevitable. Collective feeling will be about an issue and its effects can be generalized to other social issues. This is not intrinsic social issue for a society but is resulted by situations. Based on this introduction, it can be said that public issues have two subjective and objective dimensions (Lowspa, 2004), and it is not personal and it is collective and will be solved by human intervention and the benefits resulted by changes in social issue for the society is relative.

Public Issues and Public Policy

All of the public issues are not understood the same by policymakers, groups of stakeholders and people and variables including: the salience of issues from the perspective of people and elites, novelty of issue, understanding costs and resulted benefits, technical, social, economic and political complexity of an issue, The as-

Table 1. Agreement on goal and mean of public problems

Complex problems	Technical problems	Low	Agreement upon mean
Ethical problems	Simple problems	High	
Low	High		
Agreement on goal			

sumption of suitable role of government all affect the understanding effective issues. Understanding an issue and finding solution for them largely depends on the agreement between goal and mean. In agreement or dis agreement between goal and mean states will be created as shown in table 1.

Lindblom (2002) stated that "policy makers are not faced with a problem but they should be able to identify and formulate the problem. The most important part of public policy is here, where the ongoing dispute between groups is for putting their own issues in ordering policy. Some issues never enter ordering state measures because they want to be far away from social norms and values (Bosso, 1994, pp.96-99).

MANAGING PUBLIC ISSUES

With regard to the importance of public issues for the organization, managing and controlling them and selecting appropriate strategies for dealing with them may be considered necessity in the organization. the definition of public issues management, It is said that: "Public issues management is a procedure by which organization can recognize public and social issues related to itself and evaluates them and prioritize them in terms of their sensitivity and importance in order to response effectively." (Buchholz, Evans, Wagley,1985, PP. 41-42) Or in another definition, "public issues management is a procedure based on which social and state issues can recognize, evaluate and control the affection on the activity of organization (Rosenthan & Buchholz,2004, p.43). Also this management is considered as an effort to forecast public issues in relation to institute and then to investigate mentioned issues in a way to choose appropriate strategy and to keep long –term benefits (Alvani & Ghasemi,1998, p.101). Based on this description, it can be claimed that public issues management caused structural changes in organizations. These structural changes show the importance of public issues than before (Alvani,1992,pp.29-30).

Managers today for decision -making, in addition to economic useful factors, should have sufficient knowledge about the factors being considered are non -economic. In current times, skills and other abilities such as political skills, communication and analyzing skills are important for managers. Nowadays public issue management has become more important than before. public issues affects the image of organization for people and this affect covers the whole levels of organization. An organization that does not care about public issues makes a bad image in public minds. Success and survival of organization mostly depends on being sensitive to environmental changes and survival and long-term efficiency of organization depends on its attention to public context.

The context of organization activity is more cleared than before and businesses are offered to public and caused to limit the maneuver space of organization. So societies are affected faster than before by dissatisfying actions and behaviors and this led to motivate governors in formulating preventive policies. Organization will move to mortality the more they show no interest in social and public issues. Future organizations should established by using sensitive frameworks to available issues. Public issues management let us to deal with issues before they reach to unpleasant and critical point and losing opportunities (Rosenthan & Buchholz, 2004, pp.43-47.).

PUBLIC ISSUES SYSTEM OF MANAGEMENT

To respond effectively to public issues we should be take regular and systematic action. Effective response to public issues is part of the new tasks of chief executives. To do this, we require the design of public issues management. This system includes the following steps:

1. **Recognition and Identification of Issues:** In this stage, the public issues related to missions and goals of organization should be recognized. To do this, environmental issues affecting organization through public policy procedure should be recognized. Then these issues should be checked regularly and their changes should be studied and their short and long-term effects on organization performance should be recognized and investigated (Alvani & Ghasemi,1998,p.32). Many times it is seen that bureaucrats and policy makers and even media and people and as whole actors of policy will recognize consequences, effects and side effects in order to identification of issue and its introduction to policy making institution and they think that this is a consequence of issue itself, they develop solutions that their implementation does not result in solving public issues. Therefore, understanding the issue and the nature of pivotal point in this stage.
2. **Evaluation the Effects of Public Issues:** When public issues are identified. their actual and potential effects should be carefully evaluated . The reason for this assessment is prioritization of public issues for appropriate response.

In evaluating issues, their social effects, the probability of their occurrence power of organizing in response to them should be studied. The results of this action is preparation of a list of public issues and their preferences(Rosenthan & Buchholz,2004,P. 47).

3. **Public Policy Analysis:** This process involves research and analysis of public issues that had higher preferences in previous stage. To do this, to ask help from experts and professionals can be efficient and effective . In stage of research and analysis, the aim is not only to examine and explore the issues, but also strategies for handling the issues to be investigated and providing solutions for decision makers. The outcome of this stage is analysis of different dimensions of issues including status and for and against strategies and professionals should propose various strategies to deal with them(Rosenthan & Buchholz,2004, PP.47-48).
4. **Strategy Selection:** We have now to choose appropriate strategies in order to deal with public issues. In this stage, the role of organizations are more highlighted. Enforcement agencies should pay attention to their actual and potential resources and the consider the interests of society and organizations then choose the right strategy. There have been four main strategies for responding to public issues:
    a. **Reactive Strategies:** In this strategy, organization does not care to public and social issues of their territory and they resist to their own formulated policies. This strategy is called "stone wall" as well (Givarian & Rabiei, 2005, p.48).
    b. **Accommodative Strategies:** In this strategy, organization adapt itself with changes in the environment and public politics and tries to place in mainstream business rapidly .
    c. **Proactive Strategies:** The aim of this strategy is to prevent the effects of public issues. For instance, organization tries to change the environment of public issue occurrence.
    d. **Interactive Strategies:** In this strategy, organization respect the desire of society and seeks to influence it. In this strategy, organization cannot pass public issues and does not see itself to be given up toward them and does not want to affect them unilaterally but sometimes it affects public opinions and in other times this is organization that will change its behavior. Applying this strategy as the most appropriate strategy is offered to managers of organization (Rosenthan & Buchholz, 2004, pp. 54-56).
5. **Implementation of Strategy:** This process is implemented based on policies and strategies by benefiting plans, budgets and trends. In other word, the process of implementation of strategy represents the series of activities

and choices that are necessary to implement strategies and strategic policies. Implementing strategy appropriately requires efficient people. Therefore in this process, three questions should be answered:

a. Who are the performers of macro policies and related strategies?
b. What should do to implement these strategies and related policies?
c. How these performers want to implement these policies and related strategies?

The main part in this stage is to change organization performance, the effect on public opinions and changing he ideas of policy makers (Alvani,1998,p.107). In this stage, public relations has a very important role because it can explain the actions of organization in relation to control social and public issues to society and on the other hand reflect the effect of these actions on different social groups to organization.

6. **Evaluation of Strategy:** In this sage, we should evaluate strategic missions to use in order to ensure their effectiveness in achieving desired results. This stage is very difficult because success determination of organization actions in satisfying social environment is not easy. In other words, the issue of evaluating strategy is in the lack of criteria that can measure qualitative issues or all of these issues cannot be an excuse to ignore evaluating this strategy. This stage causes modification of missions, removal or addition of activities in implementation of the strategy (Rosenthan & Buchholz, 2004, pp. 49-50).

Based on above pattern if health is considered as a social and public area that is in real, the problems of this area also have social and public dimensions and require their management in pattern of public issue management. Based on this pattern, a procedure should be designed based on which health issues start with recognition of public issues and in the following goes to evaluate the effects of public issues, analysis of public issues, selection of strategy, implementation of strategy and finally ends in evaluation of strategy. This procedure is based on strategic pattern that is activated in framework of policymaking measures in health issues.

CONCLUSION

The review of politics and policy making in context of public issues and in health area was of goals of this chapter. To do this, first policy making and its background and goals were explained and concluded that this Science as one of the branches of administrative and political sciences studies policies, certain state measures in various fields. Then the concepts of policy making and public policy were discussed. In this part, different definitions of public policy were represented that included a series of state functions that were implemented directly by government or its representatives and affected public life. Since economic, social, governing political issues, structure of government and cultural norms affect public policy, we discussed contexts of public policy briefly.

Since nowadays governments in all communities involve in organizational affairs in a way and use their power and direct and indirect state policies have a determining role in affairs of organizations, managers should be accountable to external issues more than internal issues, especially society. In this regard, the new role of organizations will be mostly public issues. From this point of view, public policy making resulted from attention to public issues that are the origin of public policy making and policies are formulated in order to respond to them and solving public issues of society. Indeed, the origin of public policy making is public issues and in order to solve them, the analysis of issues and applying available strategies should be considered by organizations in addition to recognition of those issues, evaluation of their effects. In this case, those issues to be necessary to be researched by public organizations, should be considered important by policy makers and be placed in a procedure of policy making that it results in a package of policy making in line with that issue. Health issues are shown in headlines because of their importance and the extent of target population. Finding and choosing a rational framework of policy making in this area will help a lot in making healthy society and maturation of human societies to achieve a thriving and healthy community. What will be followed in this book is addressing this main issue and achieving such framework.

REFERENCES

Abdollahi, M. (2007). Developing social issues in Iran: goals and requirements. Letter of Sociology Association, 3, 12.

Alvani, M. (1992). Public issues in management. *Quarterly of Management Studies*, *2*, 29-30.

Alvani, M., & Ghasemi, A. R. (1998). *Management and social responsibilities of organization.* Education Center of State Management.

Bosso, C. J. (1994). The Practice and Study of Policy Formation. Northeastern University.

Buchholz, R. A., Evans, W. D., & Wagley, R. A. (1985). *Management Response Public Issues*. Prentice Hall.

Buchnolz, R. A., & Rosenthan, S. B. (2004). Stakeholder Theory and Public Policy: How Government Matters. *Journal of Business Ethics*, 51.

Dunn, W. (2007). *Public policy analysis: An introduction*. Englewood Cliffs, NJ: Prentice-Hall.

Dye, T. R. (1997). Understanding Public Policy. Prentice Hall.

Gholipour, R. (2008). *Organizational decision making and public policy making*. Samt Publication.

Gholipour, R., &Faghihi, M. (2014). *Policy making and public policy analysis*. Mahkame Publication.

Givarian, H., &Rabiei, M. R. (2005). *Decision making and state policy making* (2nd ed.). Yekan Publication.

Hasan. (2008). *Challenges of governmental management in Iran*. Samt Publication.

Hegel, G. W. F. R., & Wood, A. W. (1991). *Hegel: Elements of the Philosophy of Right*. Cambridge University Press.

Hofstede, G. (1980). *Culture's Consequences: International Differences in Work-Related Values*. Beverly Hills, CA: Sage Publications.

Howlett, M., & Ramesh, M. (2003). *Studying Public Policy*. Oxford University Press.

Kraft, M. E., & Furlong, S. R. (2012). Public policy: Politics, Analysis, and alternatives (4th ed.). CQ Press.

Lasswell, H. D. (1971). *A Pre-view of Policy Sciences*. New York: American Elsevier Publishing Co.

Lindblom, C. E. (2002). *The Market System: What it Is, how it Works, and what to Make of it*. Yale University Press.

LowsPa, D. (2004). *New approach in social issue analysis*. Tehran: Amirkabir Publication.

Marx, K. (2011). *Capital: volume one, A critique of political economy*. Dover Publications.

Muller, P. (1999). *Les politiques publiques*. Montchrestien.

Weber, M. (1994). *Political Writings*. University of Cambridge Press.

Weiss, C. H. (1997). *Evaluation* (2nd ed.). Prentice Hall.

KEY TERMS AND DEFINITIONS

Evaluation: Policy evaluation is conducted for checking the effects of the policies of respective ministries and for evaluating the policies in terms of necessity, efficiency, validity, etc. to improve the planning and implementation process.

Health Policy: Health policy broadly describes the actions taken by governments---national, state, and local---to advance the public's health. It is not a single action but requires a range of legislative and regulatory efforts ranging from ensuring air and water quality to supporting cancer research. Health care policy is that piece of health policy that deals with the organization, financing and delivery of health care services. This includes training of health professionals, overseeing the safety of drugs and medical devices, administering public programs like Medicare and regulating private health insurance.

Implementation: Public policy implementation consists of organized activities by government directed toward the-achievement of goals and objectives articulated in authorized policy statements.

Policy Analysis: Policy analysis is "determining which of various policies will most achieve a given set of goals in light of the relations between the policies and the goals". However, policy analysis can be divided into two major fields. Analysis of policy is analytical and descriptive—i.e., it attempts to explain policies and their development. Analysis for policy is prescriptive—i.e., it is involved with formulating policies and proposals (e.g., to improve social welfare).The area of interest and the purpose of analysis determines what type of analysis is conducted. A combination of policy analysis together with program evaluation would form policy studies.

Policy Outcomes: The outcome of what is implemented.

Public Policy: The principled guide to action taken by the administrative executive branches of the state with regard to a class of issues in a manner consistent with law and institutional customs. The foundation of public policy is composed of national constitutional laws and regulations.

Public Policy Program: An interdisciplinary program connecting the theoretical and analytical tools of economics, political science, philosophy, psychology, and law with their real-world policy applications.

Public Problem: Problem definition is a package of ideas that includes, at least implicitly, an account of the causes and consequences of undesirable circumstances and a theory about how to improve them. As such, it serves as the overture to policymaking, as an integral part of the process of policymaking, and as a policy outcome. In each of these roles it seems to exert influence on government action. Distinguishing among the roles clarifies the nature of that influence.

Chapter 2
EMS Denied 15 Minutes of Fame:
Newspaper Coverage of Pre-Hospital Healthcare Related to Policy Change

Bradley Wilson
Midwestern State University, USA

ABSTRACT

Local newspapers spend many square inches each week covering how long the fire department was on the scene of the most recent house fire or how many burglaries the police department had reported. Analysis of this public safety coverage indicated that, as in prior agenda-setting studies, it is correlated with policy change if only minimally yet continues to shed insight into a seldom-examined area of public health policy. Analysis of hundreds of news articles over a 10-year period in dozens of cities revealed that only about 1 percent of community newspaper coverage was devoted to pre-hospital healthcare — EMS. Subsequent qualitative investigation, which included interviews with EMS officials and newspaper reporters in cities identified with both high levels of coverage and low levels of coverage, found five potential reasons for the minimal coverage including that reporters simply were more interested in police/fire coverage and EMS simply was not on the radar screen of the citizens.

DOI: 10.4018/978-1-4666-9944-1.ch002

INTRODUCTION

When Face the Nation moderator Bob Schieffer closed his program the weekend before the 13th anniversary of 9/11, one of the worst days in American history, he recalled how Congress came together to sing "God Bless America" and how people waved and honked, carrying signs that read "I love America." He also recalled the first responders who put their lives at risk. "Most of all, I remember the heroic firefighters and police officers," he said on the Sunday program (Schieffer, 2014). Not a mention of EMS, despite 12 medics dying in the collapse of the World Trade Center that day (National EMS Memorial Service, 2001). And CBS News is not alone. It was not even close. Barely a mention. When it came to coverage of local emergency medical systems in community newspapers, readers would barely know the EMS system existed. Given that media coverage, including coverage of public safety issues, is correlated with public opinion and policy change, that lack of coverage may have impact on how such systems operate.

BACKGROUND

That media coverage leads to public opinion and then to policy outcomes has been well-documented in a growing body of academic research. In 1993, Rogers, Dearing and Bregman found 223 publications that explicitly or implicitly concerned agenda setting. Of the publications they examined, 59 percent concerned mainly the relationship between the media and its corresponding public agenda. In 1996, Dearing and Rogers discussed the results of more than 350 publications on agenda setting. Eight years later, McCombs summarized more than 400 "empirical studies" of agenda setting. All of these studies expanded upon the basic idea that McCombs and Shaw, who wrote "The Agenda-Setting Function of Mass Media" in 1972, developed and popularized — at least when it comes to national issues — the idea that by ignoring some problems and attending to others, the mass media profoundly affect which problems readers, viewers and listeners take seriously (Cohen, 1963; Funkhouser, 1973; Weaver, McCombs & Spellman, 1975; Page & Shapiro, 1992; McCombs & Valenzuela, 2014).

Despite all these studies, while national issues make headlines every day and are continually the focus of research, comparatively little research has been done about what impact local media can have on policy. Ithiel de Sola Pool (in Schramm, 1963, p. 136) argues that media outlets would be more effective if they covered local contests more often and more in-depth so they could mobilize the community's sluggish but basically more persuasive oral communication system:

The press pays great attention to a presidential campaign. It gives thousands of columns of space to it. Yet the net effect of the press on the voter's choice is small. It gives very little attention to contests for minor local offices. Yet its net effect on the voter's choice for these is substantially greater. The press in the United States is much more influential in local than in national elections.

Covering such local campaigns and issues falls not to national papers such as *USA Today* or to regional newspapers such as the *Dallas Morning News* or *Seattle Times*. "CNN is not coming to my town to cover the news, and there aren't a whole lot of bloggers here either," said Robert M. Williams Jr., editor and publisher of *The Blackshear Times* in Georgia. "Community newspapers are still a great investment because we provide something you can't get anywhere else" (Liedtke, 2009). Local newspapers, and local issues, do not draw the attention of the larger newspapers, television stations, the Huffington Post or Jon Stewart. "We still think community newspapers have an audience and it's not going away," Richard Connor, publisher of *The Times Leader* in Wilkes-Barre, Pa., (weekday circulation of about 36,000), said. "There will always be an audience for local news" (Liedtke, 2009). Indeed, as McCombs (2006, e-mail) notes, "There is very little work in the entire field of political communication on state and local elections and public opinion." As a review of agenda-setting patterns found in case studies, cross-sectional studies and experiments shows, more research into how and if newspaper agenda-setting works at the local level is warranted. (Wilson, 2012)

Ray Funkhouser (1973) wrote that the news media are our only way of knowing, at the time, what is happening in the world outside our immediate experience. Without the media, residents may not think about topics, including pre-hospital healthcare and EMS, when it comes time to advocate for policy change, to recruit volunteers or to change budget allocations. As part of a local bureaucracy or a publicly funded agency, how EMS agencies function can be just as distant to most residents as how the roads are repaired or how water is delivered to their tap. Headlines such as "Richlands EMS suspended from medical calls" after the state EMS agency received a complaint against the agency (Pippin, 2014) or "EMS Run by Idiots" (Mills, 2013) when concerns caused by delays in EMS response times after a 2-year-old was accidentally killed when his father hit him by a car, at least increase awareness of EMS, influencing public opinion if not, ultimately, policy.

RESEARCH QUESTIONS

- Does media coverage of public safety correlate with policy change?
- To what do reporters and public safety officials attribute the lack of EMS coverage in the media?

METHODOLOGY

To determine the agenda-setting impact of local newspapers on local governments, 19,494 "local governments" — as opposed to state and federal entities — were selected from a list of cities, towns, townships and boroughs and village provided by the U.S. Census Bureau. Of them, 5,221 (26.8 percent) filed their Web site URL with the Bureau and this pool served as the initial sample to be matched with towns that had newspapers in the EBSCO Newspaper Source Pro database, a database of 906 media outlets. Any media outlet that had fewer than three years of data online, data necessary to study longitudinal implications of agenda-setting, was then eliminated, leaving 241 outlets. Finally, any duplicates or large, regional papers were removed, leaving 162 media outlets that met all the criteria. The percentage of the newspapers kept in the study closely reflected the percentage of the population in each region. Over a 10-year period, a content analysis of each newspaper was conducted, looking for coverage of various aspects of public safety, including fire department, police departments and EMS agencies.

FINDINGS

The relationship between coverage of public safety and change in the line-item budget for public safety (including police, fire and EMS) (table 1) illustrated that the agenda-setting relationship between newspaper coverage and policy change was more complex than what simple correlation could describe. Descriptively, while the budgets did see an increase over the period studied (1.98 percent on average), newspaper coverage of public safety increased 10.01 percent on average. During the five years between 2005-2010, while public safety budgets increased marginally, less than the 4.7 percent increase in population, news coverage increased five times as much. For every unit increase in newspaper coverage, the town's budget increases by 0.15 ($p<0.1$) holding all other variables constant. Local ownership of the newspaper also seemed related to changes in the public safety budget. Local newspaper owners, like all residents of a community, have a vested interest in the safety and security of that community. In addition, the change in newspaper coverage was also related to the online presence of the newspaper.

The third model, including all the independent variables and excluding subregion 4.9 provided the best insight into the relationship between public safety budgets and public safety coverage. The subregion that includes California, Oregon and Washington (4.9) was omitted to unique effects of the 2008 economic downturn and well-documented over-spending and poor fiscal management of numerous local governments in that area. As table 2 indicates, the model was statistically significant,

Table 1. Correlations of newspaper and city variables on 2005-2010 public safety budget excluding subregion 4.9

	Mean	Standard Deviation	Content Analysis	Local Ownership	Market Saturation (log)	Web Coverage	Staff Size
Budget change (DV)	11.55	15.49	0.15*	0.16**	0.06	0.07	-0.11
Content analysis	13.37	9.93		0.01	-0.16**	0.15**	0.06
Local ownership	0.33	0.47			0.13*	-0.06	0.25***
Market saturation (log)	-0.75	0.70				-0.06	0.14*
Web coverage	3.59	0.76					-0.04
Staff size	21.46	12.55					

*Correlation is significant at the 0.10 level (2-tailed)
**Correlation is significant at the 0.05 level (2-tailed)
***Correlation is significant at the 0.01 level (2-tailed)

but only at the $p<0.1$ level and then with a small effect size ($r^2 = 0.08$). Media coverage of public safety does correlate with policy change if only minimally. However, the overall model showed three significant independent variables, including coverage (content analysis) ($B=0.25$, $p<0.1$), local ownership ($B=6.36$, $p<0.05$) and staff size ($B=-0.22$, $p<0.1$) in relation to budget change. Given that it is the most significant, the contribution of local ownership to a positive change in public safety coverage is especially worthy of further discussion.

By far, public safety was the largest single portion, nearly one-third (32.49 percent) on average, of most town's budgets. Despite being such a large portion of the budget — or perhaps because public safety was a large portion of the budget — public safety budgets showed less correlation between change in coverage and change in budget over time. That media had little influence on budget changes could also have been because bureaucrats and politicians see the dangers of cutting public safety in a post-9/11 era when public safety is seen as an essential, governmental function.

Beyond the empirical examination of public safety generally, a content analysis of the 70 newspapers showed that of the public safety coverage in those community newspapers, papers that were generally the sole media outlet in their city, about 53 percent of it was related to police coverage, about 24 percent was devoted to fire coverage, but only 1 percent was devoted to EMS and pre-hospital healthcare.

Table 2. Regression of change in newspaper coverage and change in public safety budget, 2005-2010 (Unstandardized coefficients)

	Model 1	Model 2	Model 3
Content analysis	0.23 (0.13)	0.22* (0.13)	0.25* (0.14)
Local ownership		4.50 (3.23)	6.36** (3.04)
Market saturation (log)		1.18 (2.06)	1.84 (2.04)
Web coverage		2.05 (1.95)	1.13 (1.85)
Staff size		-0.27** (0.13)	-0.22* (0.12)
Constant	9.10*** (2.20)	7.07 (7.91)	8.10 (7.38)
R^2	0.02*	0.07*	0.08*
Adjusted R^2	0.01	0.03	0.04
N	139	143	122
Standard error of estimate	17.38	17.10	15.16

NOTE: Standard errors are in parenthesis
Model 1: No control variables
Model 2: Control variables with all regions
Model 3: Control variables excluding region 4.9
* Significant at the 0.10 level (2-tailed)
** Significant at the 0.05 level (2-tailed)
*** Significant at the 0.01 level (2-tailed)

The remainder of the public safety coverage was devoted to a smattering of topics including budget and management coverage. An empirical examination of the content correlated with policy change (budget) found minimal effects at the level, effects that were more significant over time. In addition, locally owned media and newspaper outlets with larger newspaper staffs have more impact on public safety policy change.

QUALITATIVE FINDINGS

Using the findings from the first part of this study as a starting point and funded by a Midwestern State University internal grant, the second part of this study began by identifying cities appropriate for further discussion, cities on either end of the spectrum of EMS coverage, those with more coverage than average and those with less coverage than average. Of 162 cities initially studied, only 70 made the next cut because no coverage of EMS agencies could be found or because the database did not contain at least three consecutive years of data. The cities were ordered based on the amount of coverage in each paper. Three cities with high coverage and three cities with low coverage were selected in the same census region. In each, both EMS officials and newspaper reporters/editors were asked a series of questions approved by the Institutional Review Board as part of this qualitative analysis.

The subsequent interviews with EMS professionals and reporters revealed five possible reasons for lack of coverage: (1) EMS was not on the radar screen of reporters; (2) public information officers were more likely to serve police and fire, not EMS; (3) legislation such as HIPAA precludes coverage of EMS while other legislation makes information particularly related to police work more accessible; (4) how EMS systems are managed often means they are not publicly accountable; and (5) EMS was not on the radar screen of the citizens in the towns they serve.

EMS Not on Radar Screen of Reporters

When originally scheduling the interviews with reporters and editors, it was clear the study was about coverage of EMS. A few minutes into every interview, it was also clear that the reporters would rather talk about the police response to a recent shooting and how reporters were treated or how they evaded notice at a natural disaster. It took continual re-directing to have any discussion of EMS.

Everyone wants to know the most horrific of crimes.

Back to EMS.

We also have people who pay attention to residential concerns, vandalism, break-ins, things like that.

What about other public safety issues such as fire department and EMS?

Most of (our area fire departments) have developed websites, and it seems like a good majority of them have people who take pictures of fires. So we've been able to use more fire photos in recent years.

What about EMS?

EMS is a little harder. I'm not really sure how EMS works. Typically we don't do a lot with that. We're a small staff, and we really can't chase ambulances.

One reporter put it rather bluntly.

Actually, I can't even remember that we've tried. I mean truly. We have a story that the fire department will tell us that three people were taken to the hospital for treatment of smoke inhalation. Or burns. We'll get the information from the fire department or from the police department that there was a car wreck and one died and three people went to the hospital, two with life threatening injuries. We get it from the cops or the fire department. EMS is not part of our reporting.

It's pretty simple. "We don't get a lot of media calls about EMS," she said.

But when it came to coverage of the police department, one reporter said the newspaper relies at least initially on press releases and press briefings provided by the police department. Since neither fire nor EMS provide information so conveniently, EMS agencies do not get as much coverage. Since such coverage is positively correlated with policy change, EMS officials may find more challenges when needing new equipment, more personnel or a new station simply because EMS is not on the radar screen of reporters and, subsequently, not visible to ordinary citizens or decision makers.

Public Information Officers

Rather than EMS chiefs, division chiefs or street-level medics, three of the agencies used public information officers as the primary point of contact and part of the research. However, unlike police department public information officers, which are often commissioned police officers, or fire department PIOs, who may be firefighters or former firefighters. None of the public information officers representing EMS agencies interviewed had any prior experience in EMS. The Journal of Emergency Medical Services' own Salary and Workplace Survey didn't even include a job description that included public information as a key job duty. One PIO said, "Part of my job is to help promote a better understanding of the industry and how it will work and how the community can work with us to make what we do more effective and safer for everyone." But with lack of specific knowledge about what goes on in the back of an ambulance, the PIOs acknowledged that sometimes their job is challenging.

All of the public information officers had additional duties. Two were public information officers for the county and also did PIO work, including producing publications, supervising special projects and maintaining media relations from city departments as diverse as parks and recreation, public works and the library system in addition to serving the elected commissioners. Doing media relations for public safety generally and EMS specifically was clearly only a small part of their daily duties, often an afterthought. One public information officer said she spent 10 to 15 percent on all of public safety. One, while dedicated to the private EMS company, also handled media relations for nine counties, coordinated CPR classes, managed social media and planned company events. "Anything that falls under the marketing umbrella or the PR umbrella tends to fall on my desk."

However, she said sometimes a specific incident will spark media attention requiring her expertise. For example, she cited the time students on spring break stole an ambulance. "We are not sure if it was the kid on a joyride or what, but the thing was missing for almost 24 hours. Fortunately, we recovered it, completely intact. I was pretty involved in dealing with the media."

One reporter, however, cited an instance where having a public information officer worked against getting information out in a timely fashion, a story of when a tornado hit his area. He recounted how he was standing a quarter- or half-mile away from the scene without being able to get any images or anything. "I wanted to get in there to get some photos while it was going on. I could have told a better story about how emergency responders were actually working to help people." Instead, he said no one wanted to talk because they all need to go through the PIO and it was hours before a PIO arrived on the scene. "They want to control every bit of the situation and scene rather than it being a friendly working environment understanding that we have a job to do as well." In that case, the reporter said he was able to talk to some of the volunteer fighters who also expressed concern since they depend on public support and donations. "They want everyone to know what they're doing."

That same reporter said the main problem working with public information officers is that they rarely have experience that provides readers with useful details. "I will never be one to say that PIOs are the greatest thing ever." He said his first response is often to question: What does he know about saving lives? It is the same approach he would use with the PIO for the highway department. "You're asking a question about design on the roadway when your first thought is: What do you know about engineering on the roadway?"

While occasionally reporters said they talked to EMS personnel in the field, most agencies discourage or prohibit it. "We have a policy against our associates speaking to the media. That is for their protection and for the protection of our patients," said one EMS official. "A lot of folks, not just in EMS, but generally speaking, are scared to death of the media." Another said, "Our EMS people don't talk to reporters. But, if it's something like a fire and we have chief on scene, then they have the authority to go ahead and describe what happened, what's going on, what we're doing."

HIPAA and General Ethics of Privacy

Repeatedly, one thing both reporters and EMS officials noted that restricted their ability to cover EMS was the Health Insurance Portability and Accountability Act of 1996 (HIPAA) and the changes made in 2013. Originally designed to protect information shared electronically between medical professionals, HIPAA makes it illegal for covered healthcare providers, including EMS agencies, to disclose individually identifiable health information.

"I'm very careful, we're very careful from an organizational perspective, about scene safety and HIPPA and protecting the rights of our patients. So typically if news media is on scene it's not because we have reached out to them," said one public information officer. The law clearly allows the disclosure of personal health information needed for patient care and other important purposes between anyone involved in providing healthcare. Only healthcare providers are covered by the law, not other public safety officials not involved in the care of injured or sick personnel. Information that would otherwise be public information, such as radio traffic such as dispatch information and information regarding hospital destination for sick or injured people, is still public information and is generally readily accessible. However, certain implications of the legislation are still unclear.

However, the interpretation of these rules has often been confusing and inconsistently applied at a number of levels. As recently as January, following the tragic mass shooting in Newtown, Conn., Leon Rodriguez, director of the HHS Office for Civil Rights, felt compelled to send a message to the nation's healthcare providers clarifying HIPAA policy regarding disclosing patient information, including information from a patient's mental records.

"The rule does not prevent your ability to disclose necessary information about a patient to law enforcement, family members of the patient or other persons, when you believe the patient presents a serious danger to himself or other people," the letter reads.

It went on to say that patient health information can be shared "when necessary to treat a patient, to protect the nation's public health and for other critical purposes, such as when a provider seeks to warn or report that persons may be at risk of harm because of a patient." (McCallion, 2013)

Still reporters found HIPAA to be an impediment specifically to on-scene coverage. Said one reporter: "They're not going to talk to you. The obvious cause is HIPAA. They're not going talk about the condition of the patient. They can't say very much to the media about a patient or a situation." As *St. Louis Post-Dispatch* reporter Deborah Shelton said in a 2007 report by the Reporters Committee for Freedom of the Press, "HIPAA is an excuse."

Said another, "EMS just invokes HIPAA, and that's it. They can't say anything. We just loaded them in the bus and took them to the hospital. There's only two hospitals. If it's a fire, we get the information from the fire department. If it's a car wreck, we get the information from the police department. We have almost no contact with EMS."

Beyond an emergency scene, one of the ways that reporters provide insight into public safety agencies is by embedding themselves within the agency, including doing ride-alongs with police officers, fire fighters or ambulance crew members. However, HIPAA has provided administrators with an excuse to stop such ride-alongs denying citizens with insights into their public safety agencies. Even when reporters gain patient authorization, some cities such as Washington, D.C. no longer allow media ride-alongs on medical calls generally citing HIPAA as the reason (Reporter's Guide to Medical Privacy Law, 2007).

While HIPAA prevents pre-hospital healthcare providers from talking about the specific conditions of a patient, other legislation puts police agencies constantly out in front of the media. At universities, for example, the Jeanne Clery Discloure of Campus Security Policy and Campus Crime Statistics (20 USC § 1092(f), also known as the Campus Security Act, mandates that institutions of higher education be open and transparent regarding crimes on and near campus. Nowhere does the report mention disclosure of any information related to emergency medical incidents on campus, including incidents such as suicide, students who die from undiagnosed or pre-existing medical conditions or students who are injured or die related to athletic events or physical plant problems, such as repeated auto/pedestrian accidents or falls.

While not as readily accessible, many state health departments maintain aggregated records of health statistics. While the records do not contain specific information, they do contain aggregated data down to the level of the city. Reporters can use data about common causes of death over time. The information is aggregated into categories such as accidents, diseases of the heart and cerebrovascular diseases. While useful for comparing general trends, the information is generally useless for specific reporting. Obtaining information on deaths to which pre-hospital care providers contributed would be almost as impossible as obtaining similar information about emergency room physicians. The *Journal of Emergency Medical Services* annual surveys pre-hospital healthcare providers regarding types of calls, salaries and management, again grossly aggregated. The National EMS Database contains more specific data on all types of EMS calls, including data on delays, patient demographics and patient disposition, but the data is all but inaccessible by non computer programmers in an online database — nemsis.org.

Management (Privately-Owned, Hospital-Operated)

While almost all police departments and most fire departments are public entities, and therefore subject to all the requirements of state and federal open meetings / open records legislation, the management of EMS agencies is inconsistent. As one EMS official noted, "It's very, very different in every county and in every city." About 28 percent are part of the city-run fire department or a unique city/county department (23 percent). Some (about 11 percent) are hospital based. Some (about 30 percent) are private either for-profit or not-for-profit companies. That means at least one-third of EMS agencies would have no legal obligation to report call numbers, types, staff salaries or any information to media outlets or local residents (Greene, 2014). As one of the EMS officials said, "The majority of the public has no idea how EMS works. And they don't really care."

EMS Not on the Radar Screen of Citizens

In 2013, emergency medical technicians and paramedics, more than 237,660 of them nationwide, earned $34,870, a mean hourly wage of $16.77. Firefighters, $48,270; police officers, $58,720; the average news reporter, $44,360; the average postsecondary teacher, $74,620 (Bureau of Labor Statistics, 2013; Greene, 2013). The pre-hospital healthcare industry is a significant industry nationwide, particularly when considering all the employees in management at the local level and continuing education and certification at the state and national levels. It seems,however, it is still poorly understood by average citizens and not valued as highly in the marketplace of wages.

"The average person probably sees or notices very little difference between the fire department and EMS. I don't think they really notice," said one public information officer. "Most medics and EMTs are so-called ambulance drivers to the average person." That description, however, is offensive to those working in pre-hospital healthcare. As Rod Brouhard (2015), a paramedic, said on his blog, "When you call 911, a highly trained crew, usually consisting of a paramedic (or two) along with an EMT (or two), will respond with professional, compassionate medical care. Depending on the circumstances, they might even save your life. It's no secret that somebody had to drive to your location and somebody will also need to drive away, but their driving won't (and shouldn't) be the defining characteristic of their service."

Another public information officer attributed this lack of understanding to two things: the relative age of the profession compared to police and fire and the lack of marketing. "People understand fire trucks. And they see scenes of firemen holding babies and the American flag. And it's understood among the public because the fire association has done an excellent job promoting its industry. EMS is a relatively new industry. EMS has a disadvantage in the sense that it's not marketed."

Indeed, EMS is a young industry when compared to other types of public safety agencies: police and fire. It is a result, generally, of the need in wartime to take care of injured military personnel and, specifically, as a result of the increased use of automobiles and death by automobile, what John F. Kennedy in 1960 called one of the greatest, perhaps the greatest, of the nation's public health problems. In 1966, the National Traffic and Motor Vehicle Safety Act created standardized EMS training, promoted state involvement, encouraged community oversight, recommended radio communication and stressed a single emergency number. It also put EMS under the control of the Department of Transportation, where it remains today as part of the National Highway Traffic and Safety Administration.

In 2005, Congress mandated the creation of the Federal Interagency Committee on Emergency Medical Services to encourage cooperation between the Department of Homeland Security and the Department of Health and Human Services when dealing with EMS matters, including certification ("A Brief History of Emergency Medical Services," "The History of EMS at NHTSA").

The development of the modern EMS system, which occurred mostly since the late 1960s, makes it the new kid on the block. Even the word police dates back as early as 1530 and the earliest of societies, such as those in Ancient China, Ancient Greece and Rome, had officials who provided security. Fire brigades date back almost as far, certainly back to the time of the Roman Empire and coming of age with the development of the city in Europe with London insurance companies forming private fire brigades and developing the first fire engines in the 17th century.

LIMITATIONS

As with any research project, this one had its limitations. First and foremost of these was the method of data collection. No pre-existing data set existed either for the content analysis portion of the study of local newspapers or the budgetary data of local communities. While the EBSCO Newspaper Source Plus database did provide an efficient manner for searching the content of local newspapers, it was time-consuming and limited in scope. Over time, more newspapers will move their entire archive on to their own websites increasing the possibilities for research. In addition, there remains no central clearinghouse for local government budgets so each town's budget had to be obtained and analyzed.

A second limitation of this research included the timeframe of the study, 2005-2010. The time frame was chosen to maximize the amount of data available for each town and each media outlet in comparison to several one-year periods. However, in the middle of this timeframe lies 2008, the beginning of the Great Recession. Although town budgets did not appear to be showing the impact of the Great Recession until 2011 or 2012, the economic downturn inevitably had an impact on politicians, bureaucrats, reporters and editors even when they were not faced with short-term decisions about what to cut from the budget.

Finally, the methodology itself presented challenges. Correlations do not show direction of causation. In this short term, other pieces of literature have shown that media coverage precedes public opinion change and policy outcomes at least in isolated instances. However, the significant piece of this study examined policy outcomes over a five-year period. Inevitably over that length of time multiple factors will help bureaucrats and politicians determine policy outcomes, only one of which will be media coverage. Indeed, media coverage might follow the policy process as much as precede it.

The qualitative portion of the study served to provide insight and to generate ideas for future research. Characteristic as part of the qualitative method, the study allowed detailed and in-depth examination of the issues surrounding coverage of EMS in local newspapers. Since the questions were used as a guide and not a rigid rubric, the direction of the questioning was different based on what each person felt was important to discuss. The interviews made for a more compelling initial examination of the topic than would a cursory survey when the variables are difficult to ascertain.

Inevitably, however, the methodology also faced limitations not the least of which was that it was time-consuming with initial interviews lasting up to 45 minutes and transcription of those interviews taking hours. Initial interviews for both EMS personnel and newspaper reporters/editors were difficult to schedule often due to being short-staffed. "I do not have anyone who can assist you at this time," said one clearly over-worked news editor rather tersely. Interpretation of the transcription data and the questioning itself could easily have been influenced by the researcher's personal biases and interview style. While the qualitative method may not always be well understood or accepted, it was perfect in this case to serve as a foundation for future research.

AREAS FOR FUTURE RESEARCH

While this qualitative research identified at least five areas for further examination, it also pointed to one clear question: If media coverage is related to public awareness of an issue and public awareness changes policy or political outcomes as prior agenda-setting research has repeatedly shown (McCombs & Shaw, 1972; Funkhouser, 1973), what does lack of coverage do for EMS in an administrative or political set-

Table 3. List of cities and papers included

Newspaper	City	State	Circulation 2010	Market Saturation
American News	Aberdeen	SD	15,258	58.5%
Times Union	Albany	NY	68,114	69.6%
Telegraph	Alton	IL	22,873	82.1%
Amarillo Globe-News	Amarillo	TX	39,276	20.6%
Athens-Banner Herald	Athens	GA	23,853	12.6%
Augusta Chronicle	Augusta	GA	66,335	33.9%
Kennebec Journal	Augusta	ME	12,862	67.2%
Bakersfield Californian	Bakersfield	CA	49,414	14.2%
Bangor Daily News	Bangor	ME	57,245	173.3%
Desert Dispatch	Barstow	CA	3,259	14.4%
Belleville News-Democrat	Belleville	IL	50,967	114.6%
Bellingham Herald	Bellingham	WA	19,277	23.8%
Bulletin	Bend	OR	33,798	44.1%
Sun Herald	Biloxi	MS	37,817	85.8%
Bismarck Tribune	Bismarck	ND	26,129	42.6%
Pantagraph	Bloomington	IL	39,333	51.3%
Herald-Times	Bloomington	IN	28,408	35.3%
Daily Camera	Boulder	CO	26,698	27.4%
Bowling Green Daily News	Bowling Green	KY	22,062	38.0%
Bradenton Herald	Bradenton	FL	41,120	83.0%
Connecticut Post	Bridgeport	CT	46,388	32.2%
Buffalo News	Buffalo	NY	170,079	65.1%
Times-News	Burlington	NC	24,359	48.8%
Montana Standard	Butte	MT	13,178	39.9%
Gazette	Cedar Rapids	IA	61,247	48.5%
Post and Courier	Charleston	SC	81,821	68.1%
Charleston Gazette	Charleston	WV	55,691	108.3%
Chattanooga Times/Free Press	Chattanooga	TN	81,031	48.3%
Wyoming Tribune-Eagle	Cheyenne	WY	14,340	24.1%
Eagle Times	Claremont	NH	7,737	57.9%
Clovis News Journal	Clovis	NM	5,996	15.9%
Columbus Ledger-Enquirer	Columbus	GA	42,875	22.6%
Columbus Dispatch	Columbus	OH	237,357	30.2%
Dayton Daily News	Dayton	OH	99,121	70.0%
Decatur Daily	Decatur	AL	20,312	36.5%

continued on following page

Table 3. Continued

Newspaper	City	State	Circulation 2010	Market Saturation
Herald and Review	Decatur	IL	30,263	39.8%
Walton Sun	Destin / Santa Rosa Beach	FL	12,000	97.5%
**Delaware State News*	Dover	DE	12,720	35.3%
Erie Times-News	Erie	PA	52,758	51.8%
North County Times	Escondido	CA	63,565	44.2%
Register Guard	Eugene	OR	66,496	42.6%
Fayetteville Observer, The	Fayetteville	NC	56,238	28.0%
Arizona Daily Sun	Flagstaff	AZ	10,417	15.8%
Northwest Florida Daily News	Fort Walton Beach	FL	28,407	145.6%
News-Sentinel	Fort Wayne	IN	21,543	8.5%
Frederick News-Post	Frederick	MD	35,324	56.4%
Free Lance-Star	Fredericksburg	VA	46,558	191.7%
Grand Forks Herald	Grand Forks	ND	26,001	38.9%
Greeley Tribune	Greeley	CO	18,985	20.4%
Record	Hackensack	NJ	158,637	368.8%
Journal-News	Hamilton	OH	18,699	29.9%
**Valley Morning Star*	Harlingen	TX	17,332	26.7%
Patriot-News	Harrisburg	PA	77,378	156.2%
Havelock News	Havelock	NC	2,521	12.2%
Hesperia Star	Hesperia	CA	20,000	22.2%
High Point Enterprise	High Point	NC	17,940	17.2%
Cape Cod Times	Hyannis	MA	45,353	100.4%
**Daily News*	Jacksonville	NC	19,155	25.2%
Janesville Gazette	Janesville	WI	19,010	29.9%
Tri-City Herald	Kennewick	WA	36,048	48.8%
Free Press	Kinston	NC	11,143	51.4%
La Crosse Tribune	La Crosse	WI	34,073	66.3%
Ledger	Lakeland	FL	59,838	61.4%
Lancaster New Era	Lancaster	PA	83,427	140.6%
Las Cruces Sun-News	Las Cruces	NM	20,566	21.1%
Journal-World	Lawrence	KS	17,225	19.7%
Lexington Herald-Leader	Lexington	KY	96,556	32.6%
Lima News	Lima	OH	30,438	78.5%
Press-Telegram	Long Beach	CA	74,250	16.1%
Sun	Lowell	MA	37,508	35.2%

continued on following page

Table 3. Continued

Newspaper	City	State	Circulation 2010	Market Saturation
News and Advance	Lynchburg	VA	28,615	37.9%
**Macon Telegraph*	Macon	GA	48,402	53.0%
Wisconsin State Journal	Madison	WI	98,326	42.2%
Florida Keys Keynoter	Marathon	FL		0.0%
Appeal-Democrat	Marysville	CA	17,679	146.4%
Monitor	McAllen	TX	32,013	24.6%
Mail Tribune	Medford	OR	25,916	34.6%
Tribune	Mesa	AZ	49,126	11.2%
Middletown Journal	Middletown	OH	16,249	33.4%
Monterey County Herald	Monterey	CA	26,226	94.3%
Times	Munster	IN	81,062	343.4%
Sun News	Myrtle Beach	SC	46,264	170.7%
Telegraph	Nashua	NH	20,745	24.0%
Sun Journal	New Bern	NC	14,202	48.1%
New Haven Register	New Haven	CT	52,371	40.4%
Day	New London	CT	29,471	106.7%
Daily Press	Newport News	VA	74,825	41.4%
Hour	Norwalk	CT	16,253	19.0%
Ocala Star-Banner	Ocala	FL	44,422	78.9%
**Odessa American*	Odessa	TX	16,258	16.3%
Standard-Examiner	Ogden	UT	60,884	73.5%
Daily Oklahoman	Oklahoma City	OK	134,175	23.1%
Olympian	Olympia	WA	28,858	62.1%
Omaha World-Herald	Omaha	NE	149,539	36.6%
Times and Democrat	Orangeburg	SC	14,899	106.7%
Messenger-Inquirer	Owensboro	KY	23,902	41.7%
Paducah Sun	Paducah	KY	21,219	84.8%
**News Herald*	Panama City	FL	23,773	65.2%
Journal Star	Peoria	IL	61,122	53.1%
Sun	Port Charlotte	FL	35,544	65.3%
Portales News-Tribune	Portales	NM	2,955	24.1%
Porterville Recorder	Porterville	CA	9,118	16.8%
Portland Press Herald	Portland	ME	60,149	90.9%
Pueblo Chieftain	Pueblo	CO	46,253	43.4%
Reading Eagle	Reading	PA	58,832	66.8%

continued on following page

Table 3. Continued

Newspaper	City	State	Circulation 2010	Market Saturation
Roanoke Times	Roanoke	VA	77,938	80.3%
Post-Bulletin	Rochester	MN	44,494	41.7%
Daily Record	Rochester	NY	145,065	68.9%
Herald	Rock Hill	SC	26,765	40.5%
Salina Journal	Salina	KS	28,300	59.3%
Tribune	San Luis Obispo	CA	35,573	78.8%
Santa Barbara News-Press	Santa Barbara	CA	27,044	30.6%
Santa Fe New Mexican	Santa Fe	NM	22,219	32.7%
Savannah Morning News	Savannah	GA	39,656	29.1%
Sedalia Democrat	Sedalia	MO	10,184	47.6%
Star	Shelby	NC	14,164	69.7%
South Bend Tribune	South Bend	IN	67,085	66.3%
Herald-Journal	Spartanburg	SC	36,357	98.2%
Advocate	Stamford	CT	24,949	20.3%
Centre Daily Times	State College	PA	22,510	53.6%
Record	Stockton	CA	49,611	17.0%
Telegram	Superior	WI	8,180	30.0%
News Tribune	Tacoma	WA	88,288	44.5%
Blade	Toledo	OH	93,641	32.6%
Arizona Daily Star	Tucson	AZ	102,405	19.7%
Tulsa World	Tulsa	OK	111,641	28.5%
Northeast Mississippi Daily Journal	Tupelo	MS	33,896	98.1%
Times-News	Twin Falls	ID	18,717	42.4%
Tyler Morning Telegraph	Tyler	TX	31,784	32.8%
Columbian	Vancouver	WA	36,347	22.5%
Victoria Advocate	Victoria	TX	30,228	48.3%
Contra Costa Times	Walnut Creek	CA	171,100	266.6%
Waterbury Republican-American	Waterbury	CT	46,049	41.7%
Waterloo-Cedar Falls Courier	Waterloo	IA	39,229	57.3%
Watertown Daily Times	Watertown	NY	22,111	81.8%
Morning Sentinel	Waterville	ME	15,434	98.2%
Mountaineer	Waynesville	NC	9,312	94.4%
San Gabriel Valley Tribune	West Covina	CA	33,056	31.2%
Wichita Eagle	Wichita	KS	79,938	20.9%

continued on following page

Table 3. Continued

Newspaper	City	State	Circulation 2010	Market Saturation
Times Leader	Wilkes-Barre	PA	34,372	82.8%
News-Herald	Willoughby	OH	34,905	156.7%
Winston-Salem Journal	Winston-Salem	NC	72,186	31.4%
York Daily Record	York	PA	60,708	138.9%
Sun	Yuma	AZ	15,461	16.6%
	Average		**44,437**	**1**
	Median		**33,896**	**0**
**Cities selected for additional qualitative analysis*				

ting? Almost all current agenda-setting research examines the relationship between media coverage and reader priorities of importance or how media coverage helps change the frame in which readers view certain issues. While police and fire may change because of media coverage, the lack of coverage will certainly have impact on EMS, particularly in a country with healthcare so high on the public agenda. At the least, coverage, or lack of it, may influence the way citizens frame their views of police, fire and EMS.

The research also pointed to several other areas worth examining further, including the role of the public information officer. As Butch Ward (2014) said, “Journalists must keep up — no, escalate — the fight for access to information the public needs and has a right to get.” The job of the public information officer is to control access to that information. Do cities with PIOs get more coverage or better coverage? Do the PIOs release complete and accurate information that holds agencies accountable to the communities they serve or do they simply control controversial content? Do any of those PIOs have experience in pre-hospital healthcare and, if so, does that make them more successful when communicating with the public or the media? Such research could lead to better guidelines for public administrators when hiring PIOs in a world where social media may provide citizens and public safety officials with a faster way to get coverage published.

Finally, the research reinforced just how inaccessible information about pre-hospital healthcare providers and the services they provide is. Few EMS providers allow ride-alongs as do police and fire agencies, at least on occasion. Private companies do not release information regarding management, budget or individual calls. And the aggregated data maintained by state and federal government agencies is so difficult to obtain or aggregated so much it is generally useless. The lack of information about EMS calls, treatments and outcomes makes it difficult for the public, public administrators and elected officials to hold pre-hospital care providers accountable for providing quality care efficiently and effectively (table 3).

REFERENCES

2001 Notices of EMS Fatalities. (2001). National EMS Memorial Service. Retrieved from http://nemsms.org/notices01.htm

29-2041 Emergency Medical Technicians and Paramedics. (n.d.). U.S. Bureau of Labor Statistics. Retrieved from http://www.bls.gov/oes/current/oes292041.htm#(1)

A Brief History of Emergency Medical Services. (n.d.). Retrieved from http://wvde.state.wv.us/abe/Public Service Personnel/HistoryofEMS.html

Brouhard, R. (2015, March 31). *What's an Ambulance Driver*. About Health Blog.

Cohen, B. C. (1963). *The Press and Foreign Policy*. Princeton, NJ: Princeton University Press.

Dearing, J. W., & Rogers, E. M. (1996). *Agenda-setting*. Thousand Oaks, CA: Sage.

Funkhouser, G. R. (n.d.). The Issues of the Sixties: An Exploratory Study in the Dynamics of Public Opinion. *Public Opinion Quarterly*, *62*.

Greene, M. (2013). 2013 JEMS Salary and Workplace Survey. *A Journal of Emergency Medical Services*, (Oct), 8.

Greene, M. (2014). 2014 JEMS Salary and Workplace Survey. *A Journal of Emergency Medical Services*, (Oct), 6. PMID:25630146

Jordan, M. M. (2003). Punctuations and Agendas: A New Look at Local Government Budget Expenditures. *Journal of Policy Analysis and Management*, *22*(3), 345–360. doi:10.1002/pam.10136

Liedtke, M. (2009, August 9). Small Is Beautiful (and Successful) for Newspapers. *Palestine (Texas) Herald*.

McCallion, T. (2013). Feds Make Sweeping Changes to HIPAA Privacy and Security Rules. *A Journal of Emergency Medical Services*.

McCombs, M., & Valenzuela, S. (2014). *Agenda-Setting Theory: The Frontier Research Questions*. Retrieved from http://www.academia.edu/8239537/Agenda-Setting_Theory_The_Frontier_Research_Questions

McCombs, M. E. (2004). *Setting the Agenda: The Mass Media and Public Opinion*. Malden, MA: Blackwell Publishing.

McCombs, M. E., & Shaw, D. L. (1972). The Agenda-Setting Function of Mass Media. *Public Opinion Quarterly*, *36*(2), 176–187. doi:10.1086/267990

Mills, C. (2013, July 8). EMS Run by Idiots. *WRDW*.

Mortensen, P. B., & Serritzlew, S. (2006). Newspapers and Budgeting: The Effects of Media Coverage on Local Expenditure Decisions. *Scandinavian Political Studies*, *29*(3), 236–260. doi:10.1111/j.1467-9477.2006.00151.x

Page, B. I., & Shapiro, R. Y. (1992). *The Rational Public Fifty Years of Trends in Americans' Policy Preferences*. Chicago: University of Chicago Press. doi:10.7208/chicago/9780226644806.001.0001

Pippin, J. (2014, August 8). Richlands EMS Suspended from Medical Calls. *The Daily News*. Retrieved from: http://www.jdnews.com/news/local/richlands-ems-suspended-from-medical-calls-1.356331

Reporter's Guide to Medical Privacy Law. (2007). Reporters Committee for Freedom of the Press.

Rogers, E. M., Dearing, J. W., & Bregman, D. (1993). The Anatomy of Agenda-Setting Research. *Journal of Communication*, *43*(2), 68–84. doi:10.1111/j.1460-2466.1993.tb01263.x

Scheiffer, B. (2014, September 7). Remembering 9/11, when Americans Came Together. *Face the Nation*.

Schramm, W. (1963). *The Science of Human Communication; New Directions and New Findings in Communication Research*. New York: Basic Books.

The History of EMS at NHTSA. (n.d.). NHTSA EMS. Retrieved from http://www.ems.gov/history.htm

Ward, B. (2014, September 1). *Journalists Are Losing Access, but the Public Still Expects the Story*. Academic Press.

Weaver, D., McCombs, M., & Spellman, C. (1975). Watergate and the Media: A Case Study of Agenda-Setting. *American Politics Research*, *3*(4), 458–472. doi:10.1177/1532673X7500300407

Wilson, B. (2012). *The Impact of Media Agenda Setting on Local Governments*. (Dissertation). North Carolina State University, Raleigh, NC. Retrieved from http://repository.lib.ncsu.edu/ir/bitstream/1840.16/7870/1/etd.pdf

KEY TERMS AND DEFINITIONS

Agenda-Setting: Ability of the media to influence the salience of topics on the public agenda (McCombs & Shaw).

EMS: Emergency Medial Services; pre-hospital healthcare.

Health Insurance Portability and Accountability Act (HIPAA): U.S. Pub. L 104-191, 110 Stat. 1936 enacted in 1996 by the U.S. Congress to improve the portability and continuity of health insurance coverage; defines policies for maintaining the privacy and security of individually identifiable health information.

PIO: A communications coordinator or spokesperson that provides information to the media and public.

Chapter 3
Health Policy Implementation and Its Barriers:
The Case Study of US Health System

Augustine Nduka Eneanya
University of Lagos, Nigeria

ABSTRACT

The chapter describes policy implementation components of a health system in United States of America and explains how they affect health outcomes (service delivery). It argues that implemented policies affect various components of a health system in terms of service delivery, workforce, information, financing, medical products, technologies, leadership and governance. Using health system as framework of analysis, the paper explains that the outcome of health policy implementation determines the availability, quality and equitability of program service delivery. The chapter goes on to argue that policy implementation barriers, such as demand-and supply-side barriers, market, insufficient resources, cultural barriers, imperfect communication, information, education, coordination, leadership and governance affect the poor and vulnerable groups in developed and developing countries from benefitting from public spending on public health policies and programs.

DOI: 10.4018/978-1-4666-9944-1.ch003

BACKGROUND

An important factor in socio-economic development of any nation is the extent to which that country is involved in healthcare delivery system. Good health is a vital factor of quality of life as well as a pre-requisite for achieving socially and economically productive lives of a nation. No government can function effectively without an appropriate health care system. Health care system is one of the basic institutions that is universal in nature and without which a society cannot survive. The World Health Organization Report, (2000) defines health system as comprising all the organizations, institutions and resources that are devoted to producing health actions. Health action in this context entails any effort, whether in personal healthcare, public health services or through inter-sectional initiatives, whose primary purpose is to improve health. Healthcare institutions consist of formal and informal organizations where preventive, social and clinical services are rendered to the members of the society. Each of the institutions has specific aims and objectives even though they all exist to promote health, to prevent the occurrence of diseases, to bring about a peaceful end for those suffering from terminal disease, and to treat human illness. Most healthcare institutions form an arm of the government. Their social structure, therefore, follows the same pattern as other government institutions. Healthcare institutions form a large social system, and within this system are other large sub-systems. The systems vary from one country to another and even slightly within the same country.

The purpose of this paper, therefore, is to examine policy implementation by institutions of health care service delivery and barriers to effective outcomes. Specifically, the paper attempts to investigate how health policies support program activities of health institutions, such as; elimination of healthcare inequities; access to healthcare facilities, products and services; availability of finance infrastructures and other resources; provision of information and education to individuals and communities to medical products, facilities and services.

Consequent upon this, the paper is structured into five parts. Part one examines the introduction, purpose, clarification of concepts and underpinning theories of health policy implementation. Part two examines the inputs required in healthcare systems, such as; finance, structures and power relationships, equipment, personal and clients. Part three discusses the processes or series of activities that transform resources (inputs) into a desired product, service or output. Part four examines the outputs – direct result of the interaction between inputs and processes in the system, the types and quantities of goods and services produced by an activity, program or project.

Finally, part five identifies the barriers to effective health policy implementation and its implications.

CONCEPTUAL CLARIFICATIONS

Health System

Health system comprises all organizations, institutions and resources that are devoted to producing health actions. Health actions in this context refers to any efforts, whether in personal healthcare, public health services or through inter-sectional initiatives whose primary purpose is to improve health. It is an open system with three components of input, processes and outputs. Inputs required in a healthcare system include: finance, physical structure, equipment personnel and clients. The process refers to a series of activities that transform inputs (resources) into a desired product, service or output. The term output is used to describe the direct result of the interaction of inputs and processes in the system, the types of and quantities of goods and services produced by any activity, program or project. On the other hand, the term outcome refers to the result of the outputs, the effects or impacts. All these depend on how efficiently the system within the operating environment is administered and how the resources are managed.

Health Policy

According to WHO, it is the approach to medicine that is concerned with the health of the community as a whole. Health policy, in other words, refers to decisions, plans, and actions that are undertaken to achieve specific health care goals within a society. An explicit health policy can achieve several things: it defines a vision for the future which in turn helps to establish targets and points of reference for the short and medium term. It outlines priorities and the expected roles of different groups; and it builds consensus and informs people.

In fact, the mission of health policy is to "fulfill society's interest in assuring conditions in which people can be healthy." The three core public health policy functions are:

- The assessment and monitoring of the health of communities and populations at risk to identify health problems and priorities;
- The formulation of public policies designed to solve identified local and national health problems and priorities;

- To assure that all populations have access to appropriate and cost-effective care, including health promotion and disease prevention services, and evaluation of the effectiveness of that care.

To be more precise, Health policy means more than a national law or intervention. Operational policies are the rules regulations, guidelines and administrative norms that governments use to translate national laws and polices into programs and services. Health policy can be defined as the decisions, plans and actions that are undertaken to achieve specific healthcare goals in a society. Health policy can also support program activities, such as elimination of inequities in healthcare delivery services or mobilization of community health workers.

Policy Implementation

Implementation, viewed broadly, means administration of law in which various actors, organization, states, local authorities, procedures and techniques work together to put adopted polices into effect in an effort to attain policy or program goals. For our purpose, implementation can be conceptualized as a process, outputs (series of activities) and outcome. As a process, it is viewed as a series of decisions and actions directed toward putting a prior authoritative federal legislative decision into effect by the state or local authorities or organizations. As an output, implementation can be defined in terms of the extent to which programmatic goals are supported, such as the level of expenditures committed to a program or the number of violations issued for failure to comply with the implementation directive. Policy implementation can be conceptualized as some measureable change in the large problem that was addressed by the program, public law, or judicial decisions (outcomes).

Implementation can be considered from Fullan(2007) glasses;Fullan (2007: 14) rightly notes that many change attempts fail because 'no distinction is made between theories of change (what causes change) and theories of changing (how to influence those causes)'. Therefore, it is important to point out that policy change goes hand in hand with policy implementation. Mazmanian and Sabatier (1983: 20) define implementation as 'the carrying out of a basic policy decision, usually incorporated in a statute but which can also take the form of important executive orders or court decisions'. A policy decision 'identifies the problem(s) to be addressed, stipulates the objective(s) to be pursued and structures the implementation process' (Sabatier and Mazmanian 1980: 540). Passing policies does not guarantee success on the ground if policies are not implemented well. Pressman and Wildavsky (1984) were the first ones to show that implementation dominates outcomes.

It is difficult to say which factors or conditions facilitate successful implementation since so much depends on the political, economic and social context. For instance, local factors (e.g. size, institutional complexity) matter for policy responses (McLaughlin 1987). In this vein, Payne (2008) argues that only looking for general solutions and not acknowledging the particular context can lead to incoherent implementation efforts. Therefore, no 'one-size–fits-all' policy exists. However, this has not stopped some scholars from trying to come up with the most important factors for certain policy areas. To take the example of education policy, according to Payne (2008), successful implementation has been evidenced in schools where there is:

- Coherence
- Stability
- Peer support
- Training
- Engagement.

Successful system reform means that a small number of powerful actors are interacting to produce substantial impact (Fullan 2009: 108). Successful implementation implies that 'agencies comply with the directives of the statues, agencies are held accountable for reaching specific indicators of success, goals of the statute are achieved, local goals are achieved or there is an improvement in the political climate around the programme' (Ingram and Schneider 1990). Local capacity and will matter for policy success; adequate resources and clear goals are important too (McLaughlin 1987). In addition, the implementation process is characterised by a 'multi-staged, developmental character' (McLaughlin 1987: 176).

Even if policy implementation appears to be successful, Fullan (2000) points out that there is no guarantee that success will last. In terms of the change process in schools, there has been strong adoption and implementation, but not strong institutionalisation. Fullan (2000; 2007) further notes that both local school development (which engage teachers and students) and quality of surrounding infrastructure are key for lasting success. But successful examples of policy change (in schools) are still in the minority (Fullan 2007). Changing policies is not sufficient if there is no 'reculturing' of classrooms (Fullan 2000; 2007). As a result, a number of conditions need to be satisfied to enhance the change of successful and sustainable implementation, though these conditions vary across systems. This adds to the difficulty of the whole process.

Top-Down and Bottom-Up Approaches

A widely used concept in the policy implementation (and change) literature distinguishes between top-down and bottom-up approaches. The two approaches vary in a number of areas, such as the role of actors and their relationships and the type of policies they can be applied to.

Top-Down Approach

Top-down theorists see policy designers as the central actors and concentrate their attention on factors that can be manipulated at the central level (Matland 1995). The most detailed top-down approach was presented by Sabatier and Mazmanian (1979), who identified a number of legal and political variables and then synthesised them into six conditions needed for effective implementation ranging from clear objectives, causal theory, legal structure of the implementation process, committed officials, supportive interests groups to no undermining of changing socio-economic conditions (for more detail on these conditions, see Sabatier 2005: 19). In terms of policy areas, 'top-downers' usually prioritise clear policies (Matland 1995: 155).

Strengths and Weaknesses

One strength of the top-down approach is that it seeks to develop generalisable policy advice and come up with consistent recognisable patterns in behaviour across different policy areas (Matland 1995). But top-down approaches are criticised for only taking statutory language as a starting point and hence do not consider the significance of previous actions. The approach may be said to consider implementation as an administrative process and ignores or eliminates political aspects. The emphasis on statute framers as key actors is another source of criticism (i.e. local actors are not taken into consideration).

Bottom-Up Approach

Bottom-up theorists emphasize target groups and service deliverers, arguing that policy is made at the local level (Matland 1995: 146). These scholars (e.g. Hjern and Hull 1982, Elmore 1979) thus criticize top-down theorists for only taking into consideration the central decision-makers and neglecting other actors. The bottom-up approach, developed by Hanf, Hjern and Porter (1978), identifies the networks of actors who are involved in service delivery in one or more local areas and asks them about their goals, strategies, activities and contacts. It then uses the contacts in order to develop a networking technique to identify the local, regional and national actors involved in the planning, financing and execution of relevant governmental and non-governmental programs. This provides a mechanism for moving from local actors and decision-makers such as teachers or doctors up to the top policy-makers in both the public and private sectors (Sabatier 2005: 23). In terms of policy areas, bottom-uppers examine policies with greater uncertainty in the policy (Matland 1995: 155).

Strengths and Weaknesses

Among the benefits of the bottom-up approach is its focus on centrally located actors who devise and implement government programs, thus contextual factors within the implementing environment are important. Actors and their goals, strategies and activities need to be understood in order to comprehend implementation. Bottom-up approaches do not present prescriptive advice, but rather describe what factors have caused difficulty in reaching stated goals (Matland 1995). It is significant that strategies are flexible so that they can adapt to local difficulties and contextual factors. Nonetheless, bottom-up approaches have been criticised on two counts. First, policy control should be exercised by actors whose power derives from their accountability to sovereign voters through their elected representatives, but the authority of local service deliverers does not derive from this. Second, this approach tends to overemphasise the level of local autonomy (Matland 1995).

Combined Approach

Increasingly, the literature has focused on combining (micro-level variables of) bottom-up and (macro-level variables of) top-down approaches in implementation research in order to benefit from the strengths of both approaches and enable different levels to interact regularly (Elmore 1985, Fullan 2007, Matland 1995, Sabatier and Jenkins-Smith 1999). Building on Matland (1995), Suggett (2011) develops a framework distinguishing areas by the level of political conflict about goals or intent of a policy, and the level of uncertainty about the means or actions to achieve the goal. The two-by-two typology captures how top-down and bottom-up approaches can vary according to policy areas.

For instance, strategies that use bottom-up approaches (e.g. networks and devolution) are more common in areas of low conflict but high uncertainty and lack of consensus about the means to achieve a goal – such as educational disadvantage (Suggett 2011:8). In contrast, strategies that use such top-down approaches as strong political direction and sound governance are more likely in areas of high conflict about the goal but relatively high certainty on how it might be implemented (e.g. taxation for a specific industry sector) (Suggett 2011: 8).

Strengths and Weaknesses

Combining the two approaches might thus draw on their main strengths while minimising their weaknesses. Policy implementation often takes place because a wide range of stakeholders interact between different levels – thus both central policy-makers and local actors on the ground are important for successful implementation. In addition, this combined approach allows for differentiating between various policy areas. For instance, while the suggested framework by Suggett (2011) in its current form could be further elaborated, it is a good start for differentiating between implementation strategies. It matters whether health care, taxation or education policies are considered. Even within policy sectors, implementation strategies are not the same for higher education and secondary education policies, for example (see Gornitzka, Kyvik and Stensaker 2005). As a result, implementation varies according to different content and type of policies.

Rational-Choice Theories

At times, researchers have looked for more sophisticated ways of theorizing about implementation by applying rational-choice approaches. In a nutshell, rational choice theories are based on the assumptions that actors have a fixed set of preferences and act rationally in order to maximise the attainment of these preferences. Politics is seen as a series of collective action dilemmas due to the lack of institutional arrangements to encourage cooperation. In addition, strategic interactions between actors determine political outcomes (Hall and Taylor, 1996, pp. 944-945).

Game Theory

One example of a rational choice approach is game theory which is 'a mathematical treatment of how rational individuals will act in conflict situations to achieve their preferred objectives' (Firestone 1989: 18). It is in particular helpful for theories that seek to clarify how coalitions build and pass legislation. The literature on implementation and game theory is still rather sparse in the political science literature (for exceptions, see Bardach 1977, Koremenos and Lynn 1996, O'Toole 1995). For example, Bardach (1977) considers implementation as a continuation of a political game from the policy adoption stage, but with other actors and other relations between actors. He analyses the type of games that actors apply in the implementation process in order to pursue their own interests. But these games distort implementation from the legislative goals (Winter 2003: 213). Despite limitations, game theoretic models are helpful for exposing points of leverage for implementation managers.

O'Toole (1995) examines the use of rational choice theories (in particular game theory) in implementation research. He argues that while game theory might enhance inter-organizational management, it has some serious practical limitations which constrain what might be theoretically possible (O'Toole 1995: 43). There are several challenges in rational-choice approaches to implementation, such as uncertainty across different areas and the lack of institutionalization in the implementation setting (since many implementation networks are not highly institutionalized). But active and skilful multilateral implementation managers can successfully intervene at several points in a network context to reduce uncertainty and institutionalize cooperation. Such strategies include facilitating moves and linking games through signaling, commitment, and iteration; influencing preferences of actors and persuading them of the benefits to encourage cooperative outcomes; developing norms of trust and cooperation; and shifting the inter-unit structure to facilitate cooperation (O'Toole 1995: 47-51).

Also drawing on game theory, Firestone (1989) offers an education policy example by analyzing an ecology of games. Individuals compete in one or few available games, which can be in government, education, business, religion or news. This model borrows from ecology as species interrelate in their environment in different ways – through competition, cooperation or interdependence (Firestone 1989). Educational games are linked through flows between them: an downward flow of resources and regulation from legislature to classroom, and an upward flow of demands from educators as well as the general public (Firestone 1989: 19). Again, the temporal dimensions and context play an important role in the implementation of education policy. Local variation should be taken advantage of, and practitioners should experiment with different models at the local level (Firestone 1989).

Agency Theory

A different application of rational choice is *agency theory* - how principals delegate implementation to state agents - which has been applied in political science, economics and sociology (Kiser 1999). Different political science scholars such as (Kiewiet & McCubbins 1991, Weingast & Moran 1983) have focused on the monitoring of agents by principals in order to reduce drift in implementation. In contrast to the economics literature on this topic, political science pays attention to three issues: third parties, administrative procedures and multiple principals. But several questions remain unanswered, such as who exactly the principal is that is supposed to monitor the actions of the agents, and how agents are selected (Kiser 1999).

Strengths and Weaknesses

Rational choice theory proposes a parsimonious framework in which actors are rational in the pursuit of their preferences and interact strategically with other actors in the system. However, as John (2003: 485) argues, 'rational choice does not offer solutions for all cases and contexts'. The theory is better at explaining outcomes when preferences are settled, rather than clarifying the origin of preferences and the reason for change (John 2003). Game theory provides several advantages, such as a rigorous deductive theory and the potential to combine top-down and bottom-up approaches by treating all relevant actors as strategic players. But, as mentioned before, there are a few challenges, such as uncertainty and the lack of institutionalization (O'Toole 1995: 54). Overall, there is considerable potential to apply rational choice theories, including game theory, to implementation, especially when there are testable hypotheses.

CONCEPTUAL FRAMEWORK

This chapter, therefore, adopts health system as our conceptual framework of analysis as no single theory can help us explain health system variables. WHO (2000) defines health system as comprising all organizations, institutions and resources that are devoted to producing health actions. Health actions in this context refers to any efforts, whether in personal healthcare, public health services or through intersectional initiatives whose primary purpose is to improve health. Health system is an open system with three components of input, processes and outputs.

Inputs required in a healthcare system include: finance, physical structure, equipment, health information, technology, material resources, personnel, health policies and clients. The process refers to a series of actions or activities that transform inputs or resources into a desired product, service or outcome. The series of activities in the process include treatment, client education, community empowerment, official meetings and other health interventions. The term output is used to describe the direct result of the interaction of inputs and processes in the system, the types of and quantities of goods and services produced by an activity, program or project. It includes treated patient, efficient services, improved health status, community empowerment, trained staff, good quality of life and sanitation. On the other hand, the term outcome refers to the result of a process, including output, effects or impacts (Quality Assurance Project, TASC 2 Eritrea, 2003). All this depends on how efficiently the system is administered and how the resources within the operating environment. The enabling environment comprises the government, State, Local authorities, health institutions, socio-cultural and economic factors, regulatory quality control by government, rule of law, civil society, community, individuals, political stability and support, accountability and so on.

This conceptual framework is adopted because the analysis is not intended to identify causal pathway. The health system, which is an open system, is one of the basic institutions that are universal in nature and without which a society cannot survive. According to WHO,(2000), all health systems carry out the functions of providing or delivering personal and non-personal health services; generating the necessary human and physical resources; raising and pooling the revenue used to purchase services; acting as the overall steward of the resources, powers and expectations entrusted to them. The health system is, therefore, justified as our conceptual framework of analysis for this paper because large number of people and institutions are involved at different levels of health activities but are all working together to achieve the objective of improving healthcare delivery. The framework would enable us analyze and explain how different levels of government, organizations and community implement policies on health resource generation, financing, stewardship and service provision.

METHOD OF ANALYSIS

The chapter adopts qualitative research technique. The purpose is to select information that would help us describe and explain health policy implementation and barriers to its effectiveness. Data were collected from secondary sources. They include textbooks, journals, newspapers, internet and records. Data from these sources were analyzed using documentary data analysis, thematic analysis and content analysis techniques to elicit key concepts or themes. The concepts were coded and categorized into units of analyses: policy implementation of resources or inputs; policy implementation intervention process or series of activities; and policy implementation of outputs/outcomes (efficient services or improved health status) and subsequent barriers. Now, let us examine these concepts in the context of the healthcare service delivery.

HEALTH POLICY IMPLEMENTATION (RESOURCES OR INPUTS)

Formal organizations such as health institutions are made up of people and are set up to achieve specific goals and objectives. The attainment of these goals depends on the availability of resources in the right kind, quantity and mix. Ultimately, the attainment of the goals depends on proper utilization of resources. Resources are those inputs that help, support and/or have positive impact upon the achievement of organizational goals (Peretomode & Peretomode, 2005). According to them, resources can be categorized into human and non-human resources. Non-human resources can be further categorized into financial and non-financial resources. Non-financial resources include: facilities, structures, equipment, time, technology, land, transportation, organizational climate, geography, information, policies and so on.

The provision of health care services involves putting together a considerable number of resource inputs to deliver an extraordinary array of different service outputs. Finance is an important asset in healthcare delivery services. The performance of the health system depends ultimately on the knowledge, skills, and motivation of the people responsible for delivering services. It enables health institutions to train health workers, employ physicians, pharmacists, establish health clinics/hospital buildings, procure vehicles, equipment, procure vaccines, pay labor cost and invest on new program activity or project.

GOVERNMENT INTERVENTIONS IN IMPLEMENTATION PROCESS

Perhaps the most pervasive impact of government on the delivery of healthcare services in most nations is through regulation. There are many kinds of health-care regulations, namely: facilities, costs, quality and pharmaceuticals. Governments attempt to influence health-care delivery indirectly by providing financial support for certain activities, and directly attempt to move resources around in the health industry. One such attempt is through the regulation of "healthcare facilities and more comprehensive planning for the health needs of communities" (Peter, 1988:258). Another regulatory device is the control of costs in terms of making majority of expenses paid by a third party, such as "Blue Cross or Medicare or Medicaid" in America health care system (Peter, 1988: 258). For example, the regulation of health-care quality is another area of intervention by USA government in health policy implementation. The major public instruments used for regulating the quality of medical care are the Professional Standards Review Organizations (PSROs). These organizations are designed in part to monitor costs of services provided to Medicare Patients. Some PSROs have gone as far as to establish standard profiles of treatment for certain rather common conditions and then to question physicians whose treatment differs significantly from those patterns.

Furthermore, the USA government and other nations are deeply involved in the regulation of pharmaceutical industry and in the control of substances in food and water that are potentially harmful to health. The Food and Drug Administration (FDA) in USA and National Agency for Food and Drug Administration and Control (NAFDAC) in Nigeria are responsible for most of the drug regulation. The safety and effectiveness of a drug must be demonstrated by clinical trials. Associated with drug regulation in the Food and Drug Administration (FDA). Another issue relating to the regulation of pharmaceuticals is the regulation of tobacco, especially cigarettes. It has been observed that smoking cigarettes is harmful to health. It requires warning labels on to be placed on packages and forbid advertising on electronic media. Cigarettes and their regulations figure prominently in financing of health care, especially increased tax on cigarettes. Moreover, competitive mechanisms using market forces to produce desired changes in the health-service industry have been on the increase in recent times.

So, government should develop institutional capacities to ensure that appropriate uptake and integration of policies into existing activities. That is, integration of policy into private sector and community programs, such as: public-private partnership and community-based distribution network. These health policies can also support other program activities:

- Elimination of health inequities or mal-distribution of medical products or vaccines through increased mobilization and distribution of services, such as modern contraceptives and vaccines by community health workers.
- Conduct of media campaigns for improved public education and information on prevention, care and treatments; demand creation for services to marginalized populations and for population mobilization for health activities, programs or projects.
- Integration of policy can also be into sectors that contribute to health, education, agriculture, roads and so on.

HEALTH POLICY IMPLEMENTATION (OUTPUTS/ OUTCOMES)

Outcomes of these activities help increase accountability and identify implementation barriers. There have been reported cases of fraud, for example in America's health-care system. Home-health fraud, such as charging for non-existent visits to giving insulin injections- got- so bad that the "Medicare and Medicaid Centres" (CMS), which run the programs called a moratorium on enrolling new providers in several large cities in 2013. Since tighter screening was introduced under "Obamacare", the CMS has stripped 17,000 providers of their licenses to bill "Medicare"- services meant for the elderly recipients. Thousands of suppliers also quit after being acquired to seek accreditation and to post surety bonds of $50,000. It was reported that health-care fraud in America amounted to about $272 billion in 2013 (www.businessdayonline.com).

Thus, the outcome of health policy implementation is improved health status for individuals and community. According to WHO, (2000), the main objective of health action or series of health activities, whether in personal healthcare, public health services or through inter-sectoral initiatives is to improve health. Health policy implementation outcomes, therefore, can be summarized as: efficient services, improved health status, treated patients, community empowerment, trained staff, good sanitation and good quality of life.

ENABLING ENVIRONMENT IN HEALTH SYSTEM

For efficient services to emerge from health policy implementation, accountability and transparent mechanisms should be well established, so that civil society can monitor the implementation process, in terms of service coverage and quality, population coverage and equity, healthy behaviors by increased number of people.

BARRIERS TO EFFECTIVE HEALTH POLICY IMPLEMENTATION

1. **Economics:** The most commonly cited barrier to access to healthcare is economics. For example in USA, majority of medical care is still paid for privately. Those who lack the income or insurance to pay for medical care may not have that medical care. Many who are poor but not sufficiently poor to qualify are not eligible to receive Medicaid benefits. Many people do not have health insurance. The elderly poor who have access to Medicare as a result of their age must still pay for parts of their insurance, at a rate that may deter some taking full advantage of healthcare program. Even having insurance as well as not having it can present troubles. The principal problem is that it can minimize mobility in the economy. For example, if a person has a job that provides health benefits it is difficult for him or her to leave that job for one that may be better in other respects but does not offer insurance. Besides, if the new job does provide insurance, it may not cover pre-existing conditions, then moving between jobs may be possible.
2. **Demand and Supply Barrier:** On the demand side, the economic literature is dominated by adaptations of Grossman model that analyze individual investment and consumption decisions to improve health and utilize healthcare (Grossman, 2000). Demand is influenced by factors that determine whether an individual identifies illness and is willing and able to seek appropriate healthcare. The model levels to a demand for healthcare of a given quality that is determined by individual and community factors as well as the price of medical care and other similar goods. Individual (and household) factors include: age, sex and income. Demand barriers to utilization of healthcare include:
    a. **Information on Health Care Choices:** This provides lack of knowledge of the providers.
    b. **Education:** Low ability to assimilate health choices and negotiate access to appropriate providers.
    c. **Education and Knowledge about the Characteristics of and Need for Medical Treatment:** Information and education are related to failures, either in the form of knowledge of healthcare choices or in the ability to utilize this information in an effective way.

d. **Indirect Consumer Costs Barriers:** Are the result partly of income distribution and partly of lack of mechanisms to spread risk across the population or across time (so that individuals can pay for care when they can afford it rather than at the time of illness). The effect of household choices in preventing access to care to certain members is likely to be mainly the result of intra-household inequity:
   i. **Distance Cost:** Long and slow travel to facilities.
   ii. Distances to facilities imposes a considerable cost on individuals and this may reduce demand.
   iii. Opportunity cost need for patient and career to stop working for long periods in order to seek care.
e. Household preferences as a symmetric control over household resources.
f. Community and cultural preferences, attitudes and norms: reluctance to seek healthcare for women outside home; community resistance to using modern medical care to assist pregnancy. For example, cultural barriers such as cultural norms, such as "purdah" restrictions can prevent women from seeking healthcare outside the home for themselves and their children (Rashid et al. 2001). The barrier is often raised still further when men provide services and has often offered as one reason why Asian women living in Western countries often make little use of healthcare services (Whiteford & SZelag, 2000). Such restrictions may also interact with other barriers. Community factors may include cultural and religious influences and other social factors that affect individual preferences. Community barriers may also be related to information failures where they arise as a consequence of a lack of information about what constitutes medical provision and how patients will be treated once at a facility. For example, information might be used to reassure female patients that they will be treated by a female doctor.
g. **Input Prices and Input Availability:** Substitute products and services patients seek treatment through providers that are inappropriate for their condition such as drug sellers (Ensor and Cooper, 2004). Price is a complex variable and includes direct price and distance cost, opportunity(time) cost of treatment-since treatment can be time consuming and any informal payments made to the facility for commodities or to staff. Quality of staff may be absent because of the price of the wages and staff not attracted to the area.
h. **Knowledge of Technology of Treatments:** Inability to treat disease with given technology.
i. **Management Efficiency:** Poor quality of management training, lack of management systems.

The determinants of demand may generate barriers to utilization of healthcare services. Education and information assist to assimilate health messages and are important in determining demand. Finally, barriers may also interact with other demand barriers and act as important determinant of the willingness to travel long distances to obtain treatment.

Therefore, increasing demand is far more complex than simply the provision of health education advice or information but is also strongly related to the relative position and education are family members. Demand barriers present in low and middle-income countries and even richer countries can be found among vulnerable groups.

When it comes to supply, the provision of healthcare is, in many ways, a monopoly or cartel. Entry into the marketplace for potential suppliers is limited by licensing requirements and further controlled by the professions themselves, which limits the number of places available in medical schools. Thus, unlike other industries, the healthcare field makes it difficult for competition to develop among suppliers. One possible means for promoting competition is to break down the monopoly held by the medical profession by giving nurse practitioners and other para-professionals a greater opportunity to practice. The medical profession rather vigorously resists such changes. Hospitals do compete increasingly for patients, however, and with that competition has come some greater attention to the quality of care.

Moreover, price and quality of drugs and other consumables and weak cold chain may cause scarcity of supplies. Thus, supply barriers affect patients in obtaining treatments, especially for the poor and other vulnerable groups.

3. **High Medical Care Cost Barrier:** Medical-care costs are problem for government as well as for private citizens. In USA, half the total medical care bill is paid by government. Because decisions about health-care spending are made not by one government but by several, including several agencies interested in healthcare, central government attempt to control medical costs have been diffused and encountered difficulty overcoming the technical and political power of healthcare providers. A number of factors have been identified as causing at least part of the increase in medical care costs. For hospitals, one factor has been a rapid increase in the cost of supplies and equipment. This has been true of large capital investments such as CAT Scanners, as well as more mundane items, such as dressings and surgical gloves. In addition, labor costs for hospitals have been increasing rapidly, as many professional and unprofessional employees unionize to bargain for higher wages (Aaron, 1991:8-37).

   Besides, physician costs also have been rising, not as rapidly as hospital costs. In addition to general pressures of inflation in the economy as a whole, increases in equipment and supply costs, increased insurance paperwork, the increasing cost of medical malpractice insurance and the practice of "defensive medicine" to protect against malpractice suits by ordering every possible diagnostic procedure have all produced increases in doctors' fees (Aaron, 1991: 45-47) Finally, the method of payment increases the cost of medical care. Over 76 percent of the hospital costs and approximately 60 percent of all medical expenses in USA are paid by third party payers (Health Insurance Association, 1993)

4. **Quality Barrier:** In USA for example, both citizens and government must be concerned with the quality of medical care being provided. Citizens' obvious expressions of concern about quality have been the increased number of malpractices suits and complaints against physicians and hospitals. State Medical Associations and their Review Boards and other professional organizations who are supposed to discipline their fellow professionals and friends, find it difficult to do so. Government concern about quality extends from the general social responsibility for regulating the safety and effectiveness of medicines and medical devices on the market to the quality of care provided to Medicare and Medicaid patients to perhaps a more philosophical concern with the efficacy of modern medical care as a remedy for the health problems of American citizens. Medical care is still a difficult product for which to judge quality. Little information on quality of medical care is available to the consumer about the quality of services consumer about the quality of services provided by individual physicians or hospitals. The public sector has been intervening to try to make more information available, but it is still difficult for the average consumer to make choices.
5. **Unequal Access Barrier:** Medical care is mal-distributed, that is, the areas and persons with the greatest needs for healthcare are not the areas and persons with the greatest access to care. For example, in USA, Hospitals, nursing homes, clinics, doctors, dentists and other healthcare professionals are disproportionately located in well-to-do urban and sub-urban areas, as the highest fees can be generated there. The residents of these areas have better access to care than do the poor and residents of rural areas. This phenomenon is particularly true for access to specialized institutions and personnel, but it is also true to a lesser extent, for general practitioners and basic care institution. Medical care is distributed on the basis of ability to pay rather than on need. The limited access pattern contributes to the poor health and shorter life expectancy of those who are poor or live in rural communities. Black infant and maternal mortality rates are nearly twice those of whites and comparable to many countries in the Third world. The average life expectancy for blacks is six years lower than that for whites (Cochran et al, 1986).

   Unequal access is significant barrier to healthcare. Gaining equality in medical care is often difficult to the poor. Geography distantly plays a significant dual role in defining access to medical care. Urban areas are generally better served with doctors and hospitals that rural areas are. Aside from this, medical services would be even more pronounced if the areas of specialization of physicians and the standards and equipment of the hospital are considered. In some parts of USA, for example, high quality medical care may not be available even for someone who can afford it, without a substantial investment in travel. Thus, the relatively high rate of infant mortality in most low-and-middle-income countries is often taken as an indicator of poor access to medical care.

6. **Overspecialization of Healthcare:** Over specialization contributes to high cost of medical care as specialists charge more and use hospitals more than do general practitioners. For example, in USA as well as other developing countries, primary healthcare physicians, - family doctors and general practitioners constitute a small proportion of American physicians. Cardiologists Pediatricians, Urologists and other specialists are the dominant figures in the medical profession. Serious consequence from the predominance of specialists may help to account for the rather poor performance on measures of infant mortality and life expectancy relative to those of other developed nations, as these measures are more sensitive to high quality routine care than to sophisticated, exceptional procedures.
7. **Financial Inequities:** Another problem to healthcare is the financial burden imposed on many individuals and families by its high cost. The gaps in public and private health insurance are wide enough to let millions fall into financial disaster. In America, five to eight percent of the population has no health insurance, public or private. Fifty to sixty million persons have no major medical coverage. The result is that nearly ten percent of all families every year have out-of-pocket medical-gross income. Most of these families are poor, so that even $1,000 out-of-pocket is a catastrophic expense. Almost half of all personal bankruptcies each year involve medical debts.

Moreover, unintended consequences are major concern, as health education policy contributes to the over-specialization of physicians and recent changes in that policy have not yet shown an effect. Public policy, again particularly Medicare and Medicaid, in American health system contributes substantially to the cost of escalation in healthcare. As health care policy reduces the financial burden on specific individual, it increases on specific individuals, and increases on the society as a whole.

Thus, the most important problem in healthcare, shared by many nations is its soaring cost to society. The chief causes of cost escalation in the United States, for example, are growing numbers of elderly, overspecialization, mal-distribution, third-party payments, modern medical technology, federal tax policy and the public's exaggerated expectations of medical science.

There are substantial problems with America healthcare policy. Many differences in quality and access to care still remain among various groups. Medicare and Medicaid have contributed to health care is inflated costs and have not challenged structural problems in its delivery. And neither regulatory policies nor Professional Standards Review Organizations (PSROs); Health Safety Agencies (HSAs); Health Maintenance Organizations (HMOs) have had the success hoped for in introducing rational coordination and cost control into the system.

CONCLUSION

Within the fundamental obligations of governments at federal, state and local authorities. The National Healthcare system should be developed to support in a coordinated manner a three-tier system of healthcare. Essential features of the system should be its comprehensive nature, multi-sectoral inputs, community involvement and collaboration with non-governmental providers of healthcare. The goal of health policy should be based on primary healthcare that is promotion-based, protective, preventive, restorative and rehabilitative to every citizen of the country within the available resources, so that individuals and communities are assured of productivity, social wellbeing and improvement of living standard.

REFERENCES

Aaron, H. J. (1991). *Serious and Unstable condition: Financing America's Healthcare*. Washington, DC: Brooking Institutions.

Akinsola, H. A. (2007). *The Principles of Health Services Administration and Management: Perspectives from Clinical and Public Health Practices*. Ibadan: College Press and Publishers Ltd.

Anderson, G., & Sotir, H. (2006). Influencing government policy. In D. Pencheon, C. Guest, D. Melzer, & J. A. Gray (Eds.), *Oxford Handbook of Public Health*. Oxford University Press.

Bardach, E. (1977). *The implementation game: what happens after a bill comes law*. Cambridge, UK: Cambridge University Press.

Buse, K., Mays, N., & Watts, G. (2005). *Making Health Policy: Understanding Public Health Series*. Open University Press.

Cochran, C. E., Mayer, L. C., Carr, T. R., & Cayer, N. J. (1986). *American Public Policy: An introduction* (2nd ed.). New York: St Martins Press.

Elmore, R. (1979). Backward mapping. *Political Science Quarterly*, *94*(4), 601–616. doi:10.2307/2149628

Elmore, R. (1985). Forward and backward mapping. In K. Hanf & T. Toonen (Eds.), *Policy Implementation in Federal and Unitary Systems* (pp. 33–70). Dordrecht: Martinus Nijhoff. doi:10.1007/978-94-009-5089-4_4

Ensor, T., & Cooper, S. (2002). *Resource Allocation and Purchasing: Influencing the demand side*. York: Centre for Health Economics, University of York. Prepared for the World Bank, Resource Allocation and Purchasing Project.

Firestone, W. (1989). Educational policy as ecology of games. *Educational Researcher*, *18*(7), 18–24. doi:10.2307/1177165

Fullan, M. (2000). The three stories of education reform. *Phi Delta Kappan*, 581–584.

Fullan, M. (2007). *The new meaning of educational change*. New York: Teacher's College Press.

Fullan, M. (2009). Large-scale reform comes of age. *Journal of Educational Change*, *10*(2-3), 101–113. doi:10.1007/s10833-009-9108-z

Gornitzka, A., Kyvik, S., & Stensaker, B. (2005). Implementation analysis in higher education. In A. Gornitzka, M. Kogan, & A. Amaral (Eds.), *Reform and change in higher education: analyzing policy implementation* (pp. 35–56). Dordrecht: Springer. doi:10.1007/1-4020-3411-3_3

Grossman, M. (2000). The human capital model. In Handbook of Health economics. Amsterdam: North-Holland.

Hall, P., & Taylor, R. (1996). Political science and the three new institutionalisms. *Political Studies*, *64*(5), 936–957. doi:10.1111/j.1467-9248.1996.tb00343.x

Hanf, K., Hjern, B., & Porter, D. (1978). Local networks of manpower training in the Federal Republic of Germany and Sweden. In K. Hanf & F. Scharpf (Eds.), *Interorganisational Policy Making: Limits to Coordination and Central Control* (pp. 303–344). London: Sage.

Health Insurance Association of America. (1993). *Source Book on Health Insurance*. Washington, D.C.: The Association.

Hjern, B., & Hull, C. (1982). Implementation research as empirical constitutionalism. *European Journal of Political Research, 10*(2), 105–116. doi:10.1111/j.1475-6765.1982.tb00011.x

Ingram, H., & Schneider, A. (1990). Improving implementation through framing smarter statutes. *Journal of Public Policy, 10*(1), 67–88. doi:10.1017/S0143814X00004682

Jenkin, R. A., Frommer, M. S., & Rubin, G. L. (2006). Translating indicators and targets into public health action. In D. Pencheon, C. Guest, D. Melzer, & J. A. Muir Gray (Eds.), *Oxford Handbook of Public Health*. Oxford University Press.

John, P. (2003). Is there a life after policy streams, advocacy coalitions and punctuations: Using evolutionary theory to explain policy change? *Policy Studies Journal: the Journal of the Policy Studies Organization, 31*(4), 481–498. doi:10.1111/1541-0072.00039

Kiewiet, D., & McCubbins, M. (1991). *The logic of delegation*. Chicago: University of Chicago Press.

Kiser, E. (1999). Comparing varieties of agency theory in economics, political science and sociology: An illustration from state policy implementation. *Sociological Theory, 17*(2), 146-170.

Koremenos, B., & Lynn, L. (1996). Leadership of a state agency. In D. Kettl & H. Brinton Milward (Eds.), The State of Public Management. Baltimore, MD: Johns Hopkins University Press.

Matland, R. (1995). Synthesising the implementation literature: The ambiguity-conflict model of policy implementation. *Journal of Public Administration: Research and Theory, 5*(2), 145–174.

Mazmanian, D., & Sabatier, P. (1983). *Implementation and Public Policy*. Glenview: Scott, Foresman.

McLaughlin, M. W. (1987). Learning from experience: Lessons from policy implementation. *Educational Evaluation and Policy Analysis, 9*(2), 171–178. doi:10.3102/01623737009002171

O'Toole, L. (1995). Rational choice and policy implementation: Implications for interorganisational network management. *American Review of Public Administration, 25*(1), 43–57. doi:10.1177/027507409502500103

Payne, C. (2008). *So much reform, so little change: the persistence of failure in urban schools*. Cambridge, MA: Harvard Education Press.

Peter, T. (Ed.). (1988). *Inequalities in Health: The Black Report*. London: Penguin.

Peteromode, V. F., & Peretomode, O. (2005). *Human Resource Management*. Lagos: Onoosomegbwho Ogbinaka Publishers.

Pressman, J., & Wildavsky, A. (1984). *Implementation* (3rd ed.). Berkeley, CA: University of California Press.

Quality Assurance Project TASC 2, Eritrea. (2003). *Quality Assurance Core Course*. Associate Student Nurses State of Eritrea, Ministry of Health.

Rashid, S. F., Hadin, A., Afsana, K., & Begum, S. A. (2001). Acute respiratory infections in rural Bangladesh: Cultural understanding, practices and the role of mothers and community health volunteers. *Tropical Medicine & International Health*, *6*(4), 249–255. doi:10.1046/j.1365-3156.2001.00702.x PMID:11348514

Sabatier, P. (2005). From policy implementation to policy change: a personal odyssey. In A. Gornitzka, M. Kogan, & A. Amaral (Eds.), *Reform and change in higher education: analyzing policy implementation* (pp. 17–34). Dordrecht: Springer. doi:10.1007/1-4020-3411-3_2

Sabatier, P., & Jenkins-Smith, H. (1999). The advocacy coalition framework: an assessment. In P. Sabatier (Ed.), *Theories of the Policy Process* (pp. 117–168). Boulder, CO: Westview Press.

Suggett, D. (2011). *The implementation challenge: strategy is only as good as its execution*. State Services Authority Occasional Paper No. 15.

Weingast, B., & Moran, M. (1983). Bureaucratic discretion or congressional control? Regulatory policy-making by the Federal Trade Commission. *Journal of Political Economy*, *91*(5), 765–800. doi:10.1086/261181

Whiteford, L. M., & Szelag. (2000). Access and Utility as reflections of culture construction of pregnancv. *Primary Care Update, 7*, 98-104.

WHO. (2000). *The World Health Report*. Geneva: WHO.

Winter, S. (2003). Implementation perspectives: status and reconsideration. In G. Peters & J. Pierre (Eds.), *Handbook of Public Administration* (pp. 212–222). London: Sage. doi:10.4135/9781848608214.n17

Chapter 4
The Political Economy of Infectious Diseases in Africa:
Ebola Virus Disease (EVD) as a Case in Point

Titilola T. Obilade
Virginia Polytechnic Institute and State University, USA

ABSTRACT

Annually, many deaths occur in Africa due to infectious diseases. African countries are predominantly low-income. A third of all deaths in low-income countries are caused by lower respiratory infections, HIV/AIDS, diarrheal diseases, malaria and tuberculosis. These preventable diseases continue to kill millions of Africans each year. More recently, Ebola Virus Disease (EVD) has killed thousands in Africa but even with the number of deaths attributable to EVD, it is still a fraction of the deaths caused by any one of the top five causes of deaths in low-income countries. This chapter examined the political economies that have enabled infectious diseases to thrive in Africa. The numerous conflicts, barriers to education, high fertility rates in the poorest countries and the privatization-tied conditions of loans were some of the factors identified. Ecological studies also suggest that changes in climatic conditions around the West African country of Guinea enabled the index case to come from Guinea. The foundational causes of the diseases have made the African nations susceptible. The chapter concludes with recommendations.

DOI: 10.4018/978-1-4666-9944-1.ch004

INTRODUCTION

Africa is the second most populous continent with over 1 billion people (Population Reference Bureau, 2014) and home to the largest number of people living on less than $1.25 per day (The World Bank, 2014). Globally, 80 percent of the world's poor can be found in Sub-Saharan Africa and South Asia. Seventy percent of the world's extreme poor are in ten countries and five of these countries are in Africa. These five countries are the Democratic Republic of Congo, Nigeria, Ethiopia, Madagascar and Tanzania. The remaining five countries are Bangladesh, China, India, Indonesia and Pakistan (The World Bank Group & International Monetary Fund, 2015). Despite these figures, Africa is viewed as a rising economy with the influx of mobile technology and an increase in Gross Domestic Product from 2.1% in 2001 to 7.1% in 2007 (WHO, "The Health of the People that Works", 2014).

BURDEN OF DISEASE IN AFRICA

The life expectancy at birth in low-income countries is much lower than in high-income countries ("Global Health Observatory Life Expectancy Situation," n.d.). People in low income countries usually die from infectious disease while people in high income countries die from chronic diseases like cardiovascular diseases, cancers, dementia, chronic obstructive lung disease or diabetes ("Global Health Observatory Life Expectancy Situation," n.d.). Table 1 shows the ten leading causes of death.

*Table 1. Ten leading causes of death in 2012**

Rank	Diseases
1	Ischaemic Heart Disease
2	Stroke
3	Chronic Obstructive Pulmonary Disease
4	Lower Respiratory Infections
5	Trachea, Bronchus and Lung Causes
6	HIV/AIDS
7	Diarrhoeal Diseases
8	Diabetes Mellitus
9	Road Injuries
10	Hypertensive Heart Disease

*Tuberculosis was the 15th leading Cause of Death in 2012

Sources: WHO. The Top Ten Causes of Death; WHO (2014) Top ten causes of death: How has the situation changed in the past decade?

Table 2. Global deaths from infectious diseases

Infectious Disease	Deaths	Year/Time Period
Malaria	584 000	2013
Diarrhea	1.5 Million	2012
HIV/AIDS	1.5 Million	2012
Tuberculosis	900 000	2012
EVD	10 907	December 2013- April 29, 2015
EVD	11317	1976- April 29, 2015

Sources: World Bank (2015). Malaria; WHO (2014) Top ten causes of death: How has the situation changed in the past decade?

In low-income countries, a third of all deaths are caused by infectious diseases; lower respiratory infections, HIV/AIDS, diarrheal diseases, malaria and tuberculosis (WHO, 2014 Media Center: The 10 Leading Causes of Death; World Bank, "Malaria," 2015). These five diseases are all preventable and yet cause a heavy disease burden in Africa.

The deaths caused by any one of these five diseases in a year are more than all the deaths caused by the Ebola Virus Disease (EVD) since the current outbreak. The total number of deaths caused by EVD since the disease' first occurrence in 1976 till 29 April, 2015 was 11317. The number of deaths from the ongoing outbreak as of April 29, 2015 is 10907 (CDC, 2015 Outbreaks Chronology) which is still a fraction of the deaths caused by lower respiratory infections, HIV/AIDS, diarrheal diseases, malaria or tuberculosis in one year (CDC, 2015 Outbreaks Chronology; WHO, "Ten Leading Causes of Death," 2014; World Bank, "Malaria," 2015). Table 2 shows the global number of deaths due to infectious diseases.

In 2013, the global deaths from HIV-related causes world-wide were over 1 million (WHO, 2014 Media Center: The 10 Leading Causes of Death). In the same year, about 584 000 died from malaria (World Bank, "Malaria," 2015), and 90% of the malaria deaths were from Sub-Saharan Africa. Most of the deaths from malaria were from children less than five years old. Tuberculosis was responsible for 1.5 million world- wide deaths in 2013. About 360000 of those that died from tuberculosis also had HIV ("MDG 6," 2014). The sixth Millennium Development Goals (MDG) is to combat HIV/AIDS, malaria and other diseases and even though some of the moderate goals are being achieved, there is still plenty of room for improvement ("MDG 6," 2014).

Globally, Human Immuno Deficiency Virus/Acquired Immuno Deficiency Syndrome (HIV/AIDS) is the sixth leading cause of death but the leading cause of death in Africa (World Bank Group & International Monetary Fund, 2015; WHO,

2014 Media Center: The 10 Leading Causes of Death). Sub-Saharan Africa has 13 percent of the world's population (Population reference Bureau, 2014) but is home to 71 percent of all People living with HIV/AIDS (PLWHA) (UNAIDS, 2013 Global Report).

Nigeria is the seventh most populous country and the only African country in a list of the ten most populous nations (Population Reference Bureau, 2014). It has the largest number of HIV/ AIDS cases in West Africa (UNAIDS, 2013 Global Report) and the second largest number of infected persons in Sub-Saharan Africa. South Africa has the highest number of PLWHA in sub-Saharan Africa (UNAIDS, 2013, Global Report).

The burden of infectious diseases creates a toll on a nation's economy and reduces the economic earning power. School absenteeism due to malaria interrupts the child's education which in turn interrupts the employment when a parent has to stay with the sick child. Malaria reduces the Gross Domestic Product of a country. A high prevalence of malaria has been associated with a 1% decrease in economic growth (WHO, "The Health of the People that Works," 2014). The World Bank estimates that the Gross Domestic Product of some African nations is reduced by around 1.3% due to malaria (World Bank, "Malaria," 2015). The PLWHA in Africa aged between 15 to 24 years constitute around 42% of newly acquired infections (WHO, "The Health of the People that Works," 2014).

This young age group is the future of the continent and depending on the direct and indirect cost of living with HIV/AIDS, it leads to stagnation of their generation. Some employers do not employ PLWHA and some are let go when their employers know of their status (Obilade, 2015 b). Studies have also shown that when PLWHA are kept in employment, they live longer (Dray-Spira et al., 2005). When PLWHA lose their jobs or are unable to find employment, their families suffer especially when children drop out of school, take up risky health behaviors or when the children are orphaned. Ultimately, the families are left in poverty.

EBOLA VIRUS DISEASE (EVD) AS A CASE IN POINT

The EVD was first reported to have been identified in Africa in 1976 when it occurred in south Sudan and Zaire (now Democratic Republic of Congo) (WHO, 1978a; WHO, 1978b). Its first occurrence in West Africa was in a 1994 lone infection of an ethnologist in Côte d'Ivoire (Le Guenno et al., 1995) but in 2014, there was an outbreak in West Africa stemming from an index case in Guinea. After more than a year, the outbreak is still ongoing.

Although EVD has affected African nations before, the ongoing outbreak has proved to be more devastating than previous outbreaks. It is not enough to view

Figure 1. Countries that have had EVD outbreak and enabling factors

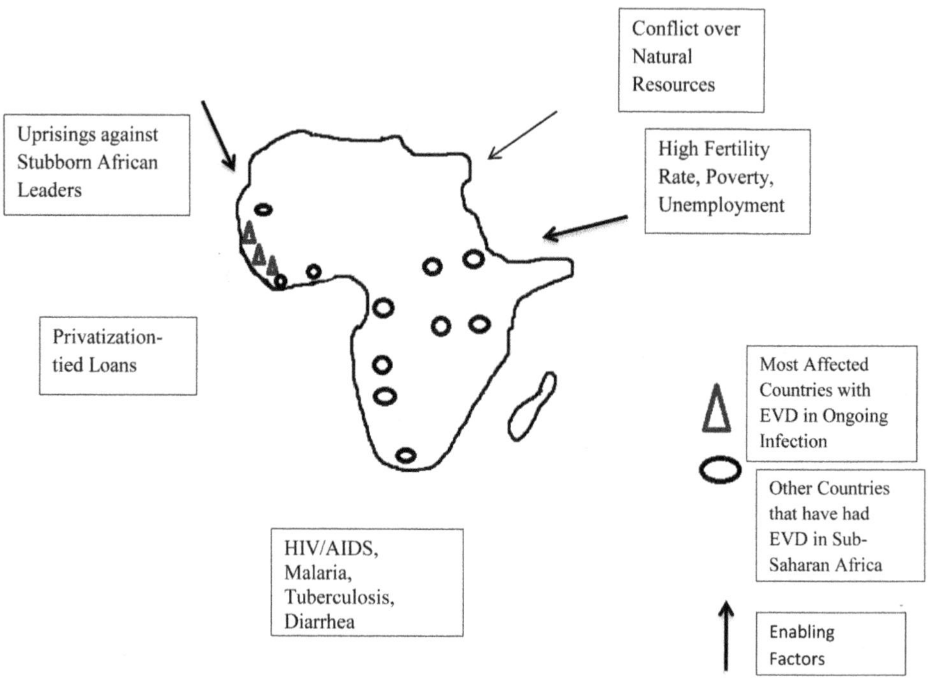

the outbreak from the lens of the media sensationalism but to delve into the foundational causes of the current outbreak. The rest of this chapter would examine the enabling factors that have allowed preventable infectious diseases to thrive. Some of the enabling factors that would be examined are the political economies over natural resources in African nations, civil unrest against African leaders that refuse to relinquish power, changing ecological climate and World Bank and International Monetary Fund loans to African nations (figure 1). The chapter would examine how these factors have provided a thriving climate for infectious diseases.

The countries most affected by EVD rank the lowest in the 2013 United Nations Development Program (UNDP) Human Development Index (UNDP Report, 2013). Guinea ranked 179 out of 187 countries, Liberia ranked 175 out of 187 countries and Sierra Leone ranked 183 out of 187 countries. Liberia beat only twelve other countries; Mali, Guinea-Bissau, Mozambique, Guinea, Burundi, Burkina Faso, Eritrea, Sierra Leone, Chad, Central African Republic, Democratic Republic of the Congo and Niger. The twelve countries that had lower rankings than Liberia are from Africa and six of these countries are from West Africa (UNDP Report, 2013). More than half of the countries in Africa are among the list of the least developed nation (tables 3 and 4) (UN List of Least Developed Nations, 2015).

*Table 3. List of countries between the 171st and 187th position in the 2013 UNDP Human Development Index **

Country	UNDP Human Development Index
Côte d'Ivoire	171
Gambia	172
Ethiopia	173
Malawi	174
Liberia	175
Mali	176
Guinea-Bissau	177
Mozambique	178
Guinea	179
Burundi	180
Burkina Faso	181
Eritrea	182
Sierra Leone	183
Chad	184
Central African Republic	185
DRC	186
Niger	187

* All the countries listed are from Africa

Source: Adapted from UNDP Human Development Reports. Table 1: Human Development Index and Its Components (UNDP Human Development Report, 2013).

PUBLIC HEALTH EMERGENCY DECLARATION OF EVD

A recent global threat of a highly infectious disease was the Severe Acute Respiratory Syndrome (SARS) outbreak in 2002. However, a public health emergency was declared earlier for SARS than in the time it took EVD to be declared a public health emergency. In 2003, SARS spread to people in over 24 countries in Asia, North America, South America and Europe before it was curtailed (CDC, 2013 SARS Response Timeline). The SARS outbreak started in November 2002 as atypical pneumonia in East Asia and WHO was not alerted until February 2003 (CDC, 2013 SARS Response Timeline). In the current EVD outbreak, a Public Health Emergency was not declared until the 8th of August 2014, almost nine months after the index case occurred showing a lapse in communication.

This lapse in communication at several levels of authority allowed the EVD to spread from porous remote borders to densely populated urban areas. Several factors

Table 4. List of African countries that are members of least developed country

Member of Least Developed Country
Benin
Burkina Faso
Gambia
Guinea
Guinea-Bissau
Liberia
Mali
Mauritania
Niger
Senegal
Sierra Leone
Togo
Angola
Burundi
Central African Republic
Democratic Republic of Congo
Djibouti
Equatorial Guinea
Eritrea
Ethiopia
Lesotho
Madagascar
Malawi
Mozambique
Rwanda
Somalia
South Sudan
Sudan
Uganda
Tanzania
Zambia
Comoros
Sao Tome and Principe

Source: United Nations (2015)

stemming from poverty and the political economies of the countries also allowed the disease to spread (Obilade, 2015a). The people's cultural practices, mistrust between the government and the people and fear were some of the other factors that allowed the disease to spread (Obilade, 2015a).

THE ZAIRE EBOLA VIRUS SPECIES

The Ebola virus is one of the causative pathogen of the viral hemorrhagic fevers (figure 2) (Paessler & Walker, 2013). Viral hemorrhagic fevers are caused by 23 enveloped RNA viruses from four distinct taxonomic families of viruses: *Filoviridae, Arenaviridae, Bunyaviridae* and *flaviviridae* (Paessler & Walker, 2013). The *Filoviridae* family is home to three virus genera: Marburgvirus (MARV), Ebolavirus (EBOV) and Cuevavirus (Negredo et al., 2011; Paessler & Walker, 2013).

The Zaire Ebola virus species is responsible for the current outbreak that has been devastating the countries of Guinea, Sierra Leone and Liberia. Non-human primates, bats, rodents, humans, mosquitoes and ticks can transmit the disease (Paessler & Walker, 2013). Infection is usually by contact with body fluids of infected humans or animals. From Guinea, the disease was able to spread to neighboring Sierra Leone and Liberia through infected persons and through weak infection control systems. The incubation period is 4 to 21 days (Paessler & Walker, 2013).

Ebola virus disease was formerly called Ebola hemorrhagic fever but the name was changed because it is not all cases of the Ebola virus infection that gives rise to hemorrhage. Since 1976 when the virus was first identified from simultaneous infections in south Sudan and Zaire (now Democratic Republic of Congo) (WHO, 1978a; WHO, 1978b) a licensed cure or treatment still does not exist (Paessler &

Figure 2. Illustration of taxonomic family, genera and species of Ebola virus

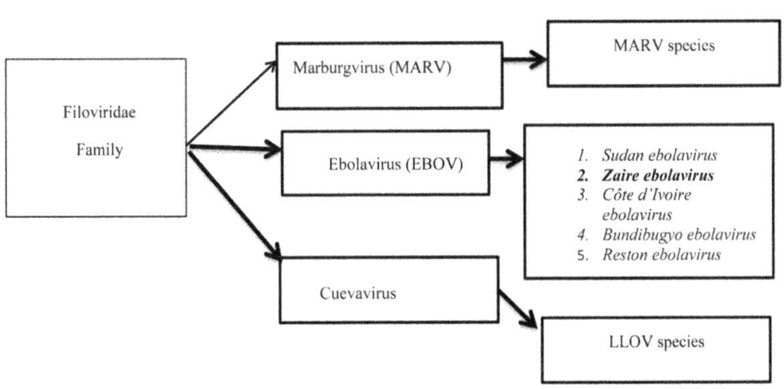

Walker, 2013). Therefore, treatment is mainly supportive but prevention of EVD is achievable through intensive infection control.

ENABLING FACTORS FOR INFECTIOUS DISEASE IN AFRICA

The rest of this chapter will examine different enabling factors that have contributed to the spread of infectious diseases in Africa.

Natural Resources and Conflict

Africa is home to natural resources like bauxite, iron ore, crude petroleum, diamonds and aluminum and export products like cocoa beans and cotton (African Development Bank Report, 2007). All the African nations have natural resources. For brevity, Table 5 shows only the list of West African nations with their main exports. Natural resources like diamond and crude petroleum are sources of main exports in countries like Sierra Leone and Nigeria.

Despite the natural resources and other valuable exports in the West African nations, about three-quarters of them are among the lowest ranked in the UNDP Human Development Index (African Development Bank Report, 2007; Obilade, 2015 b). Armed conflicts usually occur around the regions of natural resources (Balestri & Maggioni, 2014; Ross, 2008). Five civil conflicts occurred in the Mano region between 1989 and 2004 (Balestri & Maggioni, 2014). The Mano region straddles Guinea, Liberia and Sierra Leone (Ross, 2008).

The term *resource curse* is a paradox of plenty and was first used by a British Economist, Richard Auty in 1993 (Auty, 1993; Perry, 2010). It describes how nations that have abundant resources tend to become impoverished while countries that have scarce resources tend to become rich (Auty,1993). It is not all African countries with abundant resources that tend to become impoverished. Botswana has avoided conflicts despite its resources in diamonds (Sachs & Warner, 1999).

A 2007 report by the African Development Bank identified several factors associated with the paradox of plenty in countries with natural resources (African Development Bank Report, 2007). There were exacerbations of inequalities in the people, enhanced corruption and rent seeking, governments making poor investment decisions, poor governance, less prudent policies, lack of transparency and poor macroeconomic management (African Development Bank Report, 2007). It is not all conflicts that are related to natural resource as can be seen from violent government changes in African countries.

Table 5. List of West African nations and their main exports including their natural resources

Country	Main Exports
Benin	Cotton, Edible nuts, Non-ferrous Metal Waste
Burkina Faso	Cotton
Cape Verde	Fish
Côte d'Ivoire	Cocoa Beans, Crude Petroleum, Cocoa Paste
Gabon	Crude Petroleum, Wood, Manganese Ores
Gambia	Edible nuts,
Ghana	Cocoa beans, Manganese Ores,
Guinea	Aluminum Ore, Aluminum Oxide, Copper Ores
Guinea-Bissau	Edible Nuts
Liberia	Ships, Boats, Natural Rubber Latex
Mali	Cotton
Mauritania	Iron Ore, Molluscs, Fish
Niger	Radio Active Chemicals
Nigeria	Crude Petroleum
Senegal	Inorganic Acid
Sierra Leone	Diamonds, Cocoa Beans, Cultivating Machinery
Togo	Cocoa Beans, Natural Calcium Phosphates, Cotton

Source: Adapted from: African Development Report 2007

Conflicts over natural resources impoverish the people. It displaces the people, disrupts their education and increases unemployment. It also leads to political instability and infrastructures that can support the health and educational systems are destroyed or weakened. In countries where there are already existing barriers to education, the conflicts compound these barriers even further.

Political Instability and African Leaders Holding on to Power beyond Term Limits

A study of coups and attempted coups in Africa between 1990 and 2000 showed that there were 25 successful coups and 71 coup attempts. It also showed that 17% of the African countries had been plunged into civil war (Stone, 2004). Another study showed that there were more than 80 violent changes in governments in African countries between 1960 and the 1990's (Adedeji, 1999).

Several African leaders refuse to leave when their terms are up or they manipulate the constitution to extend their terms. Several African leaders that are currently in power have served for at least 15 years ("How Long Are African Leaders Staying in Power", 2015). The presidents of Algeria, Chad, Congo-Brazzaville, Djibouti, Sudan, Gambia, Uganda and Eritrea have ruled for at least 15 years. In addition, presidents of Zimbabwe, Angola and Cameroon have served for more than thirty years ("How Long Are African Leaders Staying in Power", 2015). Robert Mugbage of Zimbabwe has been in power since 1980. He is Africa's oldest president at 90 years and has ruled for 34 years (African Leaders Who Choose Power", 2015). Teodoro Obiang Nguema of Equitorial Guinea is Africa's longest serving President. He has been in power for 36 years. He came into power through a bloody coup by executing his uncle that was the president at the time (African Leaders Who Choose Power", 2015). Teodoro Obiang Nguema's son is the vice president (African Leaders Who Choose Power", 2015).

John Kabila of Democratic Republic of Congo has been in power since 2001. The next elections are due in 2016 and the citizens are anxious to see if he will seek an extension contrary to term limits (African Leaders Who Choose Power", 2015). There are already suggestions by the government that the 2016 elections could be delayed because of a proposed national census that could take three years (African Leaders Who Choose Power", 2015).

In 2014, the president of Burkina Faso, Blaise Compaore sought to extend his rule (after being in power for 27 years) through a third term but was battled out by the citizens (African Leaders Who Choose Power", 2015). Former Senegalese leader, Abdoulaye Wade also sought to rule for a third term contrary to the constitution and he was also battled out by the populace (African Leaders Who Choose Power", 2015). On the 1st of May 2015, the Burundians protested against President Pierre Nkurunziza's bid for a third term ("Burundi,"n.d").

On the 29th of April, 2015, Togo's Faure Gnassingbe was elected for a third term. The opposition had failed to stop his third term bid for the presidency. President Faure Gnassingbe took over power from his late father who had ruled the country for 38 years ("Togo's Faure Gnassingbe Wins," 2015; "Togo Profile," 2015).

In 2010, former Côte d'Ivoire's President Laurent Gbagbo's refusal to accept defeat in the elections claimed thousands of lives. In 2015, Mrs. Gbagbo was sentenced to 20 years for her role in the loss of lives during the post-election violence. Mr. Gbagbo is still awaiting trial ('Laurent Gbagbo," n.d.).

Countries in North Africa are not immune from leaders holding on to power. The former presidents of Tunisia, Egypt and Libya were toppled by popular uprisings against their almost permanent hold on to power ("Arab Uprising," 2013; "Egypt Under Sisi," n.d. ; "Libya Country Profile, 2015"). Altogether, combining the number of years ruled by Tunisia's President Zine al-Abidine Ben, Libya's Colonel

Gaddafi and Egypt's Mubarak gives a total of 95 years. All three presidents were overthrown by popular uprisings.

Sudan's President Omar al-Bashir was recently reelected in April 2015. The 71 year old president has been in power since 1989. He has been implicated in the Darfur crisis in which an estimated 300 000 people died and more than 2 million were displaced ("Omar al-Bashir Wins," 2015). South Sudan gained independence from Sudan in 2011 but has been engaged in internal and external conflicts arising from accusations between the president and the vice president as well as land disputes and conflicts over oil ("South Sudan Profile," 2015).

Selfish ambitions for power by African leaders must be overcome in order for their governments to be stable. Across Africa, the leaders strive to remain in power against the best interests of their countries. Many of the countries highlighted above have been impoverished. The conflict also paves the way for internally displaced persons and refugees. The people that are left in the impoverished situations resort to dangerous means to leave their countries in search of a more stable life. Many heads of households leave their families behind in search of better opportunities. And some of them die before they realize their dreams. This can be exemplified by thousands of migrants who attempt to cross from Africa to Europe through unsafe shipping vessels. Thousands of them drown. The families left behind are sometimes left in severe hardship leading them to undertake risky, health behaviors culminating in the spread of HIV/AIDS and other diseases. As unemployment increases crime would also increase. The governments of these countries frequently remain unstable.

Conflicts from Religious and Ethnic Interests

Some conflicts also arise from religious interests and others from both religious and ethnic interests. When people flee from areas of conflict, it can give rise to internally displaced persons or to refugees. The structures that are destroyed during the conflicts may never be rebuilt. Jobs are lost. Families are destroyed. The education of children is interrupted and any form of development stalls. When they are placed in camps, it makes it easy for infectious diseases to break out.

A total of 38 million people were internally displaced because of conflict and violence according to a new report by the Internal Displacement Monitoring Center (IDMC, 2015). Sixty percent of the newly displaced people were from Democratic Republic of Congo, South Sudan, Nigeria, Iraq and Syria (IDMC, 2015). These internally displaced persons have been forced out of their homes due to conflicts arising from political or religious interests. Some of the internally displaced remain in temporary camps for years making it impossible for stability that they need for employment and their children's education and other basic necessities that would improve their lives.

Some people become refugees in other lands and choose to remain in the countries they have sought refuge in. Therefore, their own countries of origin lose massive manpower which in turn leads to loss of production and goods which also tips the country into poverty. When large numbers of people are forced to leave their homes because of conflicts, it also means any development in the areas that they have left behind become stagnated. Any form of prolonged conflicts would lead the affected countries into poverty which makes it easy for infectious diseases to thrive.

Barriers to Education, Unemployment and Poverty

The 2005/2010 primary school completion for females was 66% in Africa, 99% in Europe and 97% in Northern America (Population Reference Bureau, The World's Women & Girls, 2011). The completion of primary school education is not enough to prevent poverty especially in this digital age. The first of the eight millennium development goals are centered on poverty reduction and a universal primary education (United Nations, We Can End Poverty, 2015) because the long term approaches to getting out of poverty include education, provision of basic infrastructure and employment.

Vulnerable employment is usually self-employment with or without a contributing family member and usually people in vulnerable employment do not have a safety security net in a crisis. People in vulnerable employment are more likely to fall into poverty (ILO, 2010). According to the 2013 global employment trends, 77% of workers in Sub-Saharan Africa were in vulnerable employment and 12% of the youth were unemployed (ILO, 2013). The challenge in Sub-Saharan Africa is not the lack of people in the work force but an inadequate production of goods and services (ILO, 2013).

Apart from the labor force contributing to the mental and physical health of the workers, it helps in building the economy of the country. An increase in the work force leads to a rise in the production of manufactured goods which amplifies the country's purchasing power, ultimately fueling the economic growth (Njoku & Ihugba, 2011). Barriers to education must be removed before families and generations can be lifted out of poverty.

High Population and Fertility Rate

The first ten countries with the highest fertility rates are from Africa. Niger has the highest fertility rate of 7.4 and Liberia, one of the West African countries that suffered severe losses from EVD comes tenth with a fertility rate of 5.9. Although the global fertility rates have fallen to an average 2.5 lifetime births per woman, the rates in Africa remain high. The average fertility rate in sub Saharan Africa is 5.

Table 6. Countries with the highest fertility rate and their human development index

Country	Children Per Woman	UNDP Human Development Index
Niger	7.4	187
Mali	6.6	176
Somalia	6.5	***
Uganda	6.5	164
Congo, Democratic Republic	6.4	185
Zambia	6.2	141
Chad	6.2	184
Burkina Faso	6.0	181
Malawi	6.0	174
*Liberia	5.9	175
**Afghanistan	5.7	169
**Yemen	5.5	154

*Liberia is one of the three countries most hit by the current EVD.
**Apart from countries in Africa, Afghanistan and Yemen are the countries with the highest fertility rate.
*** Somalia was not ranked.
Sources: UNDP Human Development Reports and Population Reference Bureau.

Not counting any African country, Afghanistan and Yemen have the highest fertility rate with 5.7 and 5.5 children per woman respectively. The lowest fertility rates are in East Asia and Europe (Population Reference Bureau, The World's Women & Girls, 2011). Table 6 shows countries with high fertility rate alongside their Human Development Index.

A high fertility rate increases the number of people. When populations increase without a corresponding increase in schools, hospitals and food production, any achievement made in education would be lost. An increase in population without a corresponding increase in produce and infrastructure would lead to food scarcity, water shortage, lack of infrastructure and political instability because the large populations would consume natural and financial resources. Youth unemployment is also another major cause of conflict, increase in armed robbery and disorder (Ajaegbu, 2012).

Ecology of the Most Affected Nations in the EVD Outbreak

It has been suggested that climatic changes in temperature was another contributory factor in the index case coming from Guinea and for the spread of EVD in West Africa (Bausch & Schwartz, 2014; Ng, Basta & Cowling, 2014). The index case in the current EVD outbreak was from Guinea. Prior to the current outbreak, EVD had never been reported in any West African country apart from the single incident of an ethnologist that got infected in Tai Forest Park, Côte d'Ivoire (Le Guenno et al., 1995).

Recent research has also shown that the mean temperature in Guinea is similar to the mean temperatures in countries like DRC and Gabon (Ng, Basta & Cowling, 2014). Gabon and DRC have had several outbreaks of EVD. Sudan and Uganda have also had numerous outbreaks of EVD and research showed that the mean absolute humidity in Guinea was also similar to that of Sudan and Uganda (Ng, Basta & Cowling, 2014). Further, there have also been prolonged dry seasons in Guinea which increases the risk of humans making contact with the animal reservoir. Deforestation from logging and clearing of land for agriculture also increase the risk of humans coming in contact with the suspected animal reservoir of EVD (Bausch & Schwartz, 2014). Mining for natural resources also increase the risk of human contact with potential animal reservoirs.

Exacerbations of Poverty from Conditions of Foreign Loans: The Bretton Woods Institutions

The Bretton Woods Institutions (BWI) is comprised of the International Monetary Fund (IMF) and the World Bank (Bretton Woods Project, 2005). They were established after the meeting of forty-four nations in Bretton Woods, New Hampshire, USA to stabilize the global economy after the Second World War (IMF, 2015c; The World Bank, 2015). The International Monetary Fund (IMF) was established to promote international monetary cooperation and assist member countries with loan payments. The International Bank for Reconstruction and Development (IBRD) provides loans to middle income countries. It was originally the World Bank Institution. Today, The World Bank refers to both IBRD and the International Development Association (IDA) (IMF, 2015c; The World Bank, 2015). The World Bank Group refers to IBRD, IDA and three other financial groups.

The IDA is the arm of the World Bank that loans to the world's poorest countries (IDA, 2015). The IMF and the World Bank are made up of 188 member countries. The IBRD is represented by 20 elected executive directors and 5 appointed executive directors. The IMF has an executive board of 24 directors representing 188 countries (IMF, 2015a).

At the founding of the BWI, only 3 African countries had gained independence and so Africa did not have a role (Browne, 1987). In the early history of BWI, the focus was on industrialized countries and by 1963; it started lending to Sub-Saharan Africa (Browne, 1987).

Table 7. Percentage of votes held by the five largest shareholders in the IMF

Country	Percentage of Votes Held
United States	16.75
Japan	6.23
Germany	5.81
France	4.29
United Kingdom	4.29

Source: IMF (2015c).

The voting structure of the International Monetary Fund is based on the economic contribution of the member states (Wolff, 2013). Approximately 37.37% of the total votes are held by just five countries and the United States holds 16.75% of that 37.37% (IMF, 2015b). A combination of 23 African countries hold 3.34% voting power and another combination of 23 other African countries hold a 1.66% voting power (Eurodad, 2006). The five largest shareholders are the United States, France, Germany, Japan and the United Kingdom. The weighted voting system allows countries with a larger financial contribution to impose policies that are favorable to their home countries but not to the borrowing countries (Browne, 1987; IMF, 2015b). Table 7 shows the percentage of votes held by the largest states. The voting power of the IMF correlates with the economic contribution of the member states.

The voting powers of IBRD are also similar to the IMF. Five of the executive members are appointed and 20 are elected. The elected executive directors predominantly represent a group of countries that can be up to 12 at a time (The World Bank, 2015).

A study conducted to examine 20 poor countries that had taken loans from the BWI showed that each country was faced with an average of 67 conditions for each loan (Eurodad, 2006). Uganda faced 197 loan conditions (Eurodad, 2006). On average, 18 of the 20 countries had privatization related conditions to their loans (Eurodad, 2006).

Global free market benefits the countries that have the highest voting powers while countries that take loans from the World Bank or IMF are subjected to adjustment programs that impose privatization and free trade (Wolff, 2013). The conditions for accepting these high interest loans include privatization, trade liberalization and lower government spending on social issues. Trade liberalization undermines local African industries (Eurodad, 2006). These conditions translate to lower salaries and increase poverty for the borrowing countries. It exacerbates income inequalities that favor countries with the greatest voting powers. However, for the multinational companies, it means they can now purchase cheaper raw materials from the borrowing countries.

THE WAY FORWARD

The civil conflicts around the areas of natural resources have not led to stable governments in these countries. Areas that do not have civil conflicts but are dependent on their natural resources for export have not invested in strengthening of their infrastructures. Similarly, the people in these countries have been impoverished despite an abundance of natural resources. They have been left poor with weak and struggling infrastructures that cannot combat the EVD disease. Conflicts also arise when stubborn African leaders refuse to leave when their terms are up. Other conflicts also arise from religious and ethnic interests.

Loans should not be tied to conditions like privatization and trade liberalization. The BWI should reform their policies and give the borrowing countries more leverage. African leaders should be willing to relinquish power when their term is up. A system of incentives and disincentives should be set in place to motivate leaders to leave when their term is up and disincentives should be activated for leaders that refuse to leave.

The change in the ecological climate of Guinea to a climate similar to countries that have frequently had EVD also facilitated the index case in the ongoing EVD coming from Guinea. Access to education should be provided beyond the primary school level. Other African countries with natural resources should collaborate with countries like Botswana that have natural resources like diamond but have not had conflicts. Health education should be accessible to both men and women. Turmoils arising from religious and ethnic interests should be diffused through international collaboration and sharing of information.

CONCLUSION

Díẹ̀ díẹ̀ nimú ẹlẹ́dẹ̀ẹ́ fi ń wọgbà is a Yoruba proverb that means it is little by little that a pig's nose enters the compound. The morale of including this proverb is that big problems start little by little. The enabling political economic factors have contributed to the environment that allows infectious diseases to thrive in Africa. The EVD is a glaring example even though there are several infectious diseases that have been responsible for more deaths than the EVD. This chapter has examined the enabling political economies of infectious diseases in Africa.

The foundational structures at the time of the current EVD was grossly inadequate to manage the disease. In addition, lapse in communication by the World Health Organization, poverty, weakened and struggling health infrastructures, cultural beliefs, mistrust of the government and fear accelerated the spread of the disease. The privatization-attached conditions attached to loans by IMF and the World Bank has exacerbated poverty in poor countries.

Poverty is also exacerbated in populations with high fertility rates as six of the countries with the highest fertility rates (Niger, Mali, Democratic Republic of Congo, Chad, Burkina Faso and Liberia) ranked among the lowest in the UNDP Human Development Index. Conflicts arising from natural resources, African leaders that are reluctant to leave and turmoils from religious and ethnic interests have contributed to political instability, unemployment, poverty and poor infrastructures. All of the identified enabled factors provide an environment that nourishes poverty which facilitates the spread of infectious diseases.

REFERENCES

Adedeji, A. (1999). Comprehending African Conflicts: Sub-Sahara Africa, a violent continent. In A. Adedeji (Ed.), *Comprehending and Mastering African Conflicts: The Search for Sustainable Peace and Good Governance* (pp. 3–21). London: Zed.

African Development Bank. (2007). *Africa's Natural Resources: The paradox of plenty*. Retrieved from http://www.afdb.org/fileadmin/uploads/afdb/Documents/Publications/(E)%20AfricanBank%202007%20Ch4.pdf

Ajaegbu, O. O. (2012). Rising youth unemployment and violent crime in Nigeria. *American Journal of Social Issues and Humanities*, *2*(5), 315–321.

Arab Uprising: Country by Country-Tunisia. (2013, December). *BBC News*. Retrieved from http://www.bbc.co.uk/news/world-12482315

Auty, R. M. (1993). *Sustaining Development in Mineral Economies: The Resource Curse* (Thesis). London: Routledge.

Balestri, S., & Maggioni, M. A. (2014). Blood diamonds, dirty gold and spatial spill-overs measuring conflict dynamics in West Africa. *Peace Economics, Peace Science & Public Policy*, *20*, 551–564.

Bausch, D. G., & Schwarz, L. (2014). Outbreak of Ebola virus disease in Guinea: where ecology meets economy. *PLoS Neglected Tropical Diseases, 8*(7), e3056. Retrieved from http://journals.plos.org/plosntds/article?id=10.1371/journal.pntd.0003056

Bretton Woods Project. (2005). *What are the Bretton Woods Institutions?* Retrieved from http://www.brettonwoodsproject.org/2005/08/art-320747/

Browne, R. S. (1987). The IMF in Africa: A case of inappropriate technology in the political morality of the International Monetary Fund. In R. J. Myers (Ed.), Ethics and Foreign Policy Series (Vol. 3, pp. 65–80). Transaction: New Jersey.

Burundi. (n.d.). *The New York Times*. Retrieved from http://topics.nytimes.com/top/news/international/countriesandterritories/burundi/index.html

CDC. (2015). *Outbreaks chronology; Ebola virus disease*. Retrieved from http://www.cdc.gov/vhf/ebola/outbreaks/history/chronology.html

CDC SARS Response Timeline, SARS: Key Events. (2013). Retrieved from http://www.cdc.gov/about/history/sars/timeline.htm

Dray-Spira, R., Gueguen, A., Persoz, A., Deveau, C., Lert, F., Delfraissy, J.-F., & Meyer, L. (2005). Temporary employment, absence of stable partnership, and risk of hospitalization or death during the course of HIV infection. *Journal of Acquired Immune Deficiency Syndromes*, *40*(2), 190–197. doi:10.1097/01.qai.0000165908.12333.4e

Egypt under Sisi. (n.d.). *BBC News*. Retrieved from http://www.bbc.co.uk/news/world-middle-east-12315833

Eurodad. (2006). *World Bank and IMF Conditionality; A development injustice*. Retrieved from http://www.eurodad.org/uploadedfiles/whats_new/reports/eurodad_world_bank_and_imf_conditionality_report.pdf

Global Health Observatory, Life Expectancy Situation. (n.d.). *WHO*. Retrieved from http://www.who.int/gho/mortality_burden_disease/life_tables/situation_trends_text/en/

How Long are African Presidents Staying in Power?. (2015, May). *BBC News*. Retrieved from http://www.bbc.com/news/world-africa-32624979

IDA. (2015). *What is IDA?* Retrieved from http://www.worldbank.org/ida/what-is-ida.html

IDMC. (2015). *The Norwegian Refugee Council's Internal Displacement Monitoring Center Global Overview; People internally displaced by conflict and violence*. Retrieved from http://www.internal-displacement.org/assets/library/Media/201505-Global-Overview-2015/20150506-global-overview-2015-en.pdf

ILO. (2010). *ILO Global Employment Trends*. Retrieved from http://www.ilo.org/wcmsp5/groups/public/---ed_emp/---emp_elm/---trends/documents/publication/wcms_120471.pdf

ILO. (2013). *ILO Global employment Trends 2013*. Retrieved from http://www.ilo.org/wcmsp5/groups/public/---dgreports/---dcomm/---publ/documents/publication/wcms_202326.pdf

IMF. (2015a). *About the IMF*. Retrieved from http://www.imf.org/external/about.htm

IMF. (2015b). *IMF Executive directors and voting powers*. Retrieved from http://www.imf.org/external/np/sec/memdir/eds.aspx

IMF. (2015c). *IMF Executive Directors and Voting Powers*. Available from: http://www.imf.org/external/np/sec/memdir/eds.aspx

IMF. (2015c). *IMF Lending*. Retrieved from http://www.imf.org/external/np/exr/facts/howlend.htm

Laurent Gbagbo. (n.d.). *The New York Times*. Retrieved from http://topics.nytimes.com/top/reference/timestopics/people/g/laurent_gbagbo/index.html

Le Guenno, B., Formentry, P., Wyers, M., Gounon, P., Walker, F., & Boesch, C. (1995). Isolation and partial characterization of a new strain of Ebola virus. *Lancet*, *345*(8960), 1271–1274. doi:10.1016/S0140-6736(95)90925-7

Libya Country Profile-Overview. (2015, June). *BBC News*. Retrieved from http://www.bbc.co.uk/news/world-africa-13754897

Malaria. (2015, April). *The World Bank*. Retrieved from http://www.worldbank.org/en/topic/health/brief/malaria

MDG 6. Combat HIV/AIDS, Malaria and Other Diseases. (2014, December). *WHO*. Retrieved from http://www.who.int/topics/millennium_development_goals/diseases/en/

Negredo, A., Palacios, G., Vázquez-Morón, S., González, F., Dopazo, H., Molero, F., & Tenorio, A. et al. (2011). Discovery of an Ebolavirus-like filovirus in Europe. *PLoS Pathogens*, *7*(10), e1002304.

Ng, S., Basta, N. E., & Cowling, B. J. (2014). Association between temperature, humidity and ebolavirus disease outbreaks in Africa, 1976 to 2014. *Eurosurveillance*, *19*(35), 20892. doi:10.2807/1560-7917.ES2014.19.35.20892

Njoku, A. C., & Ihugba, O. A. (2011). Unemployment and Nigerian Economic Growth (1985-2009). *Mediterranean Journal of Social Sciences*, *2*(6), 23–32.

Obilade, T. T. (2015a). Ebola virus disease stigmatization: The role of societal attributes. *International Archives of Medicine*, *8*(14), 1-19. Retrieved from http://imed.pub/ojs/index.php/iam/article/view/1007/674

Obilade, T. T. (2015b). The political economy and stigmatization of HIV/AIDS in patients attending a clinic in Lagos, Nigeria. *The International Archives of Medicine*, *8*(26), 1-11. Retrieved from http://imed.pub/ojs/index.php/iam/article/view/997/687

Omar al-Bashir wins Sudan Elections by a Landslide. (2015, April). *BBC News*. Retrieved from http://www.bbc.com/news/world-africa-32481013

Paessler, S., & Walker, D. H. (2013). Pathogenesis of the viral hemorrhagic fevers. *Annual Review of Pathology*, *8*(1), 411–440. doi:10.1146/annurev-pathol-020712-164041

Perry, A. (2010, June 28). Brief History: The Resource Curse. *Time Magazine*. Retrieved from http://content.time.com/time/magazine/article/0,9171,1997460,00.html

Population Reference Bureau. (2011). *The World's Women's and Girls' 2011 Data Sheet*. Retrieved from http://www.prb.org/pdf11/world-women-girls-2011-data-sheet.pdf

Population Reference Bureau. (2014). *Population Reference Bureau 2014 World Population Data Sheet*. Retrieved from http://www. prb.org/pdf14/2014-world-population-data-sheet_eng.pdf

Ross, W. (2008, August 6). Guinea Turmoil Threatens Mine Deal. *BBC News*. Retrieved from http://news.bbc.co.uk/2/hi/africa/7544046.stm

Sachs, J. D., & Warner, A. M. (1999). The big push, natural resource booms and growth. *Journal of Development Economics*, *59*(1), 43–76. doi:10.1016/S0304-3878(99)00005-X

South Sudan Profile- Overview. (2015, August). *BBC News*. Retrieved from http://www.bbc.com/news/world-africa-14069082

Stone, R. W. (2004). The political economy of IMF lending in Africa. *The American Political Science Review*, *98*(04), 577–591. doi:10.1017/S000305540404136X

The African Leaders Who Chose Power above the People. (2015, January). *BBC News*. Retrieved from http://www.bbc.com/news/world-africa-30886067

The World Bank. (2014). *Country and Lending Groups; Sub-Saharan Africa*. Retrieved from http://data.worldbank.org/about/country-and-lending-groups#Sub_Saharan_Africa

The World Bank. (2015). *The International Bank for Reconstruction and Development*. Retrieved from http://www.worldbank.org/en/about/what-we-do/brief/ibrd

The World Bank Group & International Monetary Fund. (2015). *Global Monitoring Report 2014/2015; Ending Poverty and Sharing Prosperity*. Retrieved from http://www.worldbank.org/content/dam/Worldbank/gmr/gmr2014/GMR_2014_Full_Report.pdf

Togo Profile Leaders-Togo. (2015, May). *BBC News*. Retrieved from http://www.bbc.com/news/world-africa-14106787

Togo's Faure Gnassingbe Wins Third Term as President. (2015, April). *BBC News*. Retrieved from http://www.bbc.com/news/world-africa-32512615

Top Ten Causes of Death: How Has the Situation Changed in the Past Decade?. (n.d.). *WHO*. Retrieved from http://www.who.int/mediacentre/factsheets/fs310/en/index2.html

UNAIDS. (2013). *Global Report: UNAIDS report on the global AIDS epidemic 2013*. Retrieved from http://www.unaids.org/sites/default/files/en/media/unaids/contentassets/documents/epidemiology/2013/gr2013/UNAIDS_Global_Report_2013_en.pdf

UNDP Human Development Reports. (n.d.). *Table 1: Human Development Index and Its Components*. Available from: http://hdr.undp.org/en/content/table-1-human-development-index-and-its-components

UNDP Human Development Reports. (n.d.). *Table 1: Human Development Index and its components*. Retrieved from http://hdr.undp.org/en/content/table-1-human-development-index-and-its-components

United Nations. (2015). *We can end poverty; Millennium Development Goals*. Retrieved from http://www.un.org/millenniumgoals/

United Nations, UN List of Least Developed Countries. (2015). Retrieved from http://www.un.org/en/development/desa/policy/cdp/ldc/ldc_list.pdf

United Nations. (n.d.). *UN List of Least Developed Countries*. Available from: http://www.un.org/en/development/desa/policy/cdp/ldc/ldc_list.pdf

WHO. (1978a). Report of a WHO/International Study Team. (1978). Ebola Haemorrhagic Fever in Sudan, 1976. *Bulletin of the World Health Organization*, *56*, 247–270.

WHO. (1978b). Report of an International Commission. (1978). Ebola Haemorrhagic Fever in Zaire, 1976. *Bulletin of the World Health Organization*, *56*, 271–293.

WHO. (2014a). *The health of the people-what works: The African regional health report*. Retrieved from http://apps.who.int/iris/bitstream/10665/137377/4/9789290232612.pdf?ua=1

WHO. (2014b). *The 10 leading causes of death in the world 2000 and 2012*. Retrieved from http://www.who.int/mediacentre/factsheets/fs310/en/

Wolff, M. J. (2013). Failure of the International Monetary Fund and World Bank to Achieve Integral Development: A Critical Historical Assessment of Bretton Woods Institutions Policies, Structures & Governance. *Syracuse Journal of International Law & Commerce*, *41*, 71–144.

Chapter 5
The States as Generators of Incremental Change in American Health Care Policy: 1935 to 1965

Robert A. Peters
Western Michigan University, USA

Minerva Cruz
Western Michigan University, USA

ABSTRACT

The literature defines the role of interest groups and administration officials in the evolution of health care policy but does not acknowledge the impact of Congressional casework or the initial Social Security (OASI) eligibility criteria. There is, as a result, an inadequate appreciation for (1) the extent to which the initial development of federal policy was a function of Congressional delegations pursuing initiatives that would increase the flow of federal dollars their states could use to expand health services or (2) the way in which the regional cleavages created OASI eligibility criteria combined with the South's control of Congressional leadership positions to yield an expansion of health care for indigent people while intentionally delaying the creation of Medicare. This chapter addresses these gaps and provides a more complete picture of the way in which the incremental, unplanned evolution of federal health care policy was the product of using federal resources to diminish the states' fiscal needs and the south's capacity to temporarily control the health care agenda.

DOI: 10.4018/978-1-4666-9944-1.ch005

BACKGROUND

The literature relating to the evolution of federal health care financing and policy has not adequately examined the roles of the states in the growth of federal programs or the unintended effects of the initial Social Security (OASI) eligibility criteria. Although the literature has delineated the evolution of federal health care matching formulas from their origins in the public assistance programs to the establishment of the Medicaid and Medicare programs, the analyses focus on the strategies and tactics of federal officials to the exclusion of the states and their congressional delegations. There is, as a result, inadequate understanding of the financial implications of the partnership between state officials and their congressional delegations that enabled them to increase the flow of federal funds for the purpose of advancing their states' policy goals. In similar fashion, the literature acknowledges that the initial OASI eligibility criteria created regional variations in the percentage of people aged 65 and older who received OASI benefits (Corson, 1939; Sloman, 1942; Trafton & Feinroth, 1944). However, it does not examine the impact of these patterns on the origins and composition of the Kerr-Mills Medical Assistance for the Aged (MAA) program that was the precursor to the Medicaid program (Engel, 2006; Gilman, 1998; Olson, 2010; Patel & Rushefsky, 2006; Smith & Moore, 2009; Sundquist, 1968).

To address the gaps in the literature and convey lessons arising from the American experience, the next section outlines the policymaking model for the interactions between the state and national governments. The discussion is followed by descriptions of (1) the revisions of public assistance matching formulas that were initiated by the states for the purpose of increasing the flow of federal health care dollars to the states, (2) the basis for and the regional implications of the initial OASI eligibility criteria, (3) the impact of the regional patterns on Kerr-Mills, and (4) the manner in which the preceding factors affected the development and enactment of the Medicaid and Medicare programs in 1965. The chapter's final section summarizes the findings and examine their implications for health care finance and policy.

MODEL FOR THE EXPANSION OF FEDERAL HEALTH CARE FINANCING

During the thirty years between the establishment of the public assistance matching formulas in 1935 and the enactment of the Medicare and Medicaid programs in 1965, the states' pursuit of their self-interest affected the evolution of federal health care funding for elderly and indigent citizens. Kingdon's (1995) policymaking model suggests that the state's success in placing their health care financing proposals on Congress' agenda was a function of their congressional delegations' ability to merge the problem, policy, and politics streams to take advantage of windows of opportunity (Gilman, 1998). The problem component, as defined by the states, focused on minimizing welfare dependency, i.e., providing health care services that would enable public assistance recipients to become self-sufficient. Given definition of the problem and the states' desire to limit the demands on their resources and the need for state tax increases, the states' policy was to expand the flow of federal grants-in-aid via federal matching formula revisions. As an increasing share of states availed themselves of the expansion of federal funding, there was a concomitant increase in the probability of securing Congressional support for additional matching formula revisions. The process, in other words, was self-perpetuating: an expansion in the number of states benefiting from the revised federal matching formulas enhanced the feasibility of enacting additional changes that would generate further increases in federal outlays.

The probability of achieving their policy goal was also facilitated by procedural strategies: the process of adding matching formula revisions to larger bills virtually guaranteed that congressional attention would be focused on the legislation's primary components. By deflecting the lawmakers' attention in this manner, the proponents of matching formula revisions were able to minimize the number of congressional supporters that was needed to assure passage. In addition, whenever the proposal was attached to must pass legislation, the probability of a presidential veto was reduced (Gilman, 1998). Due to the preceding elements, the revisions of federal matching formulas reflected the initiatives of state governments and federal health care policy was incremental.

PUBLIC ASSISTANCE MATCHING FORMULAS: THE FOUNDATION FOR FEDERAL HEALTH CARE SPENDING

Although the American Medical Association's (AMAs) opposition to national health insurance resulted in its removal from the social security legislation that the Roosevelt Administration sent to Capitol Hill (Olson, 2010; Patel & Rushefsky, 2006; Smith & Moore, 2009), federal health care funding was not dead: the bill's public assistance matching formulas contained the seeds for the subsequent growth of federal health care expenditures. More specifically, each of the three public assistance matching formulas (Aid to the Blind (AB), Aid to Dependent Children (ADC) and Old Age Assistance (OAA)) specified the percentage of benefits that would be funded by the Federal Government, the ceiling on federal reimbursements, and a prohibition against using federal funds for payments to individuals who were in public institutions (49 Stat. 620-648 (1935)). At first glance, the final element does not appear to provide a basis for establishing and expanding the federal government's role in health care finance. However, the subsequent actions of Members of Congress clearly indicate that the prohibition provided an opportunity to dramatically increase federal health care spending.

The first instance of exploiting the opportunity occurred in 1949 when Congress undertook a major revision of the Social Security Act of 1935. The Congressional Record reveals four rationales for terminating the prohibition against using federal public assistance funds to defray a portion of the cost of providing health care to public assistance recipients. The first rationale emanated from the equitable treatment of recipients. Given that the Federal Government was covering a portion of the payments to individuals who were in private institutions, it was argued that federal funds should also match payments for those who were in public institutions. In so doing, the affected individuals would no longer have to give up their public assistance checks when they receive extended medical care in county or local facilities. The second rationale focused on the states' capacity to provide a wider array of services that would reduce dependence. More specifically, lawmakers argued that insufficient health care and chronic illness are barriers to securing a job and economic self-sufficiency. The provision of health care services therefore is an essential tool for ensuring or restoring health and thereby minimizing the citizens' reliance on public assistance programs (U.S. House of Representatives, 1949).

The third rationale is persistent and persuasive lobbying for federal financing of health care services. During the House floor debate, Representative Cooper (Democrat-Tennessee) noted that the representative from Wisconsin, for a number of years, was advocating for federal funding of health care services that were provided to public assistance recipients. The record also indicates that the House Committee on Ways and Means was "most favorably impressed by his appearance before the committee [and] . . . endeavored to take care of the situation which he so ably presented to the committee" (U.S. House of Representatives, 1949, p. 13899). The fourth and final rationale addressed the need for additional facilities to serve the chronically ill. If health care would be added to the public assistance matching formulas, then the states could use the additional federal monies to support a greater volume of health services for recipients. The additional income, in turn, would enable communities to "develop" additional facilities for chronically ill patients and thereby assist in fulfilling the need for such facilities (U.S. House of Representatives, 1949). In this respect, the liberalization of public assistance matching formulas was a forerunner of Hill-Burton (Patel & Rushefsky, 2006) which provided federal funding for hospital construction.

Congress approved the addition of medical vendor payments to the public assistance matching formulas (64 Stat 477–561, (1950)) but was not willing to approve the Social Security Administration's Wilbur Cohen (Smith & Moore, 2009) or Senator Lehman's (Democrat-New York) proposals to establish two public assistance matching formulas: one for payments to recipients and one for payments to doctors and hospitals. Senator Lehman argued that the establishment of distinct matching formulas was necessary for states in which the average public assistance payments were approaching or exceeding the ceiling on federal reimbursements. If Congress did not approve the proposal, the states would be forced to use the limited space between existing assistance payments and the federal reimbursement ceiling to increase payments to individuals or institute a program of payments to health care providers. Under these conditions, the senator argued that the matching formula would constrain the extent to which these states could provide health services that would minimize dependency emanating from "medical neglect and chronic illness" (U.S. Senate, 1950, p. 8791).

He also noted that his amendment was supported by the interassociation committee on health and its decision was "formally confirmed by the governing boards of its six constituent organizations–the American Dental Society, the American Hospital Association, the American Medical Association, the American Nursing Association, the American Public Health Association and the American Public Welfare Association" (U.S. Senate, 1950, p. 8791). The associations' support was based on the premise that the additional federal funding would stimulate the provision of quality care and the accompanying proviso that the assistance would be administered by public health departments and the administrative arrangements would be approved by the six organizations (U.S. Senate, 1950). As is the case for third party insurance, the AMAs support of Senator Lehman's amendment suggests that the organization is not opposed to all publicly-financed health care initiatives: it opposes initiatives that insert a third party, rather than members of the medical community (e.g., Blue Cross/Blue Shield insurance as initially constituted and public health departments), into the doctor/patient relationship.

As indicated by the data in Tables 1 to 4, two years after enacting the Social Security Act Amendments of 1950, the Federal Government was defraying a portion of the health care costs for two adult public assistance programs (AB and OAA) in 18 states, the adult public assistance program Aid to the Permanently and Totally Disabled (APTD) program (established in 1950) in 12 states, and the ADC program in 17 states. The data also reveal that federal health care expenditures in FY 1952 were greatest for the OAA Program ($49.6 million). Federal health care reimbursements for the other programs, in descending order, were $9.4 million for ADC, $5.9 million for ATPD, and $1.3 million for AB. By 1956, the number of states for which the Federal Government was subsidizing public assistance health care costs rose to 20 to 24 states for the adult public assistance programs and 22 states for the ADC program. The evidence also indicates that the gap between health care reimbursements for the OAA program and the remaining public assistance programs widened. Federal health care reimbursements were $130.5 million for the OAA program, between $23 and $24 million for the ADC and APTD programs and a relatively paltry $3.4 million for the AB program.

Table 1. Amount of medical vendor payments for the medical care of OAA recipients for selected years, by state

State	1952	1954	1956	1958	1960
Alabama		11,902	17,511	20,439	12,455
Alaska					
Arkansas				2,096,364	4,010,575
California			1,564,227	14,362,380	26,866,177
Colorado				2,157,471	10,071,078
Connecticut	1,981,999	2,318,567	3,265,761	3,264,386	3,633,356
Delaware					
Florida					4,178,406
Hawaii		115,210	224,972	107,772	133,930
Idaho					453,481
Illinois	8,931,585	18,498,983	22,681,883	25,351,489	25,915,059
Indiana	3,185,747	3,951,588	5,377,734	5,724,926	6,188,975
Iowa					2,745,306
Kansas	1,478,125	1,989,953	2,585,045	3,500,339	4,068,951
Louisiana	531	772	3,497	1,593,738	2,912,301
Maine			514,548	1,001,181	1,599,495
Maryland				60,047	598,662
Massachusetts	2,500,609	10,481,939	24,692,145	21,040,010	40,504,037
Michigan	298,617	1,375,499	1,887,870	4,720,536	5,140,094
Minnesota	8,368,903	11,441,907	15,201,125	6,979,084	19,483,833
Missouri					231,720
Montana					15,744
Nebraska	2,059,885	1,735,841		1,409,350	4,124,864
Nevada	18,954	41,859	78,647	168,891	188,466
New Hampshire	728,376	958,935	879,708	1,001,551	1,048,049
New Jersey				2,612,959	7,592,296
New Mexico		300,652	380,181	753,849	1,094,728
New York	14,078,448	20,788,569	25,533,901	20,499,796	32,699,781
North Carolina	102,984	150,284	357,578	786,102	1,168,436
North Dakota	266,458	339,456	1,637,844	1,314,734	2,681,646

continued on following page

Table 1. Continued

State	1952	1954	1956	1958	1960
Ohio	2,192,640	2,613,178	3,074,712	6,723,203	11,238,456
Oklahoma				6,735,336	12,451,356
Oregon				4,015,672	5,446,931
Pennsylvania			1,593,419	3,044,355	2,255,779
Rhode Island	9,524	704,470	612,672	792,261	1,145,508
South Carolina					819,206
South Dakota					
Tennessee				537,832	875,174
Utah	5,470	11,688	11,330	633,244	406,811
Vermont					298,681
Virginia					1,201,892
Washington			11,903,083	8,038,062	16,268,222
West Virginia				713,659	825,963
Wisconsin	3,439,250	4,738,523	6,468,050	6,944,504	17,494,968
Wyoming				335,025	361,396
Total	49,648,105	82,569,775	130,547,443	159,040,547	280,452,244

Source: Social Security Administration. 1951-1960. Social Security Bulletin, 14(12)-23(9), Operating statistics: Amount of vendor payments for medical care for recipients of public assistance, by program and state, month and year.

Given the dramatic increase in the number of states availing themselves of federal health care matching funds and the explosion in federal health care outlays, it is not surprising that the Senate Committee on Finance added the Kerr-George amendment that accomplished the goal Senator Lehman was unable to achieve in 1949: establishing a federal matching formula for medical vendor payments that was separate from the formulas for payments to public assistance recipients. By establishing a separate formula for health care costs, it was no longer necessary for medical vendor payments to compete against income support payments for federal dollars. They could generate federal matching funds from the new formula that obligated the Federal Government to cover 50 percent of the health care costs up to $6 for the adult public assistance programs and up to $3 for the ADC program (70 Stat. 846-848 (1956)).

The data in Tables 1 to 4 indicate that the states represented by Senators Kerr (Democrat-Oklahoma) and George (Democrat-Georgia) did not receive federal reimbursements for medical vendor spending prior to Congress's consideration of the Social Security Act Amendments of 1956. However, Senator Kerr's motivation

Table 2. Amount of medical vendor payments for the medical care of ADC recipients for selected years, by state

State	1952	1954	1956	1958	1960
Alabama		7,347	12,064	9,922	6,461
Alaska					
Arkansas				226,599	260,648
California				7,026,414	11,683,743
Colorado				380,042	474,250
Connecticut	812,872	771,334	1,168,142	1,054,920	1,940,626
Delaware	5,536	10,042			
Florida					224,642
Hawaii		197,695	74,663	369,177	295,164
Idaho					
Illinois	757,206	1,903,662	3,037,599	4,311,303	6,017,599
Indiana	553,166	542,142	881,164	1,255,103	1,605,734
Iowa					781,535
Kansas	322,642	379,613	496,271	695,618	1,033,239
Louisiana	27,031	37,797	50,617	104,051	157,416
Maine			159,201	190,566	308,962
Maryland				107,659	979,341
Massachusetts	335,136	1,011,089	1,695,599	1,607,853	2,439,737
Michigan				548,129	997,947
Minnesota	551,929	827,650	1,311,709	1,678,466	2,362,867
Missouri					40,424
Montana					481
Nebraska	108,999	64,138		49,557	109,226
Nevada					
New Hampshire	226,401	184,882	163,391	168,511	203,335
New Jersey	138,695	133,688	201,594	333,934	249,577
New Mexico		143,575	378,876	663,111	704,520
New York	4,456,819	5,690,101	8,252,545	10,189,326	13,174,185
North Carolina	58,032	94,637	166,808	425,437	631,109
North Dakota	12,143	49,343	196,070	284,595	340,626
Ohio	88,868	191,354	212,475	129,800	993,022
Oklahoma				2,506,862	51,023
Oregon				418,330	309,417

continued on following page

Table 2. Continued

State	1952	1954	1956	1958	1960
Pennsylvania			1,335,140	2,433,923	3,747,785
Rhode Island		264,761	352,009	671,949	916,385
South Carolina					224,687
South Dakota					
Tennessee				281,965	275,230
Utah	3,009	7,615	13,326	440,102	288,617
Vermont					
Virginia					
Washington			1,540,348	2,138,623	2,095,658
West Virginia				763,987	1,036,332
Wisconsin	915,942	1,129,364	1,423,262	1,759,563	2,249,787
Wyoming				52,270	72,818
Total	9,374,426	13,641,829	23,122,873	43,277,667	59,284,155

Source: Social Security Administration. 1951-1960. Social Security Bulletin, 14(12)-23(9), Operating statistics: Amount of vendor payments for medical care for recipients of public assistance, by program and state, month and year.

for introducing the amendment is suggested by the fact that Oklahoma's payments to AB, APTD and OAA recipients by the mid-1950s. Given the benefit levels, the establishment of a medical vendor program would have been financed primarily by the state's own resources. The introduction and passage of the Kerr-George amendment therefore enabled the state of Oklahoma to shift a significant portion of its medical vendor costs to the Federal Government. The validity of the assumption is supported by the fact that Oklahoma began to receive federal medical vendor payments within one year of the amendment's enactment and federal reimbursements increased from $10 million in 1958 to $14 million in 1960.

The rationale for Senator George's support is not evident because his home state of Georgia did not establish a medical vendor program during the 1950s and payments to public assistance recipients were significantly less than the federal reimbursement ceiling. His home state therefore could have established a medical vendor program under the public assistance matching formulas without resorting to the medical vendor formulas created by the Kerr-George amendment. Given that he retired slightly more than a year after the legislation was approved, there may have been a political or policy rationale for Senator George to champion the amendment.

It is noteworthy that the new medical vendor matching formulas were not beneficial for all states. In the case of 13 states whose medical vendor spending exceeded

Table 3. Amount of medical vendor payments for the medical care of AB recipients for selected years, by state

State	1952	1954	1956	1958	1960
Alabama		31	435	119	28
Alaska					
Arkansas				77,924	118,643
California			140,749	739,236	1,414,977
Colorado			2,677	25,188	29,451
Connecticut	31,234	44,859	58,423	62,992	86,959
Delaware				8,509	12,940
Florida					98,532
Hawaii		5,048	11,898	7,063	6,299
Idaho					4,872
Illinois	249,552	523,408	699,738	691,785	768,469
Indiana	115,300	131,084	218,325	251,967	315,120
Iowa					102,848
Kansas	32,356	36,872	45,861	62,900	69,569
Louisiana	1,534	2,050	6,196	32,842	44,784
Maine			19,176	36,768	43,014
Maryland				2,326	16,062
Massachusetts		3,925	26,547	231,118	234,523
Michigan	3,166	19,920	28,560	104,115	122,724
Minnesota	54,850	268,856	386,172	205,781	419,323
Missouri					
Montana				13,182	7,156
Nebraska	7,055	6,653		134,496	336,541
Nevada				8,901	12,882
New Hampshire	27,278	31,239	28,926	33,269	42,609
New Jersey			883	24,305	2,415
New Mexico		11,014	23,208	24,572	25,986
New York	574,990	801,833	1,003,189	743,462	1,245,875
North Carolina				42,492	96,721
North Dakota	1,005	3,051	8,763	10,014	16,332
Ohio	65,763	83,228	105,253	308,849	304,191
Oklahoma				137,580	228,783
Oregon				40,227	38,190

continued on following page

Table 3. Continued

State	1952	1954	1956	1958	1960
Pennsylvania			333,381	704,719	610,744
Rhode Island	60	16,702	15,566	9,480	11,424
South Carolina					27,814
South Dakota					
Tennessee				30,766	22,452
Utah	92	1,306	1,672	15,168	7,047
Vermont					2,704
Virginia					54,175
Washington			112,918	88,905	204,053
West Virginia				28,109	30,517
Wisconsin	94,265	110,119	152,550	170,058	366,896
Wyoming				6,132	5,885
Total	1,258,500	2,101,198	3,431,066	5,115,319	7,610,529

Source: Social Security Administration. 1951-1960. Social Security Bulletin, 14(12)-23(9), Operating statistics: Amount of vendor payments for medical care for recipients of public assistance, by program and state, month and year.

the new ceilings on reimbursable expenditures, switching from the public assistance formulas to the medical vendor formulas would have resulted in less federal funding. To avoid this outcome for his and the other states, Senator Douglas (Democrat-Illinois) proposed an amendment that would enable the states to use the new formula to calculate the federal share of health care costs. For any medical vendor spending greater than the ceilings set by the new formula, the states could move the unmatched health care expenditures to the matching formulas for public assistance payments. The floor manager for the bill, Senator Byrd (Democrat-Virginia), agreed to take the amendment to conference committee.

Although the 1950 and 1956 matching formula revisions were portrayed as mechanisms for assisting the states in broadening and improving their health care services for public assistance recipients (Schottland, 1956), the evidence suggests that the changes were a function of the states pursuing matching formula changes that would minimize the demand on state coffers by maximizing the flow of federal funds. The record also reveals that the success of the efforts to shift costs was a function of Congress's focus on other parts of the legislation. In 1950, most of the debate focused on the Social Security (OASI) benefits and eligibility standards. In similar fashion, the Senate debate in 1956 focused on the OASI eligibility standards and whether disability insurance should be added to the OASI program. The

Table 4. Amount of medical vendor payments for the medical care of APTD recipients for selected years, by state

State	1952	1954	1956	1958	1960
Alabama		4,442	7,128	5,643	3,491
Alaska					
Arkansas				295,267	583,403
California					1,381,039
Colorado				100,789	159,861
Connecticut		58,157	797,054	799,634	1,060,738
Delaware					
Florida					639,710
Hawaii		86,124	188,016	80,268	104,439
Idaho					34,923
Illinois	435,266	2,051,366	3,260,319	4,851,383	4,774,283
Indiana					
Iowa					
Kansas	190,119	279,908	382,765	586,069	714,805
Louisiana	13,415	16,634	23,904	340,388	615,978
Maine			30,828	136,465	204,435
Maryland				43,905	192,025
Massachusetts	1,010,978	4,246,105	5,948,127	3,928,636	6,975,199
Michigan	48,402	224,487	313,529	236,856	344,052
Minnesota		10,251	110,130	94,664	112,961
Missouri					31,305
Montana					2,765
Nebraska				148,203	421,456
Nevada					
New Hampshire	288	35,100	63,640	120,205	161,571
New Jersey				538,782	1,591,938
New Mexico		54,971	71,186	147,016	236,264
New York	4,101,017	7,101,780	9,717,901	9,661,355	13,597,663
North Carolina	17,258	47,645	113,918	430,688	678,884
North Dakota	17,382	45,862	268,871	236,582	482,029
Ohio				607,090	1,264,780
Oklahoma				568,374	1,272,068
Oregon				891,896	1,123,526

continued on following page

Table 4. Continued

State	1952	1954	1956	1958	1960
Pennsylvania			547,765	1,125,650	1,149,318
Rhode Island	60	149,050	208,756	290,112	502,605
South Carolina					241,011
South Dakota					
Tennessee				40,201	138,601
Utah	1,209	2,247	4,894	130,290	136,625
Vermont					30,533
Virginia					341,705
Washington			1,335,259	1,068,031	2,357,672
West Virginia				284,365	287,868
Wisconsin	69,301	234,569	448,903	510,605	1,781,588
Wyoming				49,090	54,159
Total	5,904,695	14,648,698	23,842,893	28,348,502	45,787,276

Source: Social Security Administration. 1951-1960. Social Security Bulletin, 14(12)-23(9), Operating statistics: Amount of vendor payments for medical care for recipients of public assistance, by program and state, month and year.

provisions relating to federal reimbursement of health care costs therefore could be entitled the “who cares” provisions.

As is the case with other policies such as public assistance (Advisory Commission on Intergovernmental Relations, 1980), the “who cares” provisions generated dramatic increases in spending. Between 1952 and 1960, the data presented in Tables 1 to 4 indicate that total medical vendor spending increased from $66.2 million to $393.1 million, which is a growth rate of more than ten times the rate of growth for all federal outlays (Office of Management and Budget, 2015). It is also evident that a disproportionate share of the expansion relating to the adult public assistance programs (AB, APTD and OAA) was due to an increase of more than 50 percent in the number of participating states. Plus, health care spending for OAA recipients generated between two-thirds and three-quarters of total expenditures. If, as was suggested by Senator Douglas (Democrat-Georgia), nursing homes were “having an increasing importance in the care of the aged” (U.S. Senate, 1956, p. 13092), then nursing homes were responsible for a significant and increasing share of the health care expenditures for OAA recipients and were a harbinger of future spending trends for the Medicaid program.

Table 5. Per capita income in 1950 and number of social security beneficiaries per 1,000 aged population for selected years (1949, 1953, 1956, 1960, and 1964), by state

	Per Capita Income	Aged Social Security Beneficiaries Per 1,000 Aged Population, End of				
State	**1950**	**1949**	**1953**	**1956**	**1960**	**1964**
United States	1510	160	338	479	638	745
Alabama	909	106	250	353	540	674
Alaska	2400	140	394	509	586	531
Arizona	1367	135	333	462	591	742
Arkansas	847	77	226	325	561	695
California	1877	189	390	515	621	733
Colorado	1521	129	299	431	565	694
Connecticut	1891	247	435	608	716	795
Delaware	2075	193	389	554	677	812
Florida	1304	162	421	546	631	747
Georgia	1065	92	222	328	512	651
Hawaii	1429	193	365	496	645	760
Idaho	1329	114	300	432	680	779
Illinois	1831	173	347	489	657	746
Indiana	1524	159	349	512	702	798
Iowa	1532	94	247	388	642	755
Kansas	1463	97	254	403	620	725
Kentucky	990	101	251	377	614	733
Louisiana	1117	99	234	332	456	603
Maine	1195	201	440	575	712	797
Maryland	1642	164	349	498	608	722
Massachusetts	1656	230	435	601	680	758
Michigan	1718	183	384	545	719	812
Minnesota	1437	114	284	424	635	739
Mississippi	770	54	165	262	529	669
Missouri	1427	121	283	431	605	724
Montana	1654	114	276	398	654	760
Nebraska	1560	83	227	376	633	751
Nevada	1991	157	329	572	583	748
New Hampshire	1348	213	439	580	719	811
New Jersey	1802	229	433	609	709	792
New Mexico	1204	73	219	334	525	651

continued on following page

Table 5. Continued

	Per Capita Income	Aged Social Security Beneficiaries Per 1,000 Aged Population, End of				
State	**1950**	**1949**	**1953**	**1956**	**1960**	**1964**
New York	1858	204	401	569	685	769
North Carolina	1077	103	236	348	628	757
North Dakota	1360	46	154	274	643	783
Ohio	1608	184	367	513	661	761
Oklahoma	1144	76	223	328	518	660
Oregon	1657	201	421	575	709	804
Pennsylvania	1552	214	409	559	686	783
Rhode Island	1553	278	486	635	736	810
South Carolina	925	91	215	313	565	699
South Dakota	1283	56	189	327	634	750
Tennessee	1028	89	230	347	568	710
Texas	1363	84	226	351	530	673
Utah	1348	135	318	485	640	734
Vermont	1169	161	348	489	676	789
Virginia	1257	119	278	424	609	726
Washington	1721	195	405	540	671	774
West Virginia	1056	166	367	488	660	761
Wisconsin	1506	151	342	497	701	799
Wyoming	1719	125	277	410	631	722
Coefficient of Variation	0.233	0.385	0.265	0.219	.0102	0.076

Source: Social Security Administration. 1956, 1960, 1964. Social Security Bulletin, 19(12), 23(11), 27(12), Individual beneficiaries: Number of aged beneficiaries receiving monthly benefits per 1,000 population aged 65 or over, by State, at end of (year).

U.S. Census Bureau. 2014. Median family income by State: 1959, 1969, 1979, 1989, and 1999.

Another harbinger of the future is the prescient statement of Senator Martin (Republican-Pennsylvania) who predicted the future track of incremental change. According to the Senator,

Once a separate fund has been established with the "Disability Insurance" label, it will be argued that temporary disability insurance benefits, hospitalization benefits, and other health benefits are not significant new departures. A full-scale health insurance program is the possible result after a few years' time.

Thus, disability benefits—particularly with the new feature of the separate health benefit fund—are the beginning of an almost inevitable chain of events. And yet, under the scheme of the George amendment [disability insurance], this is done merely by increasing the familiar Social Security tax. The real issue is not presented clearly and openly to the American people—namely, whether we wish to start down the Government health insurance road by the imposition of new compulsory taxes. (U.S. Senate, 1956, pp. 13053-13054)

Although the Senator's statement focused on the insurance side of the ledger (i.e., the eventual passage of Medicare Part A insurance for hospitalization and Medicare Part B for health care provided outside of the hospital setting), the incremental argument also applies to the subsequent changes in the public assistance health care provisions. Given the previously discussed gradual expansion in the federal financing of public assistance health care programs, Kerr-Mills, which will be addressed in the following section, and Medicaid were incremental expansions of the medical vendor payment programs established in the 1950s.

The preponderance of evidence therefore indicates that the Federal Government's role in financing health care gradually evolved from the toehold provided by the Social Security Act of 1935's public assistance matching formulas. It is also apparent that the Federal Government's expanding role was a function of members of Congress endeavoring to minimize the demands on their state's resources by proposing matching formula revisions that would enable their states to shift an increasing share of the health care financial burden to the Federal Government.

REGIONAL CLEAVAGES ARISING FROM THE SOCIAL SECURITY ACT OF 1935

The Social Security Act of 1935 not only established a toehold for the growth of federal health care expenditures but also established eligibility standards that determined regional patterns for the percentage of citizens aged 65 and older who received OASI benefits. The unintended regional impact was a function of abundant caution, i.e., President Roosevelt's warning concerning "the importance of "avoiding" any danger of permanently discrediting the sound and necessary policy of Federal legislation for economic security by attempting to apply it on too ambitious a scale before actual experience has provided guidance for the permanently safe direction of such efforts" (U.S. House, 1949, p. 13820). The legislation establishing OASI therefore limited eligibility to groups for which there was adequate documentation and that would be most likely to qualify for benefits, i.e., individuals who were full-time employees and worked most of the year so that they would fulfill the eligibility requirement within a reasonable amount of time (Smith & Moore, 2009; U.S. House, 1950; U.S. Senate, 1950). The primary group that fulfilled these prerequisites was industrial workers. Due to President's recommendation to gain administrative experience before changing eligibility requirements and Congress's subsequent focus on World War II (Advisory Commission on Intergovernmental Relations, 1980), the eligibility criteria were not appreciably altered until the enactment of the Social Security Act Amendments of 1950 (U.S. House, 1950; U.S. Senate, 1950).

The regional implications of limiting eligibility primarily to industrial workers are reflected in the data contained in Table 5. In 1949, the greatest percentages of individuals aged 65 and older who received OASI payments occurred in the industrial Northeast, Mid-Atlantic, East North Central and Pacific Regions of the country while the lesser percentages occurred in the Southern and West North Central Regions. As experience with the OASI program increased and members of Congress endeavored to cover a greater share of their constituents, eligibility standards were liberalized during the 1950s.

The effects of liberalizing the OASI eligibility criteria are evident in the increasing share of elderly citizens who received OASI benefits and the dramatic reduction in the interstate variation of the percentage of elderly citizens who received OASI benefits. More specifically, the data in Table 5 indicate that the percentage of elderly citizens receiving OASI benefits increased from 16.0 percent in 1949 to 63.8 percent in 1960 and 74.5 percent in 1964. During the same period, the coefficient of variation, which measures the extent of variation, declined from .385 in 1949 to .102 in 1960 and 0.076 in 1964. Although 2010 is beyond the study's scope, it is also noteworthy that the percentage of older individuals who received benefits rose to 89.4 percent while the coefficient of variation fell to .041. The data therefore indicate that most of the increase in the percentage of elderly citizens receiving OASI benefits and most of the decrease in the interstate variation of benefits occurred during the 1950s.

The preceding regional patterns were also reflected in the distribution of per capita income. Although the per capita incomes of northern industrial states were more widely dispersed among the top three quartiles of states than was the case for the percentage of elderly citizens receiving OASI benefits, the Southern states dominated the lowest quartile for both measures. The relatively small percentage of elderly citizens receiving OASI benefits meant the Southern states were able to shift a lesser percentage of their OAA clients to the OASI rolls than was the case in other parts of the country. Since OAA was partially funded by the states while OASI was funded entirely by the Federal Government, the shift of a relatively small proportion of the OAA clients meant that the Southern states were also able to transfer a relatively small share of the OAA financial burden to the federal OASI program. When the ability of Southern states to offload a part of the fiscal burden is combined with their less than average per capita incomes, it is evident that the states with the smallest tax base and associated capacity to fund public services also received less fiscal relief from the transfer of OAA clients to OASI rolls than was the case for their wealthier, northern industrial counterparts.

The implications of the regional patterns were voiced by Southern Members of Congress. During the Senate debate concerning the Social Security Act Amendments of 1956, Senator Long (Democrat-Louisiana) noted that

in highly industrialized States, most of the workers are covered by OASI, whereas, on the other hand, in many of the agricultural States, and particularly in quite a number of Southern States, only a small percentage of the people are covered by the social-security system, and that situation also enters into the overall picture. In many [Southern] States with low per capita income, the economy still suffers from the after effects of [post-Civil War] reconstruction days. In some of those States many people were born in poverty, and have very limited resources. Therefore more welfare assistance is needed, of course, in comparison with the amount of welfare assistance needed in wealthy States. (U.S. Senate, 1956, pp. 12875-12876)
[The low per capita incomes also means that] it is those same States which have the greatest difficulty in providing essential services of State government and raising sufficient revenues to provide adequately for the needy within their boundaries. (U.S. Senate, 1956, p. 12671)

Six years earlier, Representative Elliot (Democrat-Alabama) observed that

the coverage of the Social Security Act must be expanded. This is shown by the fact that in all of the State of Alabama with its 3,000,000 people, there are only 15,000 persons now drawing old-age pensions [OASI] under the Social Security Act. As contrasted with this figure we have some 71,000 people now receiving old-age assistance through the county and State departments of public welfare. (U.S. House, 1950, p. 13956)

A similar perspective was raised by Representative Curtis's (Republican-Missouri) questioning of Representative Boggs (Democrat-Louisiana): "Why is it that Louisiana has 8 out of 10 people on OAA, when the national average is about 2 out of 10?" (U.S. House, 1950, p. 13960).

Due to the Southern states being able to shift a smaller portion of their OAA clients to the OASI rolls and thereby accruing less fiscal relief than the northern industrial states, the regional disparities set the stage for the next iteration of federal health care policy: the Kerr-Mills component of the Social Security Act Amendments of 1960.

THE SOCIAL SECURITY ACT AMENDMENTS OF 1960

The political viability of national health insurance was set during the first half of the 20th Century. President Woodrow Wilson was the first President to propose the establishment of national health insurance (Patel & Rushefsky, 2006). Following a 20 year hiatus, health insurance was on Presidents Roosevelt and Truman's agendas. However, the combination of government policies and charges of socialized medicine during the McCarthy era reduced its political salience. More specifically, the imposition of wage and price controls during World War II forced employers to compete for scarce labor on the basis of benefits and resulted in an increasing share of the workforce securing employer-provided health insurance. The share of workers covered by employer-provided insurance was also boosted by federal tax laws that enabled employers to write off part of their health care insurance costs. Due in large part to these government policies, the percentage of public and private employees with hospitalization coverage rose from 48.7 percent in 1950 to 68.9 percent in 1960. During the same period, increases of approximately 30 percentage points were achieved for surgical and regular medical insurance coverage (Kolodrubetz, 1972). The growing pervasiveness of employer-provided health insurance, in conjunction with charges of socialized medicine during the McCarthy era, significantly diminished public support for national health insurance coverage for working people and their families. However, due to the number of workers who lost their health insurance coverage upon retirement, health insurance advocates shifted their attention to elderly citizens (Patel & Rushefsky, 2006).

The pivot toward the elderly was also motivated by the increasing share of voters who were elderly and society's positive view of the age group. Between 1950 and 1960, the percentage of Americans who were aged 65 and older rose from 8.1 percent to 9.2 percent while the share of people between the ages of 19 and 65 declined. Due to these demographic shifts, the percentage of voting age people who were elderly increased by slightly less than three percentage points (Infoplease, 2014). The clout generated by their greater numbers was enhanced by the fact that they were more likely to vote than their younger counterparts and, because of their lifetime of hard work and sacrifices, were prone to be viewed positive terms. Due to these characteristics, the elderly possessed the political clout to secure a greater share of government resources and society was likely to contend that they deserved the additional benefits (Schneider & Ingram, 1993).

Although the changing political landscape led three Democratic presidential candidates from northern states (Kennedy, Humphrey and Symington) to propose health insurance for OASI beneficiaries (Sundquist, 1968), the probability of enacting a program in the early 1960s was modulated by regional schisms. Due to the existence of safe districts and the role of seniority in selecting committee chairs,

Southern members of Congress had sufficient longevity to secure key committee and leadership positions. In 1960, four of the five Congressional leaders represented Southern states. The Speaker of the House Sam Rayburn and Senate Majority Leader Lyndon Johnson were from the state of Texas while the chair of the House Committee on Ways and Means Wilbur Mills and the chair of the Senate Committee on Finance Harry Byrd represented the states of Arkansas and Virginia, respectively.

Representatives Mills and Rayburn and Senator Johnson had strong incentives to pursue additional federal funding for medical vendor payments instead of establishing a new health insurance program. The data in Table 5 indicates that their home states were among twenty states with the lowest median household incomes. Although the rate of decline in OAA caseloads for the period 1950 to 1960 was slightly greater in the state of Arkansas than nationwide (16.5 percent versus 15.5 percent), more than one-quarter of the elderly citizens in Arkansas and Texas continued to receive OAA benefits (Social Security Administration, 1951; Social Security Administration, 1960; United States Census Bureau, 1968). Due to these factors, the states of Arkansas and Texas had less than the average tax base (incomes) to finance government programs but were among the eight states with the highest ratios of OAA caseloads to elderly citizens.

The incentives to support an expansion of medical vendor payments were further enhanced by several political factors. The first relates to the relatively weak unions. Since the states of Arkansas and Texas were among the bottom ten states for the percentage of nonagricultural union members (Hirsch, Macpherson, & Vroman, 2001), the unions were unable to exert significant political pressure for the adoption of health insurance. The second factor involved the AMAs vehement opposition to the adoption of health insurance but support for medical vendor payments. The AMA House of Delegates Proceedings suggest the divergent positions were a function of the extent to which participation in the programs was voluntary vs. mandatory, whether the programs were state or federally administered, and the extent to which doctors were included in the promulgation of rules as well as program oversight (American Medical Association, 1961). The AMA pronouncements and Arkansas Medical Society correspondence with Representative Mills suggest an additional rationale. In order to minimize the validity of the unmet need argument, the AMA encouraged its members to provide charity care. Although the option was feasible for physicians serving areas with relatively few poor people, it was not feasible for those who served areas with high proportions of people who, due to their low incomes, were unable to pay their medical bills without assistance. Medical vendor payments therefore were a mechanism for enhancing the financial viability of practices with relatively high percentages of low income patients. It is for this reason and the desire to provide assistance to indigent elderly people who "really need help" paying their health care bills that the Arkansas Medical Society unanimously supported medical vendor payments (Mills, personal communication). The final factor is the strong opposition of Southern voters to the expansion of federal power. Lawmakers who represented the states of Arkansas and Texas therefore tended to support the medical vendor programs that were state administered and therefore more palatable to their constituents than a health insurance program that would be administered by the Federal Government.

The policy implications of the preceding factors were brought into focus by the Constitution of the United States and House committee jurisdictions. Given the constitutional requirement that legislation such as medical vendor payments and health insurance must begin in the House of Representatives (U.S. Constitution. Art. I, sec. 7) and the programs were within the jurisdiction of the House Committee on Ways and Means, House Speaker Rayburn (Democrat-Texas) and committee chair Mills (Democrat-Arkansas) were in a position to be the gatekeepers for health care legislation. Their capacity to control the flow of health care legislation was enhanced by the composition of the Ways and Means Committee. The committee, in more specific terms, consisted of 10 Republicans and 7 Southern Democrats who were prone to oppose health insurance and only 8 Democrats who were likely to support the legislation. Representative Mills was able to use his persuasive powers and the committee members' policy preferences to gain support for his recommendation that a subcommittee could investigate and study the administration of existing laws but could not consider or hold hearings on health care legislation. Since subcommittee member Forand (Democrat-Rhode Island) was a proponent of health insurance and introduced a bill during each session of Congress, the action was clearly intended to prevent him from developing a bill in subcommittee and sending it to the full committee for consideration (Peters, 2004).

The legislative tactic was effective until Representative Mills and Rayburn recognized that health insurance was becoming too popular for them to continue blocking legislation that would benefit the elderly (Peters, 2004). At this point, they had two options. The first was to advance the Democratic Party's agenda by passing health insurance legislation that President Eisenhower was prone to veto several months before the 1960 election and thereby virtually guarantee the election of the Democratic presidential nominee and a greater number of Democratic Representatives and Senators (Congressional Quarterly Almanac, 1960; Congressional Quarterly Weekly Report, 1960). The second was to advance their state's interests and political philosophy by developing an alternative to health insurance that would enable them to claim they were addressing the health care needs of elderly citizens and, in the process, derail efforts to establish a health insurance program for OASI beneficiaries. Due to the previously described political factors and the limited number of their constituents who would immediately benefit from the establishment of a health insurance program, Representatives Mills and Rayburn decided to use their position as legislative gatekeepers to enact an expansion of the medical vendor program (Peters, 2004).

The capacity of Representatives Mills and Rayburn to control the legislative process was not diminished after the legislation was reported out of committee. Due to the tradition of sending Ways and Means Committee legislation to the House floor under a closed rule and the Speaker's ability to influence the House Rules Committee, the rule under which the House considered the legislation prohibited House members from introducing amendments (Peters, 2004). The actions of health insurance proponents therefore were limited to voicing their desire to establish a health insurance program and their displeasure with the prohibition against introducing amendments that would add health insurance to the bill. When casting their votes for passage, the rule also limited their options to possibly killing the bill by voting against it or voting for the bill in the hope that the Senate would add health insurance provisions to the legislation (U.S. House, 1960).

Unlike the proceedings in the House committee and on the floor, members of the Senate Committee on Finance had an opportunity to vote on an health insurance amendment. Of the 17 committee members, six Republicans joined six Democrats—five of whom represented Southern states and one was from an industrial State—to oppose the amendment while one Southern Democrat and four Democrats from other parts of the country supported the measure. During the committee's deliberations, Senator Long (Democrat-Louisiana) introduced an amendment to raise the maximum federal match rate for the second part of the OAA matching formula. Since the federal match rate for this part was inversely related to a state's median income, the proposal to increase the federal match rate for low income states from 65 to 80 percent while retaining the federal match rate of 50 percent for high income states meant that the flow of federal funds to low income Southern states would expand by 21 percent while the rate of increase for other regions of the country would be in the eight to nine percent range (Peters, 2004).

Senator Long's effort to significantly increase the flow of federal funds to his and other Southern states was based on the fact that Louisiana had the highest percentage of elderly citizens who were receiving OAA payments (51.8 percent versus the national average of 14.2 percent) and the lowest percentage of elderly citizens who were receiving OASI benefits (45.6 percent versus the national average of 63.8 percent) (United States Department of Health, Education, and Welfare, 1960). It was also based on the fact that one-half of the state's patient days were provided by state-subsidized hospitals. The proposed hike in the federal match rate therefore was intended to defray above average OAA costs emanating from the state's inability to shift a larger share of the elderly population from the state-federal OAA program to the federally financed OASI program and the rising cost of providing health care for Louisiana's elderly population (Peters, 2004).

THE SOCIAL SECURITY ACT AMENDMENTS OF 1965

The literature suggests President Johnson's 1964 landslide victory facilitated the establishment of the Medicare and Medicaid programs in two respects. First, it enabled President Johnson to claim he had a mandate to enact a major component of his Great Society program: health insurance for OASI beneficiaries. Second, Johnson's coattails carried new Democrats into the House and Senate: Democrats who were beholden to Johnson for their election and therefore were more likely to support his agenda (Johnson, 1971; Patel and Rushefsky, 2006). The data also suggest the legislative outcome was affected by a regional shift in the number of seats occupied by Democrats. Due to redistricting that reflected a westward shift of the population and the 1964 general election, the Democrats lost 13 seats in the Southern states that tended to oppose health insurance but picked up 30 seats in states that were more favorable to Medicare: 15 in the industrial states and 15 in the western states. However, the electoral effect on the Senate was less beneficial. The Democrats lost two Southern seats and three western seats but gained five industrial state seats—a net gain of only two seats in states that tended to be supportive of health insurance (Peters, 2004).

An additional, readily apparent factor was the change in the White House's occupant. President Eisenhower who opposed an expansion of federal power and endeavored to return programs and power to the states (Advisory Commission on Intergovernmental Relations, 1980) was replaced by President Johnson who was a strong proponent of federal policy initiatives. President Johnson also possessed the political skills to neutralize the potential roadblocks imposed by Southern committee members and secure the support of key Republicans. Although the House Ways and Means Committee chair recognized that Johnson's landslide victory made it impossible to block passage of the Medicare legislation, the Senate Finance Committee chair Harry Byrd (Democrat-West Virginia) continued to oppose the legislation. After the House Committee on Ways and Means reported the legislation, President Johnson summoned the Congressional leadership to the White House for the purpose of reviewing the bill's status. Following the session, he escorted the leadership into the Cabinet Room where the media was waiting. President Johnson proceeded to ask Finance Committee chair Byrd whether there was anything "that you know of that would prevent that [a thorough hearing] coming about in a reasonable time?" When Senator Byrd responded that there was "Nothing in the committee now," Johnson surmised that "when the House acts and it is referred to the Senate Finance Committee, you will arrange for prompt hearings and thorough hearings?" Under the circumstances, Senator Byrd has no option but to respond in the affirmative and thereby eliminate the option of bottling up the bill in his committee (Johnson, 1971, p. 217).

On the House side, President Johnson understood that he needed the support of a key Republican to secure a sufficient number of Republican votes to offset the votes of Southern Democrats who would oppose the legislation. Since a key Republican lawmaker was interested in securing NASA jobs for his Ohio district, Johnson contacted the NASA Administrator and communicated in clear terms that the administrator had to satisfy the lawmaker's demands. The president's skillful use of pork barrel politics therefore facilitated the enactment of the health insurance legislation (Johnson, 1971).

It is also noteworthy that the final legislation combined Johnson's program of insurance for hospitalization with the Republicans' proposal for the coverage of non-hospital medical services and the Southern states' preference for a Medicaid program that would serve the needs of their relatively large populations of poor people. Due the merger of these programs into one piece of legislation, the Social Security Act Amendments of 1965 was the culmination of incremental changes that were initiated by the Social Security Act of 1935. As previously suggested by Senator Martin (Republican-Pennsylvania), Medicare was incremental because it was an additional example of grafting a new program onto the OASI system (U.S. Senate, 1956). And Medicaid was an incremental expansion of the medical vendor and Medical Assistance for the Aged (MAA) programs.

CONCLUSION

Even though the Roosevelt Administration's decision to remove health insurance from the social security legislation appeared to doom efforts to engage the Federal Government in the financing of non-military physician and hospital services, the public assistance federal matching formulas provided a toehold for incrementally achieving the goal. The first exploitation of the toehold occurred in 1950 when Congress enabled the states to use the public assistance matching formulas to secure federal funding of medical vendor payments. Congress's next step involved the establishment of a separate matching formula for medical vendor payments and, in 1960, liberalizing the medical vendor program's eligibility criteria to create the Medical Assistance for the Aged (MAA) program. President Johnson's 1964 landslide electoral victory set the stage for the establishment of the Medicaid and Medicare programs that were extensions of health care programs for indigent citizens and Social Security programs, respectively.

The evidence therefore indicates that the evolution of American health care policy was a function of incremental change. It is also evident that the impetus for each of the revisions that preceded the establishment of the Medicaid and Medicare programs was an outgrowth of the states' desire to achieve their short-term policy goals. Even though officials in the Truman Administration advocated the establishment of separate public assistance and medical vendor matching formulas, Congress chose in 1950 to forgo the advice and simply add medical vendor payments to the public assistance matching formulas. During the ensuing two years, the fact that only 15 states established federally approved medical vendor programs suggests that the states and their Congressional delegations did not perceive a need for separate medical vendor programs and matching formulas. They were interested in relatively small matching formula adjustments that would assist them in setting up health care programs for public assistance recipients or using the additional federal funds to expand existing programs.

During the ensuing six years, however, the public assistance formulas prevented an increasing number of states from adequately providing for the income support and health care needs of their public assistance recipients. In an effort to address the problem, Congress approved the previously rejected proposal to establish separate medical vendor matching formulas. Both sets of public assistance formula revisions suggest that the states' financial needs are a useful barometer of the magnitude of change Congress is willing to support; the greater the need the greater the liberalization of the matching formulas' scope.

Congressional approval of the MAA program in 1960 indicates that an essential, additional element is control of the legislative process. Due to the unintended effects of the initial OASI eligibility criteria, a relatively large percentage of workers in the New England, Northeastern, North Central, and Pacific states were receiving OASI benefits and therefore would have benefited from the establishment of a health insurance program for OASI recipients. However, individuals aged 65 and older who resided in the agricultural states of the South were disproportionately reliant on public assistance and therefore would not have benefited from health insurance for OASI beneficiaries. As public support for health insurance for OASI recipients increased, Southern control of key Congressional leadership positions and the effective use of House rules enabled Southern Congressional leaders to address their constituents' needs by shepherding legislation through Congress that expanded the medical vendor programs rather than following public opinion and establishing a health insurance program for OASI recipients.

Although the 1964 general election produced conditions that were conducive to the establishment of a health insurance program for elderly citizens, the preceding analysis indicates that passage was facilitated by the evolution of federal health care funding for indigent individuals and the establishment of the Social Security disability insurance program during the 1950s. By the time Congress considered legislation to create the Medicaid and Medicare programs, federal financial participation in health care and the precedent for grafting programs and earmarked taxes onto OASI were established. The magnitude of change engendered by the Medicaid and

Medicare programs, and the related challenge of securing Congressional approval therefore was less than would have been the case in the absence of the incremental expansions of health care and Social Security programs.

The evidence therefore indicates that the evolution of federal matching formulas and programs was a function of the states' needs during the period in which legislation was being considered. Since the needs of the states tended to evolve at a relatively slow pace, the process was predisposed to consider and approve small incremental changes in policy. It was these incremental changes that fostered greater change over time than fundamental change. They also facilitated the enactment of initiatives such as health insurance that were initially defined as fundamental change but, at the time of Congressional approval, were incremental.

REFERENCES

Advisory Commission on Intergovernmental Relations. (1980). *The Federal Role in the Federal System: The Dynamics of Growth—Public Assistance: The Growth of a Federal Function.* Washington, DC: U.S. Government Printing Office.

American Medical Association. (1961). *House of Delegates Proceedings, Clinical Session.* Washington, DC: American Medical Association.

Congressional Quarterly Almanac. (1960). 36(76-77), 148-164. Washington, DC: Congressional Quarterly.

Congressional Quarterly Weekly Report. (1960). 18(1), 6-8, 18(29), 1236-1250. Washington, DC: Congressional Quarterly.

Corson, J. J. (1939). Wage reports for workers covered by federal old-age insurance in 1937. *Social Security Bulletin, 2*(3), 3–9.

Engel, J. (2006). *Poor People's Medicine: Medicaid and American Charity Care since 1965.* Durham, NC: Duke University Press. doi:10.1215/9780822387633

Gilman, J. D. (1998). *Medicaid and the Costs of Federalism, 1984-1992.* New York, NY: Garland Publishing, Inc.

Hirsch, B. T., Macpherson, D. A., & Vroman, W. G. (2001). Estimates of union density by State. *Monthly Labor Review*, (July): 51–55.

Infoplease. (2014). *Population Distribution by Age, Race, and Nativity, 1860-2010.* Retrieved July 2014, from http://www.infoplease.com/ipa/A0110384.html

Johnson, L. B. (1971). *The Vantage Point: Perspectives of the Presidency, 1963-1969*. Chicago, IL: Holt, Rinehart & Winston.

Kingdon, J. W. (1995). Agendas, Alternatives, and Public Policies (Second Ed.). New York, NY: Harper Collins.

Kolodrubetz, W. W. (1972). Two decades of employee-benefit plans, 1950-70: A review. *Social Security Bulletin*, *35*(4), 10–22.

Office of Management and Budget. (2015). *Historical Tables*. Retrieved July 2014, from https://www.whitehouse.gov/omb/budget/Historicals

Olson, L. K. (2010). *The Politics of Medicaid*. New York, NY: Columbia University Press.

Patel, K., & Rushefsky, M. (2006). *Health Care Politics and Policy in America* (3rd ed.). Armonk, NY: M. E. Sharpe.

Peters, R. A. (2004). The Social Security Amendments of 1960: Completing the foundation for Medicare and Medicaid. *Journal of Health and Human Services Administration*, *26*(4), 438–469. PMID:15704642

Schneider, A., & Ingram, H. (1993). Social Construction of target populations: Implications for politics and policy. *The American Political Science Review*, *87*(2), 334–347. doi:10.2307/2939044

Schottland, C. I. (1956). Social Security Amendments of 1956: A Summary and Legislative History. *Social Security Bulletin*, (September), 1956.

Slomin, H. (1942). State and Regional Differences in Covered Employment and Taxable Wages, 1939. *Social Security Bulletin*, *5*(1), 35–44.

Smith, D. G., & Moore, J. D. (2009). *Medicaid Politics and Policy: 1965-2007*. New Brunswick, NJ: Transaction Publishers.

Social Security Act Amendments of 1950, Pub. L. No. 81-734, sections 6, 323, 1006, and 1405, 64 Stat 477–561 (1950).

Social Security Act Amendments of 1956, Pub. L. No. 84-880, sections 301-304, 70 Stat. 846-848 (1956).

Social Security Act of 1935, Pub. L. No. 74-271, sections 3, 403, and 1002, 49 Stat. 620-648 (1935).

Social Security Administration. (1951). *Social Security Bulletin. Annual Statistical Supplement*, *14*(9).

Social Security Administration. (1960). *Social Security Bulletin. Annual Statistical Supplement, 23*(12).

Social Security Administration. (1951-1964). *Social Security Bulletin, 14*(12)-*27*(12).

Sundquist, J. L. (1968). *Politics and Policy: The Eisenhower, Kennedy, and Johnson Years*. Washington, DC: The Brookings Institution.

Trafton, G. H., & Feinroth, L. H. (1944). State differences in insurance status under Old-Age and Survivors Insurance. *Social Security Bulletin, 7*(8), 6–11.

U.S. Census Bureau. (1968). *Current Population Reports, Population Estimates, Series P-25, No. 384*. Retrieved July 2014, from https://www.census.gov/prod/1/pop/p25-384.pdf

U.S. Census Bureau. (2014). *Median family income by State: 1959, 1969, 1979, 1989, and 1999*. Retrieved July 2014, from https://www.census.gov/hhes/www/income/data/historical/state/state2.html

U.S. House. (1949). Congressional Record. 95(August 15), Part 9.

U.S. Senate (1950). Congressional Record. 96(June 13), Part 6.

U.S. Senate (1956). Congressional Record. 102(July 17), Part 10.

KEY TERMS AND DEFINITIONS

Aid to Dependent Children: Public assistance program for indigent children and their caretakers.

Aid to the Blind: Public assistance program for indigent individuals who are blind.

Federal Reimbursement Ceilings: The maximum amounts of public assistance and health care benefits that are eligible for federal matching funds.

Federal Share: Percentage of public assistance and medical benefits that is defrayed by the Federal Government and defined by federal statute.

Medicaid: State-Federal health care program for indigent individuals, primarily public assistance recipients.

Medical Vendor Payments: State-Federal public assistance health care programs that preceded Medicaid.

Medicare: Federal health care program for Social Security recipients.

Old Age Assistance: Public assistance program for indigent, elderly individuals.

Public Assistance: State-Federal income support programs for indigent individuals.

Social Security (OASI): Federal payments to insured individuals who are retired, disabled or offspring of insured, deceased parents. Although the OASI program became OASDI when disabled individuals were added to the list of eligible recipients, OASI is used throughout the chapter.

Chapter 6
The Study of Public Reporting in Healthcare

Ubaldo Comite
University "Giustino Fortunato" Benevento, Italy

ABSTRACT

Public reporting, intended as the public disclosure of information on healthcare performance, is linked to the improvement of the quality of care through the incentives of selection and change, which are in turn determined by the availability of comparative information that is used by those outside the system (citizens) and those from within (organizations and professionals). In the last few decades, the healthcare sector, have undergone considerable change. This change is inevitably destined to modify the way in which citizens turn to healthcare services, and the way in which hospitals are called upon to be transparent and accountable in how they provide services. It is within this context that public reporting became widespread, as a strategy geared towards promoting informed choices to consumers and stimulating the improvement of quality of care. The aim of this paper is to highlight how public reporting systems have the potential to not only support healthcare users in making informed choices, but to also foster healthcare structures in the improvement of their services.

INTRODUCTION

The business information system represents a collection of the flow of information that circulates in businesses aimed at their own management and relative operation (Camussone, 1998).

DOI: 10.4018/978-1-4666-9944-1.ch006

The notion of an information system does not necessarily implicate the use of information technology in order to function. Nevertheless, businesses characterized by high levels of organizational complexity and numerous activities and/or services rendered need a specific technological support system for the management of their information resources.

The coexistence of the technological dimension, which organizes and classifies information, along with the necessity of fueling decision-making processes, which in turn depend on the variable organizational, environmental and personal conditions of the decision maker, inherently has certain problems which are only in part resolvable by the characteristics of the design of information systems currently in use. Decision-making processes are, in fact, determined by the representative models of reality that people build and use in order to make their choices. Each model needs different information in order to be described, and each decision-maker needs different information to carry out his or her function. The information acquires usefulness only in virtue of its capacity to represent events as interpreted by the different people who make up the organization. The information system, on the other hand, has the tendency to structure flows and to standardize the content of the information. Furthermore, it requires significant investments each time modifications to its organization are needed.

The risk of creating a dichotomy between real processes and the formal information system is, therefore, a constant in complex organizations, and even more so within professional organizations such as healthcare, which are characterized by a higher autonomy of operators on individual transactions. The information surrounding healthcare, is, therefore, crucial in supplying fair, effective, and efficient services, as well as for management purposes, including that of guaranteeing and increasing the responsibility of the main stakeholders, such as professionals and managers, when offering the services (Arduini, 2010).

The numerous studies dedicated in the last few years to economics and management in healthcare all agree on the complexity of the sector, inasmuch as a comprehensive shared definition of the good being traded is still distant. It makes sense, roughly speaking, to state that healthcare services contribute to producing "good health", through prevention, diagnosis, treatment, and, when considering health as essential for the individual, the contribution of economics and business becomes fundamental in creating conditions in order to better production and distribution procedures.

If health is considered a commodity, even with its ethical and economic peculiarities, the concept of supply and demand becomes significant, and it becomes possible, as well as necessary, to introduce principles of management into the system in which it is produced. It is even more relevant in universal healthcare models under public control, aimed at guaranteeing homogenous medical care coverage to the entire community, independently from variously defined structural thresholds.

Within public healthcare systems, the intervention of economics, specifically business economics, finds solid justification in the provision of instruments oriented towards the more correct and enduring pursuit of institutional aims, since wasting wealth is indubitably contrary to the concept of solidarity in health (Onida, 1961).

The operation of the business reporting system is inserted into this context (Cuccurullo, 2003).

The business reporting system performs a strategic importance in maintaining the organizational asset at full efficiency and in permitting the distribution of information to the various levels involved.

The reporting system is the "heart" of a larger system of planning and control. This control cannot, in fact, be carried out without a timely transfer of the information on the activities being run, and planning cannot be carried out without the information and data relative to the activities, the resources used, and the results obtained previously (Pozzoli, 2001). The systems can be of varying complexity, and can perform based on the needs and resources available, however the most important concept is that they are indispensable.

Even at the micro-organizational level, reporting is fundamental. No team will be capable of operating in the long-term if the operators do not receive feedback on their activities. Such a system must provide a "just in time" understanding of whether or not the activities planned are meeting the expectations, and if the set objectives are achieved.

Reporting systems, however, despite having been the subject of numerous experiments, are not sufficiently widespread in all healthcare authorities, and are often formed in a non-systematic manner.

On the contrary, the formalization of the data collected at various levels, relative to the resources consumed / costs (input) and the activities distributed (output) (Ferrara, Pozzoli, 2006), takes place through the provision of an adequate reporting system, aimed at illustrating, in a targeted and consistent manner, the overall trend of the management of the business over time, identifying all the relevant areas and illustrating all the events that are significant for the purposes of an internal control (Cifalà, 2008).

THE MAIN FEATURES OF THE HEALTHCARE SECTOR

In order to understand the organizational models of the healthcare systems properly, it is first and foremost necessary to analyze the main features of the sector.

Economic studies, in fact, identify doctors and patients as the two main categories of stakeholders.

The former express health needs (real or perceived) and represent the potential beneficiaries of preventative healthcare services, diagnosis, and treatments in which the production of health is expressed. Their principle features reside in trust, liabilities, and in the observance of medical regulations. The ideal – although abstract would be more correct – conditions of pure and perfect competition are distant, as noted by any real case, and in an even more evident manner in the healthcare sector (Cecchella, 1971).

The individual who expresses a health need, perceiving a lower state of psycho-physical health compared to his or her expectations, cannot, in fact, make independent decisions in relation to the acquisition of *ad hoc* goods or services, since he or she is not in possession (unless of course, the person is a medical doctor) of enough information to understand the link between his or her own condition and the healthcare services needed to improve it (Ugolini, 1999). For this reason, he/she turns to the doctor, a kind of intermediary theoretically capable of interpreting the health needs expressed, and of translating that need into a request for healthcare services, through the indication of the most appropriate diagnostic-therapeutic procedures.

In other words, the individual expresses a health need, while the doctor expresses a request for services on behalf of the individual. For this reason, a model is configured in which the request appears as actually generated by the supplier.

The relationship between patient and doctor has been effectively placed in the conceptual schemes formulated by the so-called "agency theory" (Cepiku, 2006), according to which the doctor takes on the role of the agent, with the task of satisfying the objectives that the principal (the patient) cannot personally pursue due to significant informative asymmetry. Additionally, it is opportune to highlight how the quantification of the flow of prospective demand represent an crucial element for the governing of healthcare systems, since it forms the fundamental basis of a rational organization of services at a territorial level and for a proper planning of the activity (Alesani, Ancona, 2005).

It is, however, necessary to highlight the particular complexity of this type of analysis, principally attributable to a combination of factors, which can be specified concisely:

- The demand for health depends on a number of determinants, not exclusively attributable to the psycho-physical state of individuals, nor completely foreseeable with acceptable degrees of approximation; from this point of view, it is useful to remember how individuals manifest a health need that can be, at the extreme, even independent of the actual need. The question is, in other words, and more so than in other fields, subject to phenomena of accentuated distortion (in appropriateness), among other things, by the absence or partial presence of tariff mechanisms related to consumption (for example, medical and prescription charges);

- If it is true that individuals express a health need, it is not correct, however, to declare that they request healthcare services. This, instead, is expressed by the doctors, who, in fact, translate the health need into a request for diagnostic or therapeutic services (pharmacological, outpatient, inpatient). The risk of appropriateness is still present at this stage, but should be substantially lower;
- The request, in many circumstances, is dependent upon the offer, or in other words, is generated by the offer. The very fact that, for example, a service exists and a new one is established again, is in itself a condition that generates demand. The event is, in other words, connected to the exploitative powers of the request implemented by the doctors.

For this reason, it is possible to state that, without doubt, one of the crucial points in the governing of healthcare systems is represented by the lack of ability to control demand. The difficulty of predicting, with sufficient accuracy, the flow of demand that will be generated in a given period of time, makes it more difficult to plan activities in the structures, and, in general, to plan the business, with obvious consequences on the proper allocation of resources, and on the effectiveness of the mechanisms of feedback and feed-forward, the base of management control systems (Marinò, 2008). In this case, the business information system can aid in supporting the reporting system.

THE INFORMATION SYSTEM IN HEALTHCARE

As mentioned, the business information system can be described as a set of elements, which are very heterogeneous, that collect, elaborate, exchange, and archive data. The aim is to produce and distribute information to the people who need it, at the right time and in the right place to carry out their function of decision- making and control.

In particular, the information system of a healthcare authority can be defined as an ordered set of information that participates directly or indirectly in the management of the authority, associating itself in function to the specific objectives of analysis, control, measurement, etc. In other words, a well-structured and effective information system represents the support necessary for the functioning of government and the coordination of the healthcare authority, since it is the basic condition to empower professionals in regards to management processes (greater decentralization of decision-making to a more operational level), and to implement an effective control of management at both the operational, and managerial and strategic level (Del Bene, 2000).

The complexity inherent in any business information system is emphasized in healthcare, in that these authorities, be they local authorities or hospitals, contain an organizational division characterized by high autonomy and specialization. The peculiarity of the activities carried out by healthcare authorities and their "public" nature determines the need to collect, for various purposes, a very significant and composite volume of data, and to calculate it into meaningful information, thus creating a particularly complex information system.

Within the healthcare authority, an extensive network that carries a flow of information is generated among the organizational units; the degree of complexity of the system is also expanded by the need for healthcare authorities to effectively supervise the exchange of data with interlocutors, such as regional authorities and other businesses. The information systems of the local healthcare authorities and hospitals can be analyzed through a preliminary breakdown of the "macro areas" in which specific informational needs tend to coincide, and which are related to the features of the activities carried out and the objectives of each area (Fontana, Lorenzoni, 2000).

In this sense, it is essential to consider the healthcare information system as the sum of several subsystems, identifiable in:

1. An external subsystem relationship, which is responsible for data collection and the production of reports relating to the communications with users, with other businesses and with institutional government bodies;
2. A healthcare subsystem, itself divisible into a) a hospital area subsystem, tasked with collecting data and producing reports relative to hospital admissions, specialist extra-hospital admission activity, rehabilitative medicine, etc.; b) a local area subsystem, in charge of collecting data and producing reports relative to: i) management systems and procedures of the district activities (primary care, pharmaceutical activities, rehabilitative medicine, etc.); ii) management systems and procedures of the prevention department activities (hygiene, veterinary areas, forensic and industrial medicine, etc.); iii) management systems and procedures of patient mobility;
3. An administrative subsystem, relative to the collection of data and the production of reports relative to: a) systems and procedures of the administration's financial reports; b) systems and procedures of personnel management; c) systems and procedures to meet the requirements and size of the personnel; d) systems and procedures of data collection on the activities carried out for institutional aims; e) systems and procedures of the operating costs of the administration; f) systems and procedures of analytical accounting;
4. A managerial subsystem, appointed to collect data and produce reports relative to: a) systems and procedures of budget articulation; b) systems and procedures of management control; c) systems and procedures of personnel evaluation.

GENERAL CONSIDERATIONS ON THE REPORTING SYSTEM

The reporting system is a key operational mechanism in the process aimed at giving more responsibility to operators to efficiently achieve the objectives of healthcare authorities.

The term reporting means, among other things, communication between those responsible for the attribution or obligation of certain resources, for information on managerial operations, relevant to its decision-making activities (Vendramini, 2004).

The purpose of the system under consideration, found within a more general management control system, is to transmit to managers, in an unequivocal, reliable and timely way, the elements necessary to:

- Be familiar with past dynamics and/or current trends in management, valuing such information in relation to set parameters;
- Identify the reasons for any gaps and the possible corrective action to be undertaken;
- Participate in the planning process, redefining the short, medium and long-term goals and/or the appropriate management plans to follow.

In general, the communication process can be represented as a series of ordered phases: 1) definition of the message content; 2) encoding; 3) transmission; 4) reception; 5) decoding; 6) internalization or lack of internalization.

In order for these steps to be activated, two subjects must be involved: the controller and the recipient.

Not infrequently, however, more than two figures are involved. This takes place when the need to activate communication processes, such as of the horizontal type, arises. This need originates from one subject towards multiple recipients, through the involvement of the managerial control office, which represents the operating instrument in which the process of communication materializes.

These circumstances lead to a considerably more complicated situation, in that, to guarantee the achievement of the objectives (internalization of the intended message by the final recipient), the "upstream" figures of the process should trigger a complex series of interactions. Through these, they direct the activities of the "downstream" figure or figures, check the coherence of the objective and possibly readjust it towards the desired direction.

The data collection system is designed to generate data on consumption and activity levels to be allocated to those responsible for the activation or use of the resources. As the data produced by the controller are taken into account in decision-making, the abstract reliability of the data itself is not sufficient; instead, it is essential that the data becomes information. In other words, that it is consistent with the fact-finding needs of the recipient and that it be made available in an appropriate and timely manner.

This aspect, meaningful in any business context, is even more important in healthcare organizations. On one hand, the dominant culture among operators is still linked to medical or legal acts, while little attention is paid to how the productive factors are combined to obtain results. On the other hand, the lack of correspondence to a real monetary price for the services supplied to users, the heterogeneity, the personalized nature or however the difficult measurability of the services provided and the need to respect the professional autonomy of the medical constituent, make the determination of indicators of easy interpretability difficult, such as the partial results of each "area of activity" or the gaps in a shared standard cost.

The subjects that activate the communication process can be:

- The management control office;
- An individual with hierarchical responsibilities, such as the general manager, the chief medical officer, or the managing director ;
- An individual responsible for coordination, such as the decision-making co-ordinator or a surgical suite jointly used by several divisions.

On the other hand, the potential recipients of the reporting system are:

- The bodies that make up the top management of the healthcare authority (general manager, chief medical officer, managing director, statutory auditors, the board of health);
- The holders of responsibility centers, as much in relation to this as to the possible cost centers identified within it;
- The holders of functional responsibilities;
- The holders of coordination responsibilities.

An advanced reporting system allows the management control office to prepare documents of a heterogeneous nature.

Among the many classification logics, the most significant seems to be based on the type of information needed by the recipient that the document intends to satisfy. This classification is consistent with the tools that support the decision-making process of the reporting system. At the same time, it reflects the coordination of the report for possible content, that is, documents that respond to similar requirements will have comparable content.

The different information needs can be attributed to three categories of questions related to the verification of results with respect to given parameters, the identification of emerging events and trends, and the obtainment of the data necessary to make certain choices.

We can, therefore, distinguish the following three classes:

1. Control reports (verifying the results obtained, identifying events and trends);
2. Decision-making reports (obtaining data to make choices);
3. Fact-finding reports (obtaining context data).

In practice, it is possible to prepare documents that seek to simultaneously meet different information needs. In theory, a report can be related to final or preliminary data; it can be distributed with a predefined periodicity, by decision of the controller or upon the recipient's request, and it can have a predetermined structure, or be designed *ad hoc*.

1. The control report provides the opportunity to monitor both the unit(s) of performance for which the recipient is responsible, as well as the development of the context referred to.
   Such monitoring is carried out by explaining the changes using a series of indicators as benchmarks. This may be the data collected at the end of the previous period or the amounts budgeted for, for the healthcare authorities that utilize this tool. These are the types of reports, be they concise or in depth, that are used to transmit the data collected by the system of management accounting.
   The concise report summarizes, in a single document, all relevant operational events that have affected, during the period in question, the operating unit or cost center, the hospital, or the entire healthcare authority.
   The in depth report, on the other hand, is aimed at observing, in detail, a particular specific event. For example, it can offer an explanation regarding an anomalous increase of costs incurred for medical surgical devices within a hospital clinic.
   Control reports are generally final, as it is usually only considered important to provide the measure a particular event to the recipient *ex post*.
2. The decision-making report aims to provide the information necessary to make certain choices. Consider, for example, a report containing the information required to determine the tariff level to charge patients in order to obtain a particular service, or analyzing cost-effectiveness between production economics and outsourcing the service provided as part of a protected structure, or even reporting on the results of an analysis on cost-effectiveness relative to the performance of a particular medical device.
3. Fact-finding reports can be divided into trend reports which convey historical data series relative to the same reference object, and comparative reports,

which compare, at the same time, multiple similar reference objects. The data in question help to define the wealth of information upon which planning, and operational management and control activities, are based, and are often useful as a source of statistics, for example for the preparation of periodic reports.

Furthermore, the reports make the information available to different stakeholders more homogeneous, thus representing a useful tool for both vertical and horizontal organizational coordination; for this same reason, they contribute to the cultural integration of the recipients and, therefore, also to their sense of belonging to the authority (Santi, 1998).

THE CRITERIA FOR REPORT PLANNING

Based on the principle that information does not exert a neutral role but, instead, is aimed at a specific and predefined purpose, it follows that the planning and preparation of a report are closely related to the purposes set out in this document.

In general, it is possible to identify a number of criteria or requirements that must be adhered to in planning a reporting system, such as: relevance, conciseness, flexibility, hierarchization, controllability of reference variables, balance between timeliness and accuracy, reliability, comprehensibility and readability, and comparability (Vasselli, Filippetti, Spizzichino, 2005).

Relevance

The measures included in the report must be such as to allow the recipient an effective monitoring of management variables that he or she considers critical; that is, those elements which in his or her view makes it possible to effectively reach the objectives of the operating unit and the function of which he or she is responsible.

Conciseness

As a general rule, a report that claims to convey to the reader an excessive amount of figures is likely to discourage the recipient to read it, or at least to not adequately highlight the truly relevant variables.

A concise control report, in particular, is a document that is destined to be consulted rapidly, as its aim is to highlight salient facts, and not to explain the causes.

Flexibility

It is necessary that the report profiles be able to vary based on extemporaneous informational needs.

Hierarchization

This is a corollary to the first two principles, according to which the degree of conciseness of the information must reflect the distribution of responsibility defined by the organizational structure. In other words, the more the recipient occupies a top position in the hierarchy, the more the data received must be presented in aggregate form.

Controllability of Reference Variables

The measures contained in a report must gear the attention of the recipient to the variables that he or she can maneuver, in particular on the consequences to the decisions he or she has made. Given the nature of highly interdependent and open systems to external influences, more precisely healthcare authorities, it is clear that in the majority of cases, the final results of an action depend on many factors. The requirement of controllability, consequently, cannot be understood in a restrictive sense, as this would reduce the motivation to achieve specific objectives, even in the face of adverse events.

Balance between Timeliness and Accuracy

The reporting system, in fact, borrows both of these features from the management accounting system (Bruni, Di Lazzaro, Gatti, 2001). In refining the latter, however, they should not be considered variables to maximize at any cost; the objective, rather, is coherence between the characteristics of the data collection system and the need for timeliness and accuracy by the recipients of the information. This need is set during the planning stage of the report, bearing in mind that:

- In order for the information to be sufficiently timely, it is enough that is reaches the interested party with enough time to allow him or her to make any possible necessary decisions;
- In order for the information to be sufficiently precise, the value detected must allow the interested party to reliably evaluate the direction and the intensity of the event in act;

- The determination of the desired level of timeliness and accuracy cannot be separated from the comparison between the resulting benefit of having information with given characteristics, and the cost necessary to obtain it. It is clear that at the same costs, and with all other things being equal, the timeliness of the data collection is to the detriment of its accuracy.

Reliability

The opportunity to defer accuracy to timeliness is restricted by the need for reliable values. If the values are not reliable, the recipient cannot formulate judgments based on them, and the report is no longer useful. In such cases, the need to protect credibility prompts the controller to omit values whose reliability is questionable, or to postpone the delivery of the report to allow for verification.

Comprehensibility and Readability

Because of the degree of complexity of the object of communication, and that the extent of diffusion of an economic culture is not yet high in the public healthcare sector, it is necessary that, at the planning stage of the document, particular attention is paid to what may be implemented by the recipient of the information. What is needed is a language that is understandable to the recipient, and uses graphics and tables, and is discursive, which enhances the overall readability of the report, and explains the units of measure adopted, and organizes information in a logically consequential manner.

Comparability

The final values have little meaning if they are not compared to an appropriate benchmark.

In order for the report to be easily usable, this comparison cannot rely on the knowledge, memory or willingness to retrieve the source that provides the elements of comparison, but must clearly specify the existing variations.

With regards to this aspect, the controller can choose between the following options: 1) budget parameters; 2) historical parameters; 3) organizationally comparable parameters.

1. If prepared properly, the budget is, without doubt, a predictable reference, since it allows for the possibility to compare the aimed-for objectives to the actual results, which is the foundation of the feedback mechanism.

2. In the absence of budget information, a valid alternative can be made by comparing historical parameters, that is, related to the previous period, even if considered in an incremental perspective. This, though, is the logic on the basis of which the decision-maker usually acts. The use of historical parameters, moreover, has the distinction of eliminating the limits of comparability between data resulting from periodicity. All that is needed, in fact, is to take as reference the final values for the same time period as the previous year.
3. The spatial comparison is undoubtedly the most controversial. The entities considered for the comparison can be external or internal to the healthcare authority.

The first alternative can be immediately excluded, since the size, the characteristics of the staff, the strategies pursued, and the demographic and epidemiological context make each responsibility center unique. The comparison between similar operative units from different healthcare authorities remains useful as an opportunity of analysis at a regional or national level, but for the head of a single unit, it can represent the content of a fact-finding report.

PUBLIC REPORTING IN HEALTH CARE

Public reporting (Pelone, Ricciardi, 2013), intended as the public disclosure of information on healthcare performance, is linked to the improvement of the quality of care through the incentives of selection and change, which are in turn determined by the availability of comparative information that is used by those outside the system (citizens) and those from within (organizations and professionals).

In the last few decades, the healthcare sector, as well as the relative support services, have undergone considerable change. This change is inevitably destined to modify the way in which citizens turn to healthcare services, and the way in which hospitals are called upon to be transparent and accountable in how they provide services (Saita, 2007). It is within this context that public reporting became widespread, as a strategy geared towards promoting informed consumers choices and stimulating improvements in quality of care, augmenting the responsibility of care provider in respects to their services. Transparency and accountability are major drivers towards the improvement in the quality of healthcare care systems (Comite, 2013).

The public reporting method offers the greatest benefits in encouraging healthcare providers to improve through comparative analyzes, helping patients to make informed decisions and encouraging private investors and public programs to reward quality and efficiency.

To date, many Western countries, including Italy, have begun to develop models for the monitoring, measurement and management of the performance of their healthcare systems, in order to guarantee greater transparency and accountability, and to improve quality. Among these, rightfully, is public reporting. This model, based on being patient-centered, replaces the antiquated paternalistic prototypes that placed the doctor-figure at the center (doctor-centered model) (Giarelli, Venneri, 2009).

In pursuing the objective of creating a decision-making process that includes the participation of all the involved parties, the notion that individual users are entitled to consistent and reliable information is establishing itself. In fact, this assumption leads back to Hirschmann's theory. He stated that the success of healthcare organizations is dependent on the views held by its patients (Hirschmann, 1970). In this sense, public reporting systems have the potential to not only support healthcare users in making informed choices, but to also foster healthcare structures in the improvement of their services through benchmarking (Lucianelli, Danish, 2002).

DETERMINING FACTORS IN THE DEVELOPMENT OF PUBLIC REPORTING IN HEALTHCARE

The healthcare organizations in which public reporting systems were first introduced highlight elements and common trends that have contributed towards the adoption of this strategy. Among these, a central role was played by the information technology revolution and the development of mechanisms for public accountability (Biocca, 2010). Figure 1 shows the aforementioned elements, placing them in time and in relation to each other.

It is possible to distinguish between general social trends, such as the emancipation process of the user and the rise of information and communication technology, and trends characteristic of the healthcare sector, such as the need to achieve a rationalization of costs and the growing attention paid towards quality and safety. The increasing "power" of the patient, as well as market oriented reforms in light of the need to rationalize the system, have contributed to the stabilization of strategies based on the central importance of the patient, the choice of the consumer and the individual responsibility of the user. It was primarily this element that brought about the diffusion of public accountability, taking into consideration the increased availability of indicators and instruments following the growth in the information technology field, and the growing attention paid to areas such as the quality of care and the safety of patients.

The consolidation of the Internet, in particular by the late 90s, accelerated this process by offering a constant stream of information which was both interactive and easily accessible, given the Internet's tendency to continuously publish and update

Figure 1. The evolutionary pushes to the introduction of the mechanisms of public reporting

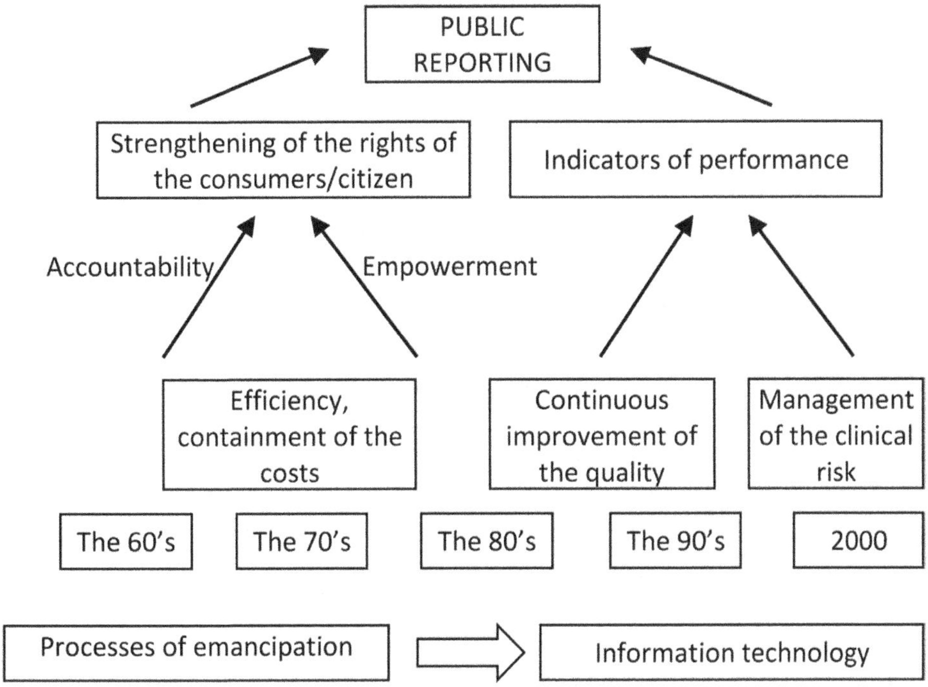

itself (Hardey, 2001). The efforts undertaken to increase the availability of transparent information has led to greater accountability, improving and rewarding quality, and increasing efficiency. Within this context there are several factors recognized as determinant in the development of public reporting, such as patient empowerment, market oriented reforms, information technology and the presentation of information.

Patient Empowerment

The orientation towards multidimensional curative approaches that are patient-centred now represents the common denominator in the themes of responsibility and social participation in the processes of promoting and protecting health. In this case, the fundamental role of the patient becomes that of a co-producer of healthcare services, whose principal prerogative is that of participation based on different levels of empowerment; that is, to have the power to influence fundamental decisions regarding the services received.

Patient empowerment is defined as the active participation of the patient in the decision-making process regarding treatments which he/she perceives as necessary.

This presupposes that the patient has access not only to the treatments but also to the pertinent information. The growing demand for healthcare-related information is one of the elements which has contributed to the increased level of individualism that has characterized recent social evolution (Census, 2013). The availability of this information, and its comparability, is by now firmly considered as one of the means by which users can affirm their role. Using this data, in fact, it is possible for users to make informed decisions, and engage in more active discussions with their healthcare professionals.

It is in this light that the doctor-patient relationship must be re-evaluated: while the fundamental roles and inherent asymmetry will always remain, changes which call for a greater participation by the patient must be adopted.

Reforms Geared towards Market Mechanism

Since the early 80s, the healthcare systems of all developed countries have faced severe structural and financial problems. These have essentially been the consequence of an increase in spending and misalignment between the services offered and those requested by citizens. The reforms that have characterized the last decade have intensified due to pressure from various sources: the growing uncertainty regarding the availability of resources, the complexity and variability that characterize the context of production, distribution and consumption of healthcare services, and the evolution and transformation of the referential epidemiological and social characteristics. In addition, healthcare policies are conditioned by the need to reconcile two categories of interest that often appear opposite: healthcare, whose interest is tightly connected the well-being of the population, and economic interests, which are conditioned by the necessity to shoulder costs through budgets and set resources.

Furthermore, it is important, both nationally and internationally, to consider that the emergence of problems relative to the restructuring of healthcare systems should be viewed within the wider context of the crisis in welfare institutions (Triassi, 2011). In the majority of cases, healthcare reforms have not occurred as isolated phenomena, but as a part of a larger debate, involving all major sectors of society in which government intervention is relevant. The basis for the reforms has been, on the one hand, the necessity to continue to provide suitable and effective services, while maintaining or improving quality, and on the other, the necessity to provide sufficient evidence that prove the degree to which the healthcare system has meet its objectives. In this regard, international comparison and the availability of information regarding the performance of healthcare systems, based on empirical evidence, is of fundamental importance. Thus, considering the growing interest towards public reporting, healthcare reforms in place in many western countries, which are aimed at reducing the costs of healthcare through the introduction of new market forces, have played a fundamental role.

Information Technology and the Presentation of Information

The recent "evolution" of the users/patients, beneficiaries of the healthcare system, who are increasingly presenting themselves as informed players within the healthcare market, as well as the healthcare system's adoption of measures for greater transparency and public reporting, would not have been possible without current information and communication technology. The ability for citizens to access and utilize information has increased vastly due to the greater availability of computers. By the 70s and 80s, computers were starting to be used in the promotion of health and education in regards to a healthy lifestyle. The diffusion of technology did not experience a rapid acceleration until the late 90s, with the advent of the Internet. This created the conditions necessary for a flow of information which was accessible, interactive and usable by different categories of stakeholders and for different purposes (Freeman, 1984). The increasing spread of technology has given citizens access to an enormous quantity of information, although, even today, not all can effectively use it, but which essentially allows anyone to increase the depth of their knowledge in all fields, including that of health. The Internet also facilitates the regular publication and updating of its contents which provides information that is accessible to the layman, and is therefore available to any and all consumers. At the same, it does not confine the user to a purely passive role, offering the possibility of interaction in the network. It is also for these reasons that the Internet has become so widespread, and the number of users continues to increase every year (Taylor, 2009).

Accountability and Patient Safety

Since the 70s, the transformation of society, characterized by factors such as increased life expectancy, an ageing population, technological development and the increased incidence of diseases of affluence, has shown the inherent unsustainability of the system and the need to rationalize the use of resources to reduce the cost of health care. The practical effect of this awareness has been, on the one hand, the expansion of technostructures which are geared towards handling, with a constantly increasing amount of information (quantitative indicators), the various aspects of accountability within healthcare systems and their organization, and on the other hand, an increased tendency towards public accountability, giving citizens access to greater amounts of information. Public accountability has experienced, in recent decades, a gradual strengthening in the mechanisms and procedures through which healthcare organizations are called to publicly report on their activities. In fact, it has been universally recognized that the responsibility of governing and administrating healthcare organizations can find a useful tool in this process in order to dialogue with citizens, make efficient use of the resources, and exploit the tension between the principle of transparency taken on as an absolute value and the possibility to develop, within the healthcare organization, effective strategies to improve quality.

CONCLUSION

As can be expected, the implementation of an information system is not an individual task, especially within a healthcare organization that wishes to treats patients as the recipient of an operating process designed to meet his or her needs. Having said this, it is necessary to balance the need for information and control with the indispensable need for quality and organizational flexibility.

Healthcare authorities turn the control systems over to highly qualified professionals with the necessary goal of economic accountability, as well as to obtain support to better decide and knowingly fulfil their assigned responsibilities. The periods of control, which find tangible implementation through reporting procedures, must be properly interpreted as opportunities to understand, formulate judgements and evaluations, and take on measures of improvement, where the data shows anomalies or problems. Rather than as opportunities for the evaluation and verification of individual skills, the periodic and recurring controls should, instead, be considered resources for those in positions of responsibility to develop problem solving skills and to foster learning processes, in view of the proper interpretation of managerial control.

During this process, communication (or rather, information) within the healthcare context plays a strategic role in favouring the appropriate access and use of services, as well as the adoption of behaviour aimed at the protection and improvement of both individual and collective health (Comite, 2004).

The growing commitment in making the results of the services provided public has transformed the quality and safety of treatments, favouring competition within the healthcare sector, and as a final outcome, allowing consumers to make informed choices. It is thus that the realization of public reporting systems is met. In fact, in order to provide effective, fair, and efficient healthcare services, accurate information is crucial, shaped by the principles of social responsibility, as well as transparency, also since accountability does not only mean being accountable for something, but also takes demand into consideration.

The public reporting of comparative information relating to the recorded performance of healthcare offered will always been seen as a tool for the improvement of quality of care.

REFERENCES

Alesani, D., & Ancona, F. (2005). *L'innovazione nei modelli di controllo delle aziende sanitarie: evidenze dall'applicazione del modello di controllo per LEA.* Mecosan, n°53.

Arduini, R. (2010). *Economia e gestione delle aziende sanitarie.* Milan, Italy: F. Angeli.

Biocca, M. (2010). *Bilancio di missione. Aziende sanitarie responsabili si raccontano.* Rome, Italy: Il Pensiero Scientifico Editore.

Bruni, G., Di Lazzaro, F., & Gatti, G. (2001). *Il reporting della performance aziendale.* Milan, Italy: F. Angeli.

Camussone, P. F. (1998). *Il sistema informativo aziendale.* Milan, Italy: Etas libri.

Cecchella, A. (1971). *Microeconomia.* Pisa, Italy: ETS.

Census. (2013). *47° Rapporto annuale sulla situazione sociale del Paese.* Retrieved from www.censis.it

Cepiku, D. (2006). L'esternalizzazione nelle amministrazioni pubbliche. Teorie, politiche ed esperienze a livello internazionale. Rome, Italy: Aracne, Roma.

Cifalà, S. S. (2008). Il sistema di reporting in sanità. Rome, Italy: Aracne.

Comite, U. (2004). *La comunicazione sanitaria: i rapporti tra personale, paziente e struttura organizzativa*, working paper n° 1, Dipartimento di Organizzazione aziendale e amministrazione pubblica, Facoltà di Economia, Università della Calabria, Italy.

Comite, U. (2013). *Accountability e bilancio sociali nei tribunali.* Padova, Italy: Cedam.

Cuccurullo, C. (2003). *Il management strategico nelle aziende sanitarie pubbliche.* Milan, Italy: Mc Graw-Hill.

Del Bene, L. (2000). *Criteri e strumenti gestionali nelle aziende sanitarie.* Milan, Italy: Giuffrè.

Ferrara, G., & Pozzoli, S. (2006). *Sistemi sanitari regionali tra razionalizzazione degli acquisti e qualità.* Torino, Italy: Giappichelli.

Fontana, F., & Lorenzoni, G. (2000). *L'architettura strategica delle aziende ospedaliere: un'analisi empirica.* Milan, Italy: F. Angeli.

Freeman, R. E. (1984). *Strategic management: a stakeholder approach*. Boston: Pitman.

Giarelli, G., & Venneri, E. (2009). *Sociologia della salute e della medicina*. Milan, Italy: F. Angeli.

Hardey, M. (2001). E-health: The internet and the transformation of patients into consumers and producers of health knowledge. *Information Communication and Society*, 4.

Hirschmann, A. O. (1970). *Exit, Voice and Loyalty: Responses to decline in firms, organizations and states*. Cambridge, MA: Harvard University Press.

Marinò, L. (2008). *La ricerca dell'economicità nelle aziende sanitarie locali. Concetti, modelli, decisioni*. Torino, Italy: Giappichelli.

Onida, P. (1961). Economicità, socialità ed efficienza nell'amministrazione d'impresa. *Stato sociale*, 3.

Pelone, F., & Ricciardi, W. (2013). Il public reporting in sanità: Riflessioni e proposte di un nuovo strumento operative. *Quaderni dell'Italian. Journal of Public Health*, *2*(10).

Pozzoli, S. (2001). *Il controllo direzionale negli enti locali*. Milan, Italy: F. Angeli.

Saita, M. (2007). Governance ed economicità nelle aziende sanitarie. Il Sole 24 Ore, Milano.

Santi, M. (1998). *I sistemi informativi per il controllo di gestione nelle aziende sanitarie. In Sanità pubblica* (p. 3). Rimini: Maggioli.

Taylor, K. (2009). Paternalism, participation and partnership. The evolution of patient centeredness in the consultation. *Patient Education and Counseling*, 74. PMID:18930624

Triassi, M. (2011). *Il management in sanità*. Rome, Italy: Società Editrice Universo.

Ugolini, C. (1999). *Libertà di scelta in sanità*. Bologna, Italy: Il Mulino.

Vasselli, S., Filippetti, G., & Spizzichino, L. (2005). *Misurare la performance di un sistema sanitario*. Rome, Italy: Il Pensiero Scientifico.

Vendramini, E. (2004). *Il sistema di budget per le aziende sanitarie pubbliche*. Milan, Italy: McGraw-Hill.

KEY TERMS AND DEFINITIONS

Accountability: *Constitutes the set of actions which have the social function of "giving account" by part of one individual or organization to another.* The concept of accountability originates from the private sector and specifies the necessity for a company to give account of its activities to all its interlocutors. The stakeholders are the individuals and groups whose support is necessary for the company's survival. The company must therefore implement the expectations of its stakeholders in the decisions and execution of its business. In order to discuss accountability, it is necessary to have a subject, the accountee, who has responsibilities towards another (the accountor), who in turn is responsible for informing the accountee of its responses. It is therefore possible to identify a "virtuous cycle" of accountability. The first step is to define what the object to be accounted for is between the accountee and accountor. The second step is for the accountor to execute the plan and provide the accountee complete, comprehensible and accessible information. The final step is for the accountee to produce an evaluation. This evaluation is used by the accountor to redefine the objectives and fix any possible errors, thus re-launching the process from the beginning. The growing need for accountability originates from the requirement of participation from various types of subjects (citizens, healthcare authorities, non-profit organizations, trade unions, consumer unions, etc.) for the success of various types of activities or projects. Obviously, to obtain participation and collaboration, it is essential to inform the various subjects on precisely what the intended goals are, the resources allocated for the project and the results. In this way, the collaborating subjects feel properly included in the project. Hence, for the organization to reach its desired goals, the communication of results obtained is necessary; consequently accounting and transparency are therefore not simply abstract societal requests, nor ethical construction with only theoretical value, but a tangible necessity for the success of any enterprise which involves different parties.

Benchmarking: The process of comparison with a known performance index. It represents the process in which an organization, either public or private, compares its services, products and procedures to examples of quality realized by other organizations. This results in the general adoption of more effective practices as innovations are emulated by the rest of the industry. This produces a virtuous cycle of innovation, as organizations borrow effective practices and then improve them further.

Business: In business administration, a company is a collection of individuals and resources aimed at the satisfaction of human needs through the production, distribution or consumption of economic goods.

Efficiency: Efficiency is given from the output/input ratio. There are several different types of efficiency, such as allocative and productive efficiency. Allocative efficiency regards the effective distribution of resources of an economic system to large-scale alternative purposes. The questions asked are the following: what to produce (pharmaceuticals or diagnostic tests); how to produce (is it better to treat a patient at home, at a clinic, or in a hospital); for whom to produce (who should receive an organ transplant). Productive efficiency occurs when, with the same output, a lower quantity of input is used. Thus, the same result is obtained while minimizing the costs. Managerial efficiency refers to the output and input of a production organization, a healthcare authority, a department, etc. In healthcare, a significant issue is the trade-off between equality and efficiency.

Managerial Accounting: An information system which is designed and founded – mainly, but not exclusively – on economic and quantitative determinants. It must be both retrospective and prospective, and both internal and external. The aim of managerial accounting is clearly to achieve long and short term goals, and ultimately, allow the business economic equilibrium over time. Moreover, management accounting achieves by absolving the functions of each measurement process in business, namely, that of information and behavioural influences, even if, obviously, the functional mix between information and influence will vary based on recipient: senior management will be provided with data with a high degree of information and moderate behavioural impact, and vice versa going down the hierarchy.

Performance: A combination of the processes, methods, criteria of measurement and systems necessary to evaluate and manage services (costs/benefits) of an organization.

Stakeholder: The term stakeholder identifies subjects which have an interest or concern in an economic initiative, be it an organization or a project. Stakeholders may be, for example, clients, suppliers, financiers (banks or shareholders), collaborators, and even groups with external vested interests, such as residents in areas neighbouring the business, or local interest groups.

Vision: The term used in strategic management to indicate a future scenario which reflects the ideals, values and aspirations of those who set goals and encourage action. The term vision implies the set of long-term goals that top management wishes to implement in their business. Its definition includes a general view of the market and the interpretation of the long-term role of the business in both an economic and social context. Even if the term is typically used in the context of companies, it can also be used in reference to associations or organizations in general, as well as individuals.

Welfare: Identified in its fullest sense as the well-being and prosperity of a population. The concept of well-being, although it is closely tied to that of health, is much wider. The World Health Organization defines it as "the emotional, mental, physical, social and spiritual condition that allows individuals to achieve and maintain their personal potential in society".

Chapter 7
A Revolutionary Look at Health Policy Analysis in Developing Countries

Rahmatollah Gholipour
University of Tehran, Iran

Khadijeh Rouzbehani
University of Tehran, Iran

Goltan Fakhteh Yavari
University of Tehran, Iran

ABSTRACT

Health policy analysis has been the focus of attention of a number of scholars, health practitioners and policy makers. However, there has been much less attention given to how to do policy analysis, what research designs, theories or methods best inform policy analysis. This study begins by looking at the health policy environment, and some of the challenges to researching this highly complex phenomenon. It focuses on research in middle and low income countries. Attention is drawn to the roles of the policy researcher and the importance of reflexivity and researcher's position in the research process and finally ways of advancing the field of health policy analysis is discussed.

DOI: 10.4018/978-1-4666-9944-1.ch007

INTRODUCTION

Health policy analysis is a multi-disciplinary approach to public policy which aims to explain the interaction between institutions, interests and ideas in the policy process. It is useful both retrospectively and prospectively, to understand past policy failures and successes and to plan for future policy implementation. This is what Walt and Gilson (1994) believed was central to health reforms. However, there has been much less attention given to how to do policy analysis, what research designs, theories or methods best inform policy analysis. Reich and Cooper (1996) designed and have updated a software tool to help researchers and policy-makers analyze the political dimensions of public policies. Others, such as Varvasovszky and Brugha (2000), have designed guidelines for undertaking stakeholder analysis, as a part of health policy analysis. Bossert (1998) developed an approach to analyze choices for the decentralization of health sectors. Sabatier (1999, 2007) has explored different theoretical frameworks of the policy process (although not focusing on health). However, it is rare to find any scholarly work that explicitly explores the methodological challenges for researchers studying the health policy process.

This chapter takes off from the conclusions drawn in the literature review by Gilson and Raphaely (2007), which identifies some of the gaps and weaknesses in the field of health policy analysis in poor and developing countries. The review notes the absence of explicit conceptual frameworks, little detail on research design and methodology, and a preponderance of single case studies on particular issues. It draws attention to the limited use of relevant theory to underpin analysis and the paucity of attempts to provide an explicit, explanatory focus. As the authors say, the main question is often 'what happened', to the neglect of 'what explains what happened'. Researchers also rarely reflect on how their own positions shape their research interpretations and conclusions.

In this study, the researchers tackle some of these issues, looking at some of the reasons for the above deficiencies identified in the Gilson and Raphaely review, and make some suggestions for advancing the field. This study, at first, begins by looking at the health policy environment, and some of the challenges to researching this highly complex phenomenon. Second, theories and frameworks are reconsidered .From there the authors move to methodology and study design, exploring the implications of case study research and temporality for health policy analysis; and then discuss the roles of the policy researcher, the importance of reflexivity and researcher's position in the research process. The final section explores ways of advancing the field of health policy analysis.

HEALTH POLICY ENVIRONMENT

It is important to contextualize the health policy environment in order to understand the challenges to methodology and theory. While drawing on ideas and concepts from general policy analysis, most of which is derived from studies on high income countries, this paper focuses on health policy, and on low and middle income countries. Much of the theory from policy analysis in high income countries has resonance for health and developing countries, and can usefully inform research in those areas.

However, transferring such concepts needs to be undertaken with caution. It is generally fair to say that the health sector has specific characteristics which affect the policy environment (and that differentiate it from other social sectors). The state may be both provider and purchaser of services, but also is involved in regulation, research and training among other functions. In service provision, it may be in competition or partnership with a private sector that it is also regulating. In undertaking its health care purchasing and regulatory functions, the state is usually heavily reliant on—and may lack—essential information that can only be provided by the sectors it is over-seeing.

Information asymmetry is often a bigger problem than with the other social sectors. Health issues are often high profile and demand public responses. Health interests, ranging from professionals to the pharmaceutical industry, have traditionally been perceived to influence the policy process significantly. They are uniquely placed to do so because of their knowledge, technology, access to political processes and stake in life and death issues. However, while these characteristics are generally typical, all scholars point out that they have to be contextualized in both place and time. Health policy environments in middle and high income countries will therefore differ from those in low income countries, where, for example, there are weaker regulations, regulatory capacity and monitoring systems; lack of purchasing power as a leverage to influence types and quality of services delivered; more patronage in political systems, and more reliance on external donor funds, among many other differences.

In spite of differences between high and low income countries, however, it is increasingly recognized that policy processes are changing everywhere. Initially policy analysis focused on the state—on the public or government sector—on politicians, bureaucrats and interest groups (Grindle and Thomas 1991). Over the past 10 years scholars have acknowledged a shift in the nature of policy and policy-making, which points to the involvement of a much larger array of actors in the policy process (Buse et al. 2005). The private sector, for example, including for-profit and not-for-profit organizations, large and small, has become an important player in health policy.

Partnerships between public and private sectors have also changed the health policy environment. Furthermore, policy is increasingly shaped and influenced by forces (such as global civil society) outside state boundaries (Keck and Sikkink 1998). The growing literature around issues of globalization which emphasize changing spatial, temporal and cognitive dimensions (Lee et al. 2002) reflects the extent to which the world is perceived to have altered. There is less geographical distance between regions, exchanges have become faster, ideas and perceptions spread rapidly through global communications and culture. This means that the policy environment is increasingly populated by complex cross-border, inter-organizational and network relationships, with policies influenced by global decisions as well as by domestic actions.

The technological revolution has facilitated communications and relationships, both between governments and their advisers as well as between many different networks of actors outside of government. While government and its hierarchical institutions remain important, all policy analysis must also take into account a range of open-ended, more ad hoc arrangements which increasingly affect decision-making. Hajer and Wagenaar (2003) talk about 'new spaces of politics' where there are concrete challenges to the practices of policymaking and politics coming from below. In their view, policy analysis has to become more deliberative: less top-down, involving expanded networks, and more interpretative, taking into account people's stories, their understandings, values and beliefs as expressed through language and behavior.

ENVIRONMENTAL CHALLENGES TO DO HEALTH POLICY ANALYSIS

These changes in the policy environment make the analysis of policy even more complex but there are conceptual and practical problems that are specific to 'doing' health policy analysis.

The first challenge is that 'policy' can itself be defined in many different ways, with consequent implications for its study. It can be useful to think of health policy as embracing 'courses of action (and inaction) that affect the set of institutions, organizations, services and funding arrangements of the health system' (Buse et al. 2005). Such policy may therefore be made within government, by non-government actors, and by organizations external to the health system.

However, such processes of 'making' policy are not necessarily overt or clearly bounded. The ways in which decisions 'emerge' rather than taking place at a single point in time, and which are often unobservable to the researcher, can be particularly difficult to unpack and explain (Exworthy 2007). On the practical level, there are often many hurdles to accessing the many different, geographically widespread, actors, individuals, groups and networks involved in policy processes. Decision making processes are often opaque, and obtaining relevant documents and papers can be problematic. Or, in contrast, an excess of information—where background documentation such as large volumes of email exchanges become available—can be burdensome and difficult to analyze. Participant observation can be difficult in practice. There is also often a tension between the long-term nature of policy development and implementation and the short-term nature both of funding for policy research and of policy-makers' demands for quick answers and remedies. Hunter (2003) has called this the curse of the temporal challenge. Much health policy research is motivated (and attracts funding) by practical concerns such as the evaluation of existing programs, and policy analysts are expected to deliver easily implementable recommendations within relatively short time horizons. The imperatives of quick policy 'fixes' may lead to reductionism. There are also many other conceptual challenges to 'doing' policy analysis. For example, capturing and measuring levels of resources, values, beliefs and power of diverse actors is difficult; also, the notion of 'power'—fundamental to policy analysis—is a highly contested concept. Yet it is often used as if there were little difficulty in agreeing what power is, where it lies, and how it is exercised. It can also be difficult to tell the story, without getting immersed in detail. Researchers have to find ways of organizing their analysis so that it provides a lens that represents but also explains a highly complex environment. As Gilson and Raphaely (2007) have shown, most health policy analysis is relatively intuitive, ad hoc, and the assumptions on which it is based are seldom identified.

In this paper researchers argue that the field of health policy analysis would be advanced if researchers approached it more systematically, developing clear and testable propositions about the issue they are studying, within explicit frameworks. Scholars have proposed a number of different theoretical frameworks to help researchers organize and focus their efforts to analyze the policymaking process. In the next section, let's look at some of them.

HEALTH POLICY FRAMEWORKS AND THEORIES

A. Frameworks

There are a number of widely used frameworks and theories of the public policy process. Brugha et al. (2002, 2004) have conducted a number of studies on global health initiatives such as the GAVI Alliance and the Global Fund to Fight AIDS, Tuberculosis and Malaria. Designed to gather and report the views of national-level stakeholders at very early stages in their implementation, the studies were sensitive. For the Global Fund, in particular, the research was perceived as premature, enabling country stakeholders to articulate criticisms, which it feared would have a deleterious effect on the need to raise significantly greater funds globally. The Global Fund Secretariat in Geneva requested that the scope of the study be widened to report its perspective, which was beyond the capacity and resources available to the researchers. In both studies, under pressure from funding agencies, the researchers reported findings within 9 months. The researchers resisted pressure from the Global Fund Secretariat to report interim findings to the Fund in late 2003, in advance of reporting back to country stakeholders. The policy environment was very fluid, and the researchers found they were tracking a moving target—one where the Global Fund itself was responding to difficulties, changing guidelines, and proving to be a 'learning organization'. Despite what the researchers viewed as rapid feedback of findings, given the need for rigour, the study funders and the Global Fund responded that the findings only confirmed what they had already learned through their own channels; and that these findings were being superseded by events. The study also found that the donor landscape had become even more complex by the time of the second phase of data collection, because of the negotiation or establishment of other new HIV/AIDS financing instruments at the country level, such as the World Bank Multicounty AIDS Program and the US President's Emergency Plan for AIDS Relief (PEPFAR). New sources of funds were being negotiated sequentially or in parallel, which was distracting countries from implementation. The dynamic nature of the policy environment made data collection and analysis difficult, and created sensitivities between the global initiatives, research funders and the researchers. One lesson was that maintaining a balance between independence and engagement with the entity being studied is difficult but key; building trust is essential if findings are to be taken on board.

We discuss some of the more enduring examples; those which have been utilized most in the published public policy literature (Gilson & Raphaely 2007). Frameworks organize inquiry by identifying elements and relationships among elements that need to be considered for theory generation (Ostrom 2007). They do not, of themselves, explain or predict behavior and outcomes (Schlager 2007). The best known public policy framework is the stages heuristic (Lasswell 1956). It divides the public policy process into four stages: agenda setting, formulation, implementation, and evaluation. Agenda setting is the issue sorting stage during which a small number of the many problems societies face rise to the attention of decision-makers.

In the formulation stage, legislatures and other decision-making bodies design and enact policies. In the implementation stage, governments carry out these policies, and in the evaluation stage impact is assessed. Analysts have criticized the stages heuristic for presuming a linearity to the public policy process that does not exist in reality, for postulating neat demarcations between stages that are blurred in practice, and for offering no propositions on causality (Sabatier 2007).Nevertheless, the heuristic offers a useful and simple way of thinking about the entire public policy process, and helps researchers situate their research within a wider framework. Walt and Gilson (1994) developed a policy analysis framework specifically for health, although its relevance extends beyond this sector. They noted that health policy research focused largely on the content of policy, neglecting actors, context and processes. Their policy triangle framework is grounded in a political economy perspective, and considers how all four of these elements interact to shape policy-making. The framework has influenced health policy research in a diverse array of countries, and has been used to analyze a large number of health issues, including mental health, health sector reform, tuberculosis, reproductive health and antenatal syphilis control (Gilson & Raphaely 2007).

As the number of actors involved in policy processes has expanded, so has interest in network frameworks. Seen largely as a tool for describing systems of interactions and interconnectedness between groups of actors, network analysis is a contested area, and there are many definitions of what a network is (Thatcher 1998). Most agree, however, that networks are clusters of actors linked together, who may be closely connected or loosely structured but are still capable of engaging in collective action. Policy networks are clusters of actors with interests in a given policy sector, and the capacity to help determine policy success or failure (Marsh 1998). There are many different ways of classifying networks. Marsh and Rhodes (1992) treat policy networks as a generic term, with policy communities at one end of a continuum and issue networks at the other. Policy communities are tight-knit networks with few participants who share basic values and share resources. There may be a strong inner or dominant core of actors, surrounded by a number of other, more peripheral members, all of whom make up a policy community. An issue network, on the other hand, brings together many different groups and individuals for a common purpose or cause, and may have little continuity in values or participation. Network analysis reflects the phenomenon of shared decision-making and exchange of resources to achieve their goals.

There is a debate among scholars as to whether the concept of networks is merely descriptive, or whether it has explanatory value, whether it is largely a Western concept, developed by looking at policy-making in the US and UK, and whether it has legitimacy for developing countries (Thatcher 1998). For some the network approach is not really a new analytical perspective, but signals rather a change in the policy environment and the political system. There are only a few empirical studies in health in developing countries which use network analysis as a lens (Schneider et al. 2006).

B. Theories

Explicit attention to theory development could benefit public policy practice by deepening our understanding of causality, and by bringing coherence to a fragmented body of knowledge. This does not imply a positivist approach to analysis, but a more thoughtful conceptualization of the policy process, that goes beyond telling the story. Influential theories of the public policy process include multiple-streams (Kingdon 1984), punctuated-equilibrium (Baumgartner & Jones 1993) and top-down and bottom-up implementation (Sabatier 1999). Theories are more specific than frameworks, and postulate precise relationships among variables that can be tested or evaluated empirically. Kingdon (1984), whose multiple-streams theory is concerned with agenda setting, argues that the public policy process has a random character, with problems, policies and politics flowing along in independent streams. The problems stream contains the broad problems and conditions facing societies, some of which become identified as issues that require public attention. The policy stream refers to the set of policy alternatives that researchers and others propose to address national problems.

This stream contains ideas and technical proposals on how problems may be solved. Political transitions, national mood and social pressure are among the constituent elements of the politics stream. At particular junctures the streams merge, and in their confluence windows of opportunity emerge and governments decide to act. Several health policy scholars have adapted ideas from Kingdon's theory to explain how particular health issues have emerged on policy agendas. Reich (1995) identified additional elements that fed into the politics stream—organizational, symbolic, economic, scientific and politician politics—all of which favored child over adult health through the 1990s, explaining the higher position of the former on the international health agenda. Ogden et al. (2003) also drew on Kingdon's ideas in their research on tuberculosis. They demonstrated that the emergence of the HIV/AIDS epidemic contributed to the opening of global policy windows, facilitating advocacy networks to promote DOTS (directly observed treatment, short-course) as a treatment of choice for tuberculosis. Baumgartner and Jones' (1993) punctuated equilibrium theory postulates that the policy-making process is characterized by periods of stability with minimal or incremental policy change, disrupted by bursts of rapid transformation. Central to their theory are the concepts of the policy image and the policy venue. The policy image is the way in which a given problem and set of solutions are conceptualized. One image may predominate over a long period of time, but may be challenged at particular moments as new understandings of the problem and alternatives come to the fore. The policy venue is the set of actors or institutions that make decisions concerning a particular set of issues.

These actors may hold monopoly power but will eventually face competition as new actors with alternative policy images gain prominence. When a particular policy venue and image hold sway over an extended period of time, the policy process will be stable and incremental. When new actors and images emerge, rapid bursts of change are possible. Thus, the policy process is constituted both by stability and change, rather than one or the other alone Shiffman et al. (2002) examined the emergence of global political attention for the control of tuberculosis, malaria and polio, finding that patterns conformed to punctuated rather than rational or incremental models of the policy process. Baumgartner and Jones themselves apply the theory to a health concern. They show that little changed in US tobacco policy in the first half of the 20th century, as the subject generated little coverage in the US media, government supported the industry through agricultural subsidies, and the product was seen positively as an important engine for economic growth. Beginning in the 1960s, however, health officials mobilized, health warnings came to dominate media coverage, and the industry was unable to counter a rapid shift in the policy image that focused on the adverse effects of tobacco on health.

Multiple implementation theories have been dominated by a discourse as to whether decision-making is top-down or bottom-up, or a synthesis of the two (Sabatier 1999). For example, Dye (2001) argues that even in a democracy like the United States, public policy is made from the top down, not from the bottom up. In his view, public policy reflects the values, interests and preferences of the governing elite. Dye separates policy development from implementation, admitting that bureaucrats may affect policy in implementation, but suggesting that all decisions are monitored to ensure they are not altered significantly. Lipsky (1980), on the other hand, describes implementation of policy as highly influenced by 'street level bureaucrats'—front-line staff who can change policies significantly—and others have developed this approach (e.g. Hjern and Porter 1981). Much of the literature focuses on the gap or deficit between policy objectives and actual implementation (Hill & Hupe 2002). Saetren (2005) reviewed all implementation literature published and concluded that while most of the studies focused on health and education, they were predominantly of high income, Western countries. There are a few notable exceptions (Kaler & Watkins 2001; Kamuzora & Gilson 2007).

Researchers have also applied a range of social science theory from outside of policy studies to health policy analysis, drawing these from disciplines such as sociology, anthropology and organizational management (Gilson & Raphaely 2007). Murray (2007), for instance, draws on sociological theory concerning consumption to understand the impact of private medical service financing mechanisms on maternity care in Chile. Others have used social construction theories to explore why public policies sometimes fail in their objectives. Ingram et al. (2007), for example, focus on how public policy-makers may construct target populations positively or negatively, leading to unfair distribution of resources that perpetuate health inequalities.

Using New Theories "Empowerment Strategies"

Researchers, however, neglected to pay more attention to empowerment strategies in healthcare sector. Empowerment strategies are supposed to help individuals link their personal struggle for improved health with the collective struggle to improve everyone's health. Individual commitment to improving other people's health improves one's own health – that is, commitment and solidarity (Navarro, 2004) are essential for good health. Commitment means a desire to serve others; solidarity means development of networks of support in joined cause to improve individual and collective health .Moreover, a collective response strengthens individual and collective health. Moreover, a collective response strengthens individual efforts to gain power, thus empowering the individual. These linkages between individual response and the collective, based on commitment and solidarity, are critical to achieving the structural determinants of good health. Linking the individual and collective struggles, which has characterized the history of labor movement, predates the faulty concept of "social capital", widely used by some researchers in the field of inequality, which trivializes the concept of solidarity and its purpose. The famous Putnam vision (Putnam, 2000) of encouraging social capitalists to be even better capitalists and to win in the competitive world is different from the concept of solidarity. it is the opposite of what healthy social behavior should be and the opposite of what is advocated here-that is, to link the struggle for individual liberation and health with the collective struggle. The objective should not be to enhance competitiveness in our societies but rather to enhance solidarity (Navarro, 2004).Something which shall be seriously mentioned here is that this concept is very much different from "social cohesion". This concept was established by the conservative and Christian Democrat tradition as a response to the labor movement's struggle to change society. In other words, social cohesion can exist side-by-side with enormous exploitation. There are many cohesive societies, where the social order is widely accepted, but where cohesiveness masks widespread exploitation and high levels of disease. In fact, a healthy intervention may be needed to facilitate a collective response, by those who are exploited, against the very cohesiveness. Therefore, solidarity refers to a hegemonic view in societies especially in the developing and poor countries.

HEALTH POLICY STUDIES' METHODOLOGY

Few health policy analyses on low and middle income countries explicitly discuss research design, and the field would benefit from more reflection on the range of approaches that could be used, and their relative benefits. Most investigations are case studies, whether or not researchers identify them as such (Gilson & Raphaely 2007). Policy decisions often have their roots in longer term processes and the choice of time frames for research is an important factor. Temporal issues thus also affect research design. Addressing these factors is an important aspect of research design.

Research Design: Case Studies

Case studies are in-depth investigations of a single instance of a phenomenon in its real-life context (Yin 1994). They are to be distinguished from other research designs, such as controlled comparisons, formal modeling, quantitative analyses and randomized-controlled experiments. A substantial body of work offers guidance on case study methodology (Yin 1994; Brady & Collier 2004; George & Bennett 2004; McKeown2004; Yin 2004).

Case study methodologists argue that asking just a few basic questions about the case can improve the value of the study considerably. First, what is it a case of (George and Bennett 2004)? Is it, say, an example of health policy implementation failure, of effective transfer of a health policy from one country to another, of health policy network influence on agenda setting, of the influence of political factors on health policy evaluation? Sometimes cases may be clearly identifiable by the researcher at the start of the study; sometimes they may be constructed or re-constructed during the course of the research as the analysis reveals their defining characteristics (Ragin & Becker 1992). The process of clarifying 'the case' enables the researcher to specify a body of knowledge to which he or she may make a contribution. Second, why is this case a useful one to study (George & Bennett 2004)? Does it offer the possibility of comparing the explanatory value of alternative theories? Is it an unusual example of policy effectiveness, potentially offering insight into factors that facilitate policy impact? It is consideration of these issues that help the researcher to select the tools and theories that might frame a study, and to determine which methods will be used.

A study on the global availability of praziquantel, a drug for the tropical disease schistosomiasis, offers clear answers to both questions (Reich and Govindaraj 1998). The researchers document how the discovery of this effective drug did not automatically result in it reaching the poor in developing countries. They identify this as a case of the gap between drug developments and drug availability for the poor—an issue of concern for many tropical disease pharmaceuticals—and highlight the usefulness of this case in revealing the influence of political and economic factors on this gap. Their careful case selection and classification enable them to suggest a set of policy prescriptions on surmounting the drug development–availability gap, recommendations that apply well beyond the case itself.

Another means of facilitating generalization is increasing the number of cases. Doing so is not always easy, since investigating even a single case is a time and resource intensive process that requires careful consideration of historical and contextual influences. Comparative case studies may introduce the further challenges of working across multiple languages and cultures. It can also be difficult to find sufficient funds for undertaking such research. Yet there are several strong examples in the health policy field. Lee et al. (1998) used matched country comparisons to investigate factors influencing the development of strong national family planning programs. They conducted four country comparisons: Bangladesh/Pakistan, Tunisia/Algeria, Zimbabwe/Zambia and Thailand/Philippines. Each pair was matched on socio-economic characteristics, but differed on the strength of the family planning program. The comparisons enabled the researchers to point to three factors that shaped the development of effective programs: the formation of coalitions among policy elites, the spread of policy risk, and the country's financial and institutional stability. Walt et al. (1999) considered individual cases of donor aid coordination in the aid-dependent countries of Bangladesh, Cambodia, Mozambique, South Africa and Zambia to develop generalizations concerning the origins and effectiveness of aid coordination mechanisms. Shiffman (2007) explored agenda-setting for maternal mortality reduction in five countries: Guatemala, Honduras, India, Indonesia and Nigeria. He identified nine factors that shaped the degree to which this issue emerged as a political priority. He found that while international donors played a role, even more critical were efforts by national champions. Collectively, these different examples highlight the value of cross-country comparative study approaches, where comparisons between similar (and different) country contexts can help disentangle generalizeable from country context-specific effects in policy adaptation, evolution and implementation. Comparisons can be incorporated into study design, ad-hoc, as in the case of Lee et al. (1998) above; researchers can select as case studies several countries with a shared feature (Brugha et al. 2005); or comparison can be made post-hoc, as in the case of Walt et al.(1999). Clearly, multi-country studies are more time and resource intensive.

HEALTH POLICY ANALYST'S POSITION

One of the issues facing health policy analysts is how they are viewed or 'situated' as researchers, their institutional base, perceived legitimacy, and prior involvement in policy communities. This is critical to their ability to access the policy environment and conduct meaningful research, especially in policy analyses that require engaging with policy elites (Shiffman 2007). Yet, in contrast to other disciplines in the social sciences (e.g. Lincoln 1995; Rose 1997), the policy analysis literature seldom explicitly discusses researcher 'positionality' and its possible impact on the research process. With respect to positionality, the classic distinction often made is between 'insiders' and 'outsiders', where insiders may be both participants and researchers (participant-observers) of the policy process, or alternatively, country-based rather than foreign researchers. Class, caste, gender, age, ethnicity and profession may also be highly relevant to insider/outsider status in some health policy research contexts. In seeking to unravel complex policy dynamics, insiders may see things quite differently to outsiders, with implications for the data collected and the interpretation of research findings. As explained by Merriam et al. (2001), 'being an insider means easy access, the ability to ask more meaningful questions and read non-verbal cues, and most importantly, to be able to project a more truthful, authentic understanding of the culture under study. On the other hand, insiders have been accused of being inherently biased - the outsider's advantage lies in curiosity with the unfamiliar, the ability to ask taboo questions, and being seen as non-aligned with sub-groups.

Policy research teams that combine both insiders and outsiders and that engage all team members in active discussions of findings during data collection and analysis may therefore yield the richest and most comprehensive understanding of the policy process (as proposed by Buse 2008, this issue). However, implementation of such a model is not easy. While policy research designs may recognize the value of this team approach, the reality is that policy analysis is only emerging and has yet to establish its legitimacy as a field within developing countries, 'insider' policy researchers are hard to recruit and 'outsider' researchers may be expensive and time-constrained.

Researcher positionality has implications not only for access to data but also for knowledge construction. Research may be based on externally imposed categories and constructs. Parkhurst (2002), for example, argues that explanations of the decline in HIV prevalence in Uganda were driven at first by the need to hold up a success story on HIV in Africa, leading to an overly simplified analysis of both the extent and the ingredients of this success by UN and donor agencies. Short timeframe policy research initiated in response to external political imperatives runs a real risk of superficial and decontextualized analyses of the policy process that reveal only part of the picture.

'Position' can influence the issues that researchers focus on and therefore the research agendas created and the research questions asked. Scholars have noted that positionality is tied to questions of power and resistance, and in the context of health policy research the North/South dynamics need to be acknowledged. Tensions can occur between northern researchers who have the funds, and southern researchers who have insider knowledge and understanding. As Staeheli and Lawson (1995) point out, 'researchers cannot escape the power relations even when they wish to do so. Western researchers are in a position of power by virtue of being able to name the categories, control information about the research agenda, define interventions and come and go as research scientists.'

National policy researchers, for their part, tend to be invested in their policy environments in some way, even if they operate from an independent research base or are not involved in the specific policy process under investigation. Researchers linked to particular policy environments will naturally be inclined to focus on specific and contemporary features of the particular policy space, rather than more universal themes that cut across policy or country contexts. They may also be more concerned with developing policy relevant conclusions than new theoretical or methodological understanding. Over time, such researchers will typically move in and out of various policy networks: sometimes directly implicated in policy communities, other times more loosely as part of issue networks or epistemic communities (Haas,1992) that provide public commentary on policy developments.

Increasingly, funders are mandating researchers to engage in research translation, forcing them to become policy actors. Being an interested actor may have both advantages and disadvantages for generating new policy knowledge. Maintaining a degree of legitimacy amongst a wide range of actors may be crucial to the ability to conduct future research. In highly contested policy spaces this may involve complicated balancing acts that limit the ability to ask certain questions. The intense polarization that has characterized HIV/AIDS in South Africa is one such example (Fassin and Schneider, 2003). Or where researchers take strong activist stands, they may become ideologically positioned in ways that may both open and close doors in the research process (Narayan, 2007).

CONCLUSION: ADVANCING HEALTH POLICY ANALYSIS

Schlager (2007) observed that the field of policy studies is characterized by 'mountain islands of theoretical structure, intermingled with and occasionally attached together by foothills of shared methods and concepts, and empirical work, all of which is surrounded by oceans of descriptive work not attached to any mountain of theory' (Sabatier 2007). We think this statement accurately characterizes the field of health policy analysis as well. Through this discussion of theory, methodology and positionality in health policy analysis, it is clear that there are a number of ways research in this field could be strengthened:

A. On Theory
   A1. More critical application of existing frameworks and theories of the public policy process to guide and inform health policy inquiry, while recognizing the need and potential to contribute to theory development as a goal of health policy analysis, with consequent benefits for practice.
   A2. Greater use of social science theories (for example, of organizations or street level bureaucrats) that come from outside of policy studies to inform health policy analysis.
B. On Methodology
   B1. Making research design an explicit concern in all health policy analyses, and identifying and justifying the type of design in published articles.
   B2. Drawing on the growing body of work on case study research methods in order to enhance the quality of case study inquiry in the field.
   B3. Clearly identifying the type of 'case' and the unit of analysis, and considering the need for multiple cases and comparators.
   B4. Making assumptions and propositions explicit, logical and interrelated, and open to being tested empirically, so as to explain general sets of phenomena.
   B5. Making the case to funding agencies to support more comparative work in health policy analysis in order to expand the generalizability of results and develop greater certainty concerning causality. This case will be strengthened by the willingness of researchers to collaborate across institutions, countries and regions.
   B6. Exploring other approaches to synthesis (e.g. through large sample studies which employ quantitative and qualitative methods) as well as retrospective studies which draw on research from different disciplines in one policy domain or set of countries.
C. On Research Position
   C1. Greater reflexivity on the part of researchers, that involves an analysis of their own institutional power, resources and positions (in much the same way they would analyze actors in the policy process) and their role in defining research agendas and generating knowledge (rather than assuming themselves to be 'objective' and 'independent').
   C2. Greater attention to policy research team composition and roles, including insiders and outsiders, which can relate to nationality but also to multiple roles. Researcher positionality may need to be negotiated and also reflected upon, considering how it may influence data collection and interpretation.
   C3. Long-term approaches to building policy analytic capacity. This would include acknowledging and providing space for different policy research

agendas arising from different researcher positionalities, and building a critical mass of policy analytic capacity to enable this. In conclusion, we argue that if those who conduct, teach, commission, fund or publish public health policy research take on board some of these points, there will be a significant improvement in research approaches to health policy analysis, especially in relation to low and middle income country settings. If applied, these recommendations will also provide lessons on the evolution of policy implementation successes and failures as well as tools to assist policy-makers in evaluating and planning current and future policies.

REFERENCES

Baumgartner, F. R., & Jones, B. D. (1993). *Agendas and instability in American politics*. Chicago: The University of Chicago Press.

Bossert, T. (1998). Analyzing the decentralization of health systems in developing countries: Decision space, innovation and performance. *Social Science & Medicine*, *47*(10), 1513–1527. doi:10.1016/S0277-9536(98)00234-2 PMID:9823047

Brady, H. E., & Collier, D. (2004). *Rethinking social inquiry: diverse tools, shared standards*. Lanham, MD: Rowman and Littlefield Publishers, Inc.

Brewer, G., & de Leon, P. (1983). *The foundations of policy analysis*. Monterey, CA: Brooks/Cole.

Brugha, R. (2005). *Global Fund Tracking Study: a cross-country comparative analysis*. Final Report. Retrieved from http://www.theglobalfund.org/en/files/links_resources/library/studies/IE13_full.pdf

Brugha, R., Donoghue, M., Starling, M., Ndubani, P., Ssengooba, F., Fernandes, B., & Walt, G. (2004). The Global Fund: Managing great expectations. *Lancet*, *364*(9428), 95–100. doi:10.1016/S0140-6736(04)16595-1 PMID:15234862

Brugha, R., Starling, M., & Walt, G. (2002). GAVI, the first steps: Lessons for the Global Fund. *Lancet*, *359*(9304), 435–438. doi:10.1016/S0140-6736(02)07607-9 PMID:11844535

Buse, K., Mays, N., & Walt, G. (2005). *Making health policy*. Milton Keynes, UK: Open University Press.

Dye, T. (2001). *Top down policy making*. New York: Chatham House.

Dye, T., & Thomas, R. (2001). *Understanding public policy*. Prentice Hall.

Edgell, S., Hetherington, K., & Warde, A. (Eds.). (1996). *Consumption matters*. Oxford, UK: Blackwell Publishers.

Exworthy, M. (2007). *Policy to tackle the social determinants of health: Using conceptual frameworks to understand the policy process*. Paper presented to a Workshop on Health Policy Analysis, London, UK.

Fassin, D., & Schneider, H. (2003). The politics of AIDS in South Africa: Beyond the controversies (Education and Debate). *British Medical Journal*, *326*(7387), 495–497. doi:10.1136/bmj.326.7387.495 PMID:12609950

George, A. L., & Bennett, A. (2004). *Case studies and theory development in the social sciences*. Cambridge, MA: MIT Press.

Gilson, L., & Raphaely, N. (2007). The terrain of health policy analysis in low and middle income countries: a review of the literature 1994–2005. Paper presented to a Workshop on Health Policy Analysis, London, UK.

Grindle, M., & Thomas, J. (1991). *Public choice and policy change*. Baltimore, MD: Johns Hopkins University Press.

Haas, P. (1992). Introduction: Epistemic communities and international policy coordination. *International Organization*, *46*(01), 1–18. doi:10.1017/S0020818300001442

Hajer, M. A., & Wagenaar, H. (Eds.). (2003). *Deliberative policy analysis*. Cambridge, UK: Cambridge University Press. doi:10.1017/CBO9780511490934

Hill, M. J., & Hupe, P. L. (2002). *Implementing public policy: governance in theory and practice*. London: Sage.

Hjern, B., & Porter, D. O. (1981). Implementation structures: A new unit of administrative analysis. *Organization Studies*, *2*, 211–227.

Hogwood, G., & Gunn, L. (1984). *Policy analysis for the real world*. Oxford, UK: Oxford University Press.

Hunter, D. J. (2003). Evidence-based policy and practice: Riding for a fall? *Journal of the Royal Society of Medicine*, *96*(4), 194–196. doi:10.1258/jrsm.96.4.194 PMID:12668712

Ingram, H., Schneider, A. L., & De Leon, P. (2007). Social construction and policy design. In Theories of the policy process. Boulder, CO: Westview Press.

Kaler, A., & Watkins, S. C. (2001). Disobedient distributors: street-level bureaucrats and would-be patrons in community-based family planning programs in rural Kenya. *Studies in Family Planning, 32*, 254-69.

Kamuzora, P., & Gilson, L. (2007). Factors influencing implementation of the Community Health Fund in Tanzania. *Health Policy and Planning*, *22*(2), 95–102. doi:10.1093/heapol/czm001 PMID:17299023

Keck, M. E., & Sikkink, K. (1998). *Activists beyond borders*. Ithaca, NY: Cornell University Press.

Kingdon, J. W. (1984). *Agendas, alternatives and public policies*. Boston, MA: Little, Brown and Company.

Lasswell, H. (1956). *The decision process*. College Park, MD: University of Maryland Press.

Lee, K., Fustukian, S., & Buse, K. (2002). *Health policy in a globalizing world*. Cambridge, UK: Cambridge University Press.

Lee, K., Lush, L., Walt, G., & Cleland, J. (1998). Family planning policies and programmes in eight low-income countries: A comparative policy analysis. *Social Science & Medicine*, *47*(7), 949–959. doi:10.1016/S0277-9536(98)00168-3 PMID:9722114

Lincoln, Y. (1995). Emerging criteria for quality in qualitative and interpretive research. *Qualitative Inquiry*, *1*(3), 275–289. doi:10.1177/107780049500100301

Lipsky, M. (1980). *Street-level bureaucracy: dilemmas of the individual in public services*. New York: Russell Sage Foundation.

Marsh, D. (Ed.). (1998). *Comparing policy networks*. Buckingham, UK: Open University Press.

Marsh, D., & Rhodes, R. A. W. (1992). *Policy networks in British Government*. Buckingham, UK: Open University Press. doi:10.1093/acprof:oso/9780198278528.001.0001

McKeown, T. J. (2004). Case studies and the limits of the quantitative worldview. In H. E. Brady & D. Collier (Eds.), *Rethinking social inquiry: diverse tools, shared standards* (pp. 139–168). Lanham, MD: Rowman and Littlefield Publishers, Inc.

Merriam, S. B., Johnson-Bailey, J., Lee, M. Y., Kee, Y., Ntseane, G., & Muhamad, M. (2001). Power and positionality: Negotiating insider/outsider status within and across cultures. *International Journal of Lifelong Education*, *20*(5), 405–416. doi:10.1080/02601370120490

Murray, S. F. (2007). *Illuminating unintended consequences: a case study using retrospective policy analysis linking the macro, meso, and micro*. Paper presented to a Workshop on Health Policy Analysis, London, UK.

Narayan, T. (2007). *Policy Processes underlying Health and Equity Initiatives in a rapidly globalizing context – a case study from Bangalore, Karnataka, India*. Paper presented to a Workshop on Health Policy Analysis, London, UK.

Navarro, V. (2004). *A critique of social capital. In Political and Economic Determinants of Population Health and well-being*. Amityville, NY: Baywood.

Ogden, J., Walt, G., & Lush, L. (2003). The politics of 'branding' in policy transfer: The case of DOTS for tuberculosis control. *Social Science & Medicine*, *57*(1), 179–188. doi:10.1016/S0277-9536(02)00373-8 PMID:12753826

Ostrom, E. (2007). Institutional rational choice: an assessment of the institutional analysis and development framework. In P. A. Sabatier (Ed.), *Theories of the policy process* (2nd ed.; pp. 21–64). Boulder, CO: Westview Press.

Parkhurst, J. O. (2002). The Ugandan success story? Evidence and claims of HIV-1 Prevention. *Lancet*, *360*(9326), 78–80. doi:10.1016/S0140-6736(02)09340-6 PMID:12114061

Putnam, R. (2000). *Bowling Alone: The collapse and Revival of American community*. New York: Simon and Schuster. doi:10.1145/358916.361990

Ragin, C., & Becker, H. S. (1992). *What is a case? Exploring the foundations of social enquiry*. New York: Cambridge University Press.

Reich, M. R. (1995). The politics of agenda setting in international health: Child health versus adult health in developing countries. *Journal of International Development*, *7*(3), 489–502. doi:10.1002/jid.3380070310 PMID:12290763

Reich, M. R., & Cooper, D. (1996). *Policy Maker* [Software tool]. Available from http://www.hsph.harvard.edu

Reich, M. R., & Govindaraj, R. (1998). Dilemmas in drug development for tropical diseases. Experiences with praziquantel. *Health Policy (Amsterdam)*, *44*(1), 1–18. doi:10.1016/S0168-8510(98)00002-5 PMID:10180198

Rose, G. (1997). Situating knowledges: Positionality, reflexivity and other tactics. *Progress in Human Geography*, *21*(3), 305–320. doi:10.1191/030913297673302122

Sabatier, P. A. (Ed.). (1999). *Theories of the policy process*. Boulder, CO: Westview Press.

Sabatier, P. A. (Ed.). (2007). *Theories of the policy process*. Boulder, CO: Westview Press.

Saetren, H. (2005). Facts and myths about research on public policy implementation: Out-of-fashion, allegedly dead, but still very much alive and relevant. *Policy Studies Journal: the Journal of the Policy Studies Organization, 33*(4), 559–582. doi:10.1111/j.1541-0072.2005.00133.x

Schlager, E. (2007). A comparison of frameworks, theories, and models of policy processes. In P. A. Sabatier (Ed.), *Theories of the policy process*. Boulder, CO: Westview Press.

Schneider, H., Gilson, L., Ogden, J., Lush, L., & Walt, G. (2006). Health systems and the implementation of disease programmes: Case studies from South Africa. *Global Public Health: An International Journal for Research, Policy and Practice, 1*(1), 49–64. doi:10.1080/17441690500361083 PMID:19153894

Shiffman, J. (2007). Generating political priority for maternal mortality reduction in 5 developing countries. *American Journal of Public Health, 97*(5), 796–803. doi:10.2105/AJPH.2006.095455 PMID:17395848

Shiffman, J., Beer, T., & Wu, Y. H. (2002). The emergence of global disease control priorities. *Health Policy and Planning, 17*(3), 225–234. doi:10.1093/heapol/17.3.225 PMID:12135988

Staeheli, L. A., & Lawson, V. A. (1995). Feminism, praxis and human geography. *Geographical Analysis, 27*(4), 321–328. doi:10.1111/j.1538-4632.1995.tb00914.x

Thatcher, M. (1998). The development of policy network analyses. *Journal of Theoretical Politics, 10*(4), 389–416. doi:10.1177/0951692898010004002

Varvasovszky, Z., & Brugha, R. (2000). How to do a stakeholder analysis. *Health Policy and Planning, 15*(3), 338–345. doi:10.1093/heapol/15.3.338 PMID:11012410

Walt, G., & Gilson, L. (1994). Reforming the health sector in developing countries: The central role of policy analysis. *Health Policy and Planning, 9*(4), 353–370. doi:10.1093/heapol/9.4.353 PMID:10139469

Walt, G., Pavignani, E., Gilson, L., & Buse, K. (1999). Health sector development: From aid coordination to resource management. *Health Policy and Planning, 14*(3), 207–218. doi:10.1093/heapol/14.3.207 PMID:10621238

Yin, R. (1994). *Case study research: design and methods* (2nd ed.). Thousand Oaks, CA: Sage Publications.

Yin, R. (2004). *The case study anthology*. Thousand Oaks, CA: Sage Publications.

KEY TERMS AND DEFINITIONS

Empowerment Strategies: A management practice of sharing information, rewards, and power with employees so that they can take initiative and make decisions to solve problems and improve service and performance.

Health Policy Challenges: Linking the health problems to larger political, cultural, and philosophical contexts, Policy Challenges in Modern Health Care offers a compelling look at healthcare service and the barriers.

Methodology: The process used to collect information and data for the purpose of making business decisions.

Multidisciplinary Approach: Combining or involving several academic disciplines or professional specializations in an approach to a topic or problem.

Policy Analysis: An applied social science discipline which uses methods of inquiry and argument to produce and transform policy relevant information that may be used in political setting to solve policy problems.

Process: A series of actions or steps taken in order to achieve a particular end.

Chapter 8
Stakeholders Engagement and Agenda Setting in a Developing Context:
The Case of the Bangladesh Health Policy

Golam Rabbani
Rajshahi University, Bangladesh

ABSTRACT

One area of focus in the study of policymaking in developing countries is the extent to which policymaking in the developing countries is similar to the interaction among stakeholder groups, including politicians, that occurs in developed countries. This paper explores this issue in the case of the development of the Bangladesh Health Policy 2011. It is found that the policymaking process has many well-organized actors with very clear and efficient roles in generating policy outputs. This study indicates that the distinctions between policymaking in western and eastern countries, at least in some countries, may be breaking down.

INTRODUCTION

Public policy making is not a simple function, but a process where different actors interact and try their best to influence the policy. The policy process and the dynamics of politics are interrelated. The main aim of this study is to uncover the

DOI: 10.4018/978-1-4666-9944-1.ch008

dynamics of politics in the agenda setting of the health policy of Bangladesh, through investigation of the role of deferent actors.

In every policy process[1] politics plays an important role in idea generation, formulation and implementation (Peterson, 1993; Cited in Reich 1995). Policy reform in the health sector is not different from other policy reforms. In the process of health policy making of any country, different actors try to make the policy favorable to them by playing a significant role in its development. This interaction of different actors in a policy process is known as the politics of public policy. In the complex political process of health sector reform, viability of special agenda, type of changes in policy reform, and vision of national politics play important role (Oberlander, 2003; Roper, 2007). Generally, different actors have their own choices and preferences which are shaped by interest group politics[2] and national politics. Yet this does not necessarily mean that only group politics play the dominant role in the policy making. Rather, public opinion and the demands of donors have a significant impact on public policy (Oliver & Dowell, 1994). The case of health policy making of Bangladesh[3] is not an exception.

In Bangladesh, health is one of the most important sectors since good health ensures more social and economic production and good quality of life. Beyond debate, priority of the health sector is forefront in the development discourse, even though, 'health sector' itself is associated with multi-sectoral factors and actors (Perry, 2000). Thus, implementation of health sector policy requires interplay of actors and factors from different sectors and levels (local, national, regional and international) (Talukder, Rob & Mahabub, 2007). Public policy making in third world countries is not merely a simple function (Rahman, 1995 cited in Panday, 2001). When it comes to making of health policy in a developing country, it is more multi-sectoral than any other policy. This is because of the huge number of health issues and associated issues which require urgent attention (CSG, 2008). Numerous actors and factors play a crucial role in the health policy process of Bangladesh (Osman, 2004). In the total policy process, agenda setting is more important since actors (individual or groups) come forward with their (policy actors) ideas and issues at this stage. Thus, different dynamics occur at this stage. Actors' expertise, access (including network), information, authoritative and influential positions and strategies to highlight the specific issues are main determinant factors in drawing serious attention by government. The main focus of this study is on the dynamics of agenda setting in making health policy in Bangladesh. In order to find out the dynamics of agenda setting, the roles of the different actors have been investigated. To make the study more specific, community health related agenda setting in developing context the National Health Policy, 2011[4]' was chosen as a case.

Osman (2004) studied the process of formulation and implementation of health sectors plans in Bangladesh up to 2000. The study finding presented a comprehensive account of the dynamics of health policy process. Perry (2000) provided an in-depth assessment of numerous health and family planning activities having particular emphasis on some factors that influenced the health service delivery in Bangladesh. Mahmud (2007) described the chronology of health services delivery in Bangladesh having particular emphasis on identification of factors causing failure in the implementation of health services delivery. This writing was more focused on causes of implementation failure in health service delivery. Jahan (2003) illustrated how advocates for gender equity succeeded in influencing the restructuring of the health system in Bangladesh in the mid-1990s. The study explored the impact of advocacies for gender equity made in the design of the reforms. Shiffman (2003) drew political science and public administration theory to evaluate the Bangladeshi reform experience in the health sector. The study did so with reference to the norms of efficiency, effectiveness, sovereignty and democracy. Reich (1995) examined the political dynamics of health sector reform in poor countries, through a comparative study of pharmaceutical policy reform in Sri Lanka, Bangladesh, and the Philippines having a special focus on political will, political factions, and political survival models.

Existing findings substantiate existence of political dynamics in the health policy process in Bangladesh. Very few researchers have emphasised political interplay among the actors in health sector of Bangladesh. Thus, the issue of dynamics in agenda setting in Bangladesh deserves special attention for further exploration.

The 'health' sector, itself is very important sector for any nation, especially for developing nation. As in other developing nations, the health situation in Bangladesh is a developmental problem and without addressing this problem development initiatives in Bangladesh cannot be successful. In the context of Bangladesh, successful policy implementation is a rare event. So, the health sector of Bangladesh is not an exception in this regard (Walt & Gilson, 1994; Grieve, 1995; Nazneen, 2001). Inequality in health service delivery is an indication of the policy failure in health sector of Bangladesh (BDHS, 2007; Osman, 2004; Jahan & Salehin, 2006; Perry 1999).

Now a pertinent question can be raised: where lie the gaps in the policy process? Different researchers have tried to unearth the causes of implementation failure of different projects and policies, but very few attempts have been made to explore the dynamics in the policy process, especially in agenda setting, where inter-group politics play the main role. It can be argued that, without considering political dynamics, it would be very difficult to understand how health policy in Bangladesh is made. The National Health Policy, developed in 2007-2010, is a starling example of this. Thus, it can be claimed that an attempt to explore the political dynamics of agenda setting in health policy of Bangladesh is essential to understanding the process. How do policy shifts occur and what factors cause these shifts? In other words, why do policies change in the health sector of Bangladesh?

The study is qualitative and explanatory in nature. Mixed method approach (both quantitative and qualitative) has been used in this study. To analyze the politics of agenda setting case study is an ideal methodology since holistic and in-depth investigation is possible through this method (Feagin, Orum & Sjoberg, 1991). In the current study's context, the sample sizes were determined on the basis of the principles of Snowball Sampling. In this study, fifteen individuals were selected as respondent. In this technique, first subject was identified with serious attention and then the respondent was asked to identify the other potential subject.

THEORETICAL FRAMEWORK AND CONCEPTUAL CLARIFICATION

Agenda-setting is the most basic stage of the public policy cycle, which is concerned with identification of policy issues and placing these issues on the agenda of government. To promote an idea to a policy agenda requires participation of different actors in a competitive process. Participation in policymaking is a central question in the discipline of Public Policy. The role of interest groups and the public[5] in shaping administrative decisions was the main theme of early pluralists' work (notably Truman 1951, Cited in, Robinson and Eller 2010). The public participate directly as interest groups and indirectly, through the influence of elected officials. Later works, popularly known as "elite theory" (Lowi, 1979; Cited in, Robinson and Eller, 2010) focused on the dominance of political elites, bureaucratic elites and business elites in the policy-making process.

As a result of the pluralist/elitist debate over participation in administrative policymaking, a new model of policy decision making emerged. Cohen, March, and Olsen (1972) mentioned that organizations do not take decisions in a rational way (Cited in, Robinson and Eller, 2010). Moreover, rational self-interest is more dominant in organizational decision-making (interests of conflicting interest groups, from the pluralistic model or the interest of elites). In the competitive environment, organizations take decisions haphazardly based on a series of "streams" (the coming together) of organizational inputs. This is popularly known as the garbage can model (GCM) of organizational decision making. Kingdon (1995) applied this model of organizational decision-making to the policymaking processes. Kingdon described that policy processes are neither elite nor pluralist in their entireties. Instead, completion was found in separate "streams" of policymaking activity among pluralist forces and elite forces. According to Kingdon's view, an issue becomes an agenda item with the confluence of three "streams": the problem stream, the proposal stream and the politics stream (Laraway & Jennings, 2002)

The agenda-setting process happens in a specific policy environment which consists of different factors, like economic, political, social, geographical, demographical, cultural, institutional, international, etc (Cochran & Malone, 2005). In this complex interaction, both actors and institutions play their roles which are shaped by different factors. Some of these are involved in the process due to their formal authority to promote the agenda, to provide technical and financial support, while others are to advocate in favour of their own interests (Rhodes, 1997). In public policy, all actors are generally divided into two parts: state/governmental actors and societal actors/non-government actors. Elected officials (executive and legislative) and appointed officials reside within the state and interest groups. Research organisation and mass media reside within societal actors or non-state actors. (Howlett & Romesh, 1995). In every country, these two actors play vital roles, but both may not present equal influence. Role and influence of actors depend on nature of interest, capability, technical knowledge, power of actors as well as intensity of the importance of the factors. Especially, the role and influence of actors depends upon the dynamics of the role of these factors and actors (Verschuere,2009). In developing countries, public policy-making goes through a complex and ambiguous process. The process is ambiguous and complex because there is no formal, established and visible process and institutional arrangement in the public policy-making of Bangladesh (Aminuzzaman, 2002).

While there is no neat way to package the policy process (especially the agenda-setting process), due to its complexity and nonlinearity, Kingdon's theory can help to capture the facts and figures in health policy making in Bangladesh. The following will be an elaborative illustration of analytical framework of this research:

PROBLEM STREAM

Policy making presents several difficulties to the decision makers, apparently which do not get equal attention from them. To shape the agenda, the most important task is agreeing on how to weigh the competing difficulties. Most of the cases have shown that issues backed by major interest groups get more policy priority.

Demand for an updated health policy is not new in Bangladesh. Since its independence (1971), every Government has tried to come up with a comprehensive health policy for Bangladesh. After a long time, the Awami League[6] Government (1996-2001) formulated a national health policy, in 2000. In the meantime, due to different national and international factors, a lot of changes have been made to the health situation of the country. Therefore, stakeholders of this sector have long been calling for an updated health policy. In spite of several attempts made by different political Governments, no initiatives were successfully carried out. According to the respondents of the study, this policy formulation process goes back to the term of the interim caretaker Government[7] (2007-09). The then Health Advisor[8] of the Caretaker Government of Bangladesh, Dr. A M M Shawkat Ali, declared the formulation of new health policy within the following three months during a meeting on the World Health Day observation to provide better health services and ensure quality education in medical and dental colleges (The Daily Star, 07 April 2008). After this declaration, different interest groups tried to influence the policy makers to highlight their problems and prioritize their interests in the policy making process.

According to the views presented by the study respondents, numerous problems were highlighted by different levels of organizations and individuals. More than 160 organizations and individuals submitted written demands to the Program Support Office (PSO), Health Nutrition and Population Sector Program (HNPSP), Ministry of Health and Family Welfare (MoHFW) prior to the preparation of the final draft. All of these demands reflected personal or professional interests. The written comments covered about 70 issues and a significant number of NGOs participated (Official documents of PSO, MoHFW and Interview, 2010). Weight of the problems and proper evidence and strategy to highlight the problems played important roles in catching the attention of the policy makers (Laraway and Jennings, 2002). Among the policy issues, some were more dominant compared to others, e g: Rural Community Health vs. Urban Community Health, Primary Health Care vs. Health Education, Female-Friendly Health Centres vs. Home Services, Preventive Care vs. Curative Care, Climate Change and Eco-Health, Communicable Diseases vs. Non-communicable Disease, Government as Regulator or Service Provider, Public Private Partnership or Privatisation, Medical Graduate vs. Health Assistant, Skill Development of Traditional Birth Attendant or Supply of New Skill Birth Attendant, Only Modern Medical Science or Modern Medical Science with Indigenous Treatment (Official documents of PSO, MoHFW,2010).

Study findings are one type of indicator that often focuses on a particular problem at a specific point in time. These studies are conducted by government agencies or nongovernment researchers or academics and may suggest that a problematic issue necessitates government attention. However, studies are not primarily used to establish whether problems exist. Instead, problems are determined through interpretation (Kingdon, 1995; Cited in Laraway & Jennings, 2002). Nevertheless, policy makers and those who work closely with them, rely on indicators to "assess the magnitude of a problem and become aware of changes in the problem" (Kingdon, 1995: 91; Cited in Laraway & Jennings, 2002). Considering this theoretical aspect as guidance for the study, the study was interested to know how community health issues were highlighted by the policy advocates. Most of the respondents considered that PSO, HNPSP, MoHFW did the ground work to prepare the draft health policy. Team Leader of PSO, HNPSP, MoHFW informed that the entire health sector of Bangladesh was visible to them and they knew which problem/s needed special attention to ensure health rights at all levels. To make the policy strategy justifiable and valid, PSO, HNPSP, MoHFW reviewed national level findings (Interview with respondents and team leader of PSO, HNPSP, MoHFW, 2010). Most of the respondents repeatedly mentioned the Bangladesh Demographic and Health Survey (BDHS, 2007)[9], Bangladesh Urban Health Survey[10] (BUHS) 2006, Multi Indicator Cluster Survey (MICS)[11] 2006 and Bangladesh State of Health[12], (BHW, 2007, 2008, 2009) as having influenced the highlighting of the community health issues (Interview and Policy Content Review, 2010).

Policy actors deal with lots of policy problems during the stage of agenda setting. A specific problem takes place as an agenda item in the process when that problem is accepted as a real problem. Diversity, extent and consequence of the problem in the life of common people were popular indicators to measure the weight of the policy problem (Dery, 2000). In every health system there are Community Health Status Indicators (CHSI), for providing an overview of community level health situation and to encourage dialogue about actions that can be taken to improve a community's health. In Bangladesh, health related Millennium Development Goal (MDG)s are taken as benchmarks to achieve the status of community health.

Most of the respondents viewed the situations of maternal health and child health, problems of health service providers, cost of health service, health services in remote area, women- friendly health service and HIV/AIDS issues to be the dominant factors for highlighting the community health issues as a problem in the agenda setting process of health service (Interview, 2010). Maternal health situation is one of the important indicators of achieving MDG-4. Presently the antenatal care[13] from a qualified contributor who has medical training has increased to 52 percent. There are disparities in urban – rural settings in antenatal care. 71 percent of mothers are getting antenatal care in urban region while it is only 46 percent in rural the areas (BDHS, 2007). Same study findings (BDHS, 2007) shows that women in urban areas are three times higher as likely as women in rural areas to give birth in a health facility. According to MICS (2009) report, Under 5 Mortality Rate in rural and urban areas are respectively 70 and 58 percent. The gap in awareness of HIV is much higher in rural area. Urban women (87% have basic knowledge) are more knowledgeable than their rural counterpart (BDHS, 2007).

Many international declarations (The International Conference on Population and Development, 1994; the Fourth World Conference on Women, 1995 and the Safe Motherhood Technical Consultation, 1997) highlighted that women's right to getting timely, affordable and good quality health care are parts of social justice and human rights (WHO/UNICEF/UNFPA, 1999). In this connection, it can be said that gender-friendly health services are the right of all classes of women in Bangladesh. BDHS (2007) illustrated that access to maternal health services is difficult because the service centers are located at places distant from client groups. On many occasions, women are not allowed to go such a long distance to avail the services. In the rural areas, social norms, values and beliefs pose major obstacles to going outside without the accompaniment of any close relatives.

Qualified health service providers, and their presence in the service-providing locations, are important indicators for providing quality health service in Bangladesh. In the rural areas of Bangladesh, absenteeism of doctors is 40% at the Upazila Health Centres (UPCs) and in the Union Health and Family Welfare Center (UHFWC) it is as high as 74% (Chowdhury and Hammer, 2004). Rural areas have a much higher density (170 per 10,000 population) than urban areas (81 per 10,000 population) when all types of providers are considered. There is also a huge urban-rural difference in the presence of different provider groups. In fact, the majority of qualified providers in addition to the physicians, such as nurses, dentists, technicians etc. practice in urban areas (BHW, 2008).

The percentage of women receiving antenatal care from a qualified provider, with medical training, has increased to 52 percent in Bangladesh. There are disparities in urban – rural settings in antenatal care. 71 percent of mothers are getting antenatal care in urban areas, while it is only 46 percent in rural areas (BDHS, 2007). National-level research findings (BDHS, 2007) show that women in urban areas are three times as likely as women in rural areas to give birth in a health facility. Women from the top wealth quintile are almost ten times more likely to deliver at a health facility than women in the bottom quintile.

Monitoring progress towards MDG 4: "reduce child mortality" is another important aspect for achieving ultimate target within 2015. The Infant Mortality Rate (IMR) is estimated at 45 per 1,000 live births, while the U5MR is around 67 per 1,000 live births (MICS, 2009). . If Bangladesh can maintain this trend, it will meet the final target well before 2015 in the term of national rate. Nevertheless, it is not high time to be satisfied, because there are, however, distinct regional variations that need to be addressed. Rural areas (according to MICS 2009 report, U5MR in rural and urban area are respectively 70 and 58), urban slums, the Chittagong Hill Tracts (CHTs), coastal belt regions and other ecologically vulnerable areas are falling far behind.

Findings of above mentioned revealed that health situation and care service scenario in Bangladesh is not good in rural areas. In evidence creation and dissemination, Bangladeshi State and non-government organisations or foreign donor agencies played vital roles. To ensure the quality of evidence, donors imposed a condition to involve international experts (organisational or individual), who played dominant roles in setting up study indicators and methodology finalisations. These decisions ultimately influenced the study findings. Donors played positive roles to involve the experts from the NGOs sector. Here, their argument is that GO-NGO collaboration or Public Private Partnership (PPP) can help to attain the desired goal by maximising both sectors' potentiality. In evidence creation, donors get feedback from stakeholders and policy-level actors from government (Interview, 2010).

In policy-level evidence creation, government bureaucrats, especially people with medical education background played important role. They have vast experience and expertise about the health sector in Bangladesh. Due to the procurement system of evidence creation and nature of health sector (sector wide approach and HNPSP pool fund invite public private partnership for donor support) government health experts are guided by a group of experts who are basically public health specialists (Interview, 2010). The study observed different BDHS reports and it was found that professionals from different INGOs, donor agencies and national NGOs are members of these study teams.

Different findings revealed that NGOs have been coming forward as vital policy actors in Bangladesh since the 1990s (Panday 2008; Rabbani, 2009). In this connection, they create evidence to promote community health issues as candidates for government action. To do this, they used some strategies to highlight their preferred issues.

NGOs ensured participation of top-level bureaucrats from National Institute of Population Research and Training (NIPORT), NIPSOM, BSMMU in evidence creation and ensured the participation of government counterparts who helped in the time of advocacy. NGOs offered key positions to the elite people in the health sector who have good access to the policy-level decision makers. NGOs collaborated with media people to disseminate the evidence to their policy community[14]. Respondents from both policy-makers and advocacy groups said that NGO advocates used personal relationships and work relationships to promote community health issues. For example, Team Leader, PSO, HNPSP, MoHFW said that senior professors and top management of NGOs talked with him over the telephone to highlight the community health issues (Interview, 2010). For the sake of in-depth probing, we investigated the reports of Bangladesh Health Watch[15] and found that they ensured the involvement of national professors, country directors of different INGOs, leading researchers and leaders from the media community to mobilise the policy community in the health sector.

Furthermore, among the professionals who are involved with party politics, DAB (Doctors' Association of Bangladesh, aligned with the BNP) and SCP (Shawdhinata Chikitshak Parishad, aligned with the Awami League) played influential roles in agenda-setting of community health issues. In this study, it is found that these members who are affiliated with SCP remained vocal from the very beginning of the policy process (Source: Interviews, 2010).

Also, actors from Civil Society Organizations (CSOs) were more vocal to highlight the community health issues. CSOs have arranged different seminars to demonstrate the stakeholders' views. For examples, Bangladesh Association of Pharmaceutical Industries (The Daily Star, 26 July 2008), Health Movement (The Daily Star, 23 September, 2008), Bangladesh Medical Associations (The Daily Star, 26 July 2008), Health Movement (The Daily Star, 13 September, 2008), Bangladesh Mohila Parisad, Health 21 (The Daily Star, 16 September, 2009)and the Health Rights Movement have raised their voices for proper allocation and utilisation of resources for ensuring the health rights of community people, especially the rural poor. Also, they repeatedly highlighted the importance of community clinics. At the time of investigation, we found that these civil society groups are not permanent organisations. After analyzing the members profile of these organisations, the study found that they had been formed with representatives from INGOs, Donor Community, BMA and NGOs.

PROPOSAL STREAM

Consistent with Kingdon's model, more than one solution emerged for addressing a high visibility problem. Advocates of specific solutions and opponents of a specific solution describe both proponent and opponent sides of a specific problem. Considering the policy solutions, policy coherence and viability of these solutions in the specific context, decision- makers take decisions (Stout & Stevens, 2000). In agenda-setting of the health policy of Bangladesh, the community health situation is a highlighted problem. To solve this problem, different policy actors came forward with different solutions.

Since 2008, different types of actors, especially the stakeholders of health sectors, have been very active to promote their policy solutions. The study asked the respondents about different solutions which had been proposed by the different policy actors to solve the community health problem in Bangladesh. Respondents expressed the view that community clinics, health education, door-to-door service, creation of semi-skilled manpower, incentives for medical professionals, use of alternative indigenous treatment along with modern medical treatment, skill development of unskilled or semi-skilled practitioners and mobile medical services, etc. were the significant proposals for improving the community health situation in Bangladesh from both state and non-state actors (Interview, 2010).

Among the policy solutions, the community clinics got priority in ensuring the health rights of the rural people of Bangladesh. The study tried to explore the reasons why community clinic issues got priority as solution. To promote the community clinic issue on the policy agenda, international policy coherence, national policy coherence, viability of the proposal, positive attitude of donors, advocacy activities of the NGOs and interest of the ruling political party (opportunity to get a share of the large funds required and distribute jobs for renovating community clinics) were dominant factors. (Interview, 2010)

In agenda-setting, good examples, models and lessons learned, from both the national and the international contexts, are the dominant factors to vitalise a policy issue as an option for policy decision making. Success examples and lessons learned from non-government sectors, as well as success examples from GO and NGOs, played important roles in considering the community clinic as solution for the health problems of community people. In this regard, the Team Leaders of PSO, HNPSP and MoHFW mentioned that this policy document was very much influenced by lessons learned from different programs, like Past Experience of HPSP, Community based intervention of NSDP and BRAC's health programme (Interview, 2010).

POLITICS STREAM

According to the Garbage Can Model, a third stream of agenda-setting is the political stream. This stream considers the factors in the political environment that have a powerful influence on the agenda-setting. Kingdon identified three major components that make up the political stream: the national mood, organised political forces, and events within the Government (Laraway & Jennings 2002). In this section we would like to discuss how political parties play a role in agenda-setting for community health. A variety of beliefs and ideologies are found in political systems in general. It is important to understand how these beliefs and ideologies shape policy-making.

Since independence, all the ruling parties have taken Primary Health Care (PHC) as one of the priority sector for national development and carried on various programs for achieving Health for All (HFA). Although, broadly, the policy priority of each political party is the same, strategically they differ. Always, Awami League (AL)[16] gives preference to establishing community-level health facilities. In the first general election, held in 1973, Awami League pledged to accelerate family planning programmes and establish rural health centres. These commitments of AL have been reflected in the First Five Year Plan (1973-1978). Accordingly, the construction of health centres at the union level and health complexes (31- bed hospitals) at the *thana* (sub-district) level began (Osman, 2005 & Osman, 2008). At first, the BNP Government were more explicit about urban hospital-based care. Although, in the 1979 election, BNP gave priority to preventive care and rural health, in the 1996 election, they gave priority to curative care (Osman, 2005).

The Third Five Year Plan (1985–90) added a new dimension in health services, by focusing on Maternal and Child Health (MCH) as an effective means of population control, and community-based services were started. The Fourth Five Year Plan (1990–95) also emphasized MCH services, along with a focus on primary healthcare and EPI (Expanded Program on Immunization) clinics. The Fifth Five Year Plan (1997–2002) added certain new strategic issues under the influence of the Health and Population Sector Strategy (HPSS) adopted in 1997 (Osman, 2005 & Osman, 2008) to provide community-based health services.

The AL Government established health institutions at the village level for providing opportunities for more-inclusive forms of representation, to bolster community acceptance and to create real pressure on community-level staff. In 1998, as part of health sector reforms, the Bangladesh government attempted to enhance community participation in the public health system. Two experimental initiatives sought to bring about more 'people-centred' public health provisioning. In one initiative, the Ministry of Health and Family Welfare set up community-owned and -managed health clinics in every village or ward. In this connection, 11,159 community clinics were built during 1999-2001, to provide Essential Service Package (ESP) services to the rural poor but, by 2004, not one community clinic was functioning (The Daily Star, 29 April, 2004). One of the major causes was that the new BNP Government (2001-2007) did not find the community clinics so valuable. It was argued that "Community clinics were considered to be ineffective and an enormous financial burden, which was getting increasingly difficult for the government to maintain." (Cited in BHW 2009).

Also, the BNP Government thought that Family Planning (FP) staff were the core of Bangladesh's health service, as they remain in closest contact with the people through their door-to-door services. By offering one-stop service points, community clinics threatened to limit door-to-door service provision, thereby weakening field-level activities and reducing contact with the people. BNP Ministers said that the clinics were built on land donated by the communities, but that the sites were not always easily accessible. The Government de-emphasised the clinics and soon there was a chronic absence of staff, basic medical supplies, etc. (Cited in BHW 2009).

After the end of the BNP regime, in 2007, a new interim Caretaker Government (CG) sought to update health policy. While the CG were formulating the policy draft, AL arranged a press conference. At this conference, AL's Health and Population Secretary, Dr Mostafa Jalal Mohiuddin, stressed the AL's commitment to the community clinics in Bangladesh. (The Daily Star, 18 September 2008). According to the majority of survey respondents, the AL includes a number of health professionals and they are very much enthusiastic to promote the community clinic issues as a means of ensuring the health rights of the village people of Bangladesh (Interview,2010). Also, as a political party, AL has a commitment to the people to establish the community clinics for the betterment of the common people. The Election Manifesto of AL in 2008 highlighted the community clinic in the following way:

In order to ensure health facilities to every citizen of the country, the health policy of the former Awami League Government will be reevaluated and adjusted according to the demands of the time. In the light of this policy, 18,000 community clinics, established during Awami League rule, will be re-commissioned. (Election Manifesto of AL in Election, 2008)

If top political leaders of the ruling Party take initiatives to promote a problem or proposal, then that problem or proposal gets priority promptly. According to the team leader of the PSO, HNPSP, MoHFW, the Party leaders of the new Awami League Government, elected in 2008, were very much interested in preparing a health policy and promoting the community clinic agenda, as well as giving direction about the strategic part of the policy content. Also, the Health Minister publicly promised that his Government would build one community clinic in each village (The Daily Star, 10 January, 2009).

In a parliamentary system, the Prime Minister is the top policy decision-maker in a country. So, the Prime Minister is the supreme policy decision maker in Bangladesh. Sheikh Hasina, the Prime Minister, back in office after an 8-year absence, took up the community clinic issue and often made promises to resuscitate the community clinics, even after the election (The Daily Star, 10 January, 2009; The Daily Star, 1 November, 2009; The Daily Star, 05 June 2010). The National Health Policy announced in 2011 was the result.

DISCUSSION AND CONCLUSION

Evidence is crucial to guide improvements in health systems and develop new initiatives. In this connection, state actors and non-state actors create evidence for highlighting the importance of a policy problem or issues. Also, in the study of agenda setting, it is important to understand how research and knowledge from various sources are produced and synthesised (Pang and et.al 2003). BDHS (2007), UHS (2006), BHW (2007, 2008, 2009), MICS (2006, 2009) etc. were main sources of evidence which highlighted the health problems of the rural community. This evidence revealed that the maternal and child health situation and services had not reached satisfactory levels due to human resource gaps at community level, absenteeism and unequal distribution of health service providers.

It was found that about 160 organizations and individuals took part in the agenda-setting process of the health policy. Among the participants, the NGOs' presence was significant considering their number. One may wonder why a significant number of NGOs took part in the agenda-setting process. The answer is a large number of NGOs are working in health sectors of Bangladesh, whose mission is to highlight the common peoples' rights and external support for doing policy advocacy (Rahman, 2006; Haque, 2002, WB 2005).

Donors provide financial support during evidence creation. While offering financial support, donors imposed some conditions, including methodology finalisation and indicators setting which, ultimately influenced the process of making evidence-based policy. In addition, donors suggested that government include NGOs in this process on the ground of GO-NGO collaboration or public-private partnerships. In the community health related evidence creation, USAID, UNICEF and WHO have played leading roles since 2000. This is not new in the health sector of Bangladesh. In case of evidence creation for a sector-wide approach, introduction of the donor community provided guidance and financial support for evidence creation. (Sundewall, Forsberg & Tomson, 2006). In other words, NGOs became powerful and influential, especially because of their external sources of financial support, cooperation, and technical support from donors.

Civil society/NGOs are potential actors to highlight health rights and social welfare goals through mobilization of citizen demand. Also, the NGOs are playing the roles of academics and professionals by monitoring and analysing contextual factors (Schurmann & Mahmud, 2009). Bangladesh Health Watch (BHW) was in the leading position to provide evidence for policy-making. BWH, located in the BRAC School of Public Health, publishes a report every year, focusing on specific themes and key indicators. The first report, published in 2006, addressed the theme of health and equity. Bangladesh Health Watch is governed by an advisory board consisting of key persons in the field of development and health. A working group carries out different activities of the Watch. BHW ensured participation of top level bureaucrats, elite people in the health sectors who have good connection with the policy makers and leaders of media community. They assumed that media can help in disseminating information and mobilizing stakeholders. They are advocating involving people from government in order to build relationships and to make the government a part of this process (Haque, 2002).

To highlight the community health issues, people from bodies composed of medical professionals, top management of NGOs and people from donor community formulated different advocacy groups. By conducting in-depth investigations, it was found that medical professionals who are affiliated with national politics, (like SCP) were in leading positions to form different advocacy groups, with assistance from the people from NGOs and donor community. Overlapping in membership was found among the advocacy groups. The main causes of such overlap lies in the fact that the same people would like to push their preferred agenda to the policy arena. In addition, some instant advocacy groups were formed by the medical professionals to promote their policy agenda. Good connections or network among the medical professionals working in NGOs, INGOs and donor agencies played important roles to formulate the advocacy groups. Sometimes, they used personal relationships during advocacy, because informal relationships[17] in Bangladesh are very active in organisational communication.

The study findings recommend that successive Governments, of all ideologies, of Bangladesh have been committed to provide basic health services to all. Moreover, socially and economically, operation of community clinics is a reasonable strategy (in this country there are some successful community health programmes) in Bangladesh.

From the historical perspective, donors played an important role in the health sector of Bangladesh (Jahan 2003, Buse 1999). While identifying good practices, donors played a vital role by providing financial and non-financial resources. The donors helped the partners in capacity-building and in mapping of success examples. It is found in the study that members of the donor community were very much positive about community clinics in Bangladesh. Green signals from the donor communities was one of the major factors that highlighted the issue. Leading donor agencies and UN bodies and WHO showed their commitment to provide support in the improvement of community clinic services (The Daily Star, 10 March 2010).

Politicians were initially influenced by the bureaucrats to reverse the reform. In this study, it is found that, as a political party, AL made a commitment, in their election manifesto of 2008, that they would restart the community-level health clinics. Moreover, top-level policy- makers, including the Prime Minister and Health Minister, were enthusiastic to promote the community health issues that they had publicly addressed.

It can be concluded that, in the problem stream, evidence production and dissemination were highly-supportive in highlighting the problems of community health issues as policy agenda. These problems were highlighted in different documents of governments, NGOs and donors. Moreover, these problems were recognised by bureaucrats, politicians, media people, donors and NGOs. In the proposal stream, national and international policy coherences, international and national good practices and positive attitudes of donors were among other factors that supported the community clinics as a policy proposal. Also, political support of the ruling party (AL) was positive, to highlight the community clinic and community health issues.

REFERENCES

Aminuzzaman, S. (2002). Public Policy Making in Bangladesh: An Overview. *Public Money and Management*, *2*, 1–7.

BDHS. (2007). *National Institute of Population Research and Training (NIPORT), Mitra and Associates, and Macro International. 2009. Bangladesh Demographic and Health Survey 2007*. Dhaka, Bangladesh: National Institute of Population Research and Training, Mitra and Associates, and Macro International.

BHW. (2007). *The Sate of Health in Bangladesh 2006: Challenges of Achieving Equity in Health, Bangladesh Health Watch (BHW)*. Dhaka: BRAC University School of Public Health.

BHW. (2008). *Bangladesh Health Watch Report 2007: How Healthy is Health Sector Governance, Bangladesh Health Watch (BHW)*. Dhaka: BRAC University School of Public Health.

BHW. (2009). *The Sate of Health in Bangladesh 2010: Health Workforce in Bangladesh, Bangladesh Health Watch (BHW)*. Dhaka: BRAC University School of Public Health.

BUHS. (2006). *National Institute of Population Research and Training (NIPORT), MEASURE Evaluation, International Centre for Diarrhoeal Disease Research, Bangladesh (ICDDR,B), and Associates for Community and Population Research (ACPR). 2006 Bangladesh Urban Health Survey*. Dhaka, Bangladesh: NIPORT, MEASURE Evaluation, ICDDR,B, and ACPR.

Buse, K. (1999). Keeping a Tight Grip in the Reins: Donor Control over Aid Coordination and. Management in Bangladesh. *Health Policy and Planning*, *14*(3), 219–228. doi:10.1093/heapol/14.3.219 PMID:10621239

Chaudhury, N., & Hammer, J. S. (2004). Ghost Doctors: Absenteeism in Rural Bangladeshi Health Facilities. *The World Bank Economic Review*, *18*(3), 423–441. doi:10.1093/wber/lhh047

Cochran, C. L., & Malone, E. F. (2005). Public Policy Perspective and Choices (3rd ed.). Academic Press.

Community H. S. I. (CHSI). (n.d.). Retrieved 22 April 2010 from: http://www.communityhealth.hhs.gov/homepage.aspx?j=1

CSG. (2008). *State Policy Guide: Using Research in Public Health Policymaking*. Retrieved from http://stacks.cdc.gov/view/cdc/5233

Dery, D. (2000). Agenda Setting and Problem Definition. *Policy Studies*, *21*(1), 37–47.

Feagin, J., Orum, A., & Sjoberg, G. (Eds.). (1991). *A Case for Case study*. Chapel Hill, NC: University of North Carolina Press.

Grieve, H. R. (1995). Health for All by 2000: Some issues of Health and Health Care in Bangladesh. In Bangladesh Strategy for Development. Dhaka: University Press Limited.

Haque, M. S. (2002). The Changing Balance of Power between the Government and NGOs in Bangladesh. *International Political Science Review*, *23*(4), 411–435. doi:10.1177/0192512102023004006

Howlett, M., & Romesh, M. (1995). *Studying Public Policy-Policy Cycles and Policy Subsystems*. New York: Oxford University Press.

Jahan, R. (2003). Restructuring the Health System: Experiences of Advocates for Gender Equity in Bangladesh. *Reproductive Health Matters*, *11*(21), 183–191. doi:10.1016/S0968-8080(03)02173-6 PMID:12800715

Jahan, R., & Salehin, M. (2006). Health Care for Rural People of Bangladesh: Overview of Some Governance Issues. In Governance and Development: Bangladesh and Regional Experiences. Dhaka: Shrabon Prokashoni.

Kingdon, J. W. (1995). *Agendas, Alternatives, and Public Policies*. New York: HarperCollins College Publishers.

Laraway, A. S., & Jennings, C. P. (2002). Health Insurance Flexibility and Accountability Demonstration Initiative (HIFA): A Policy Analysis Using Kingdon's Policy Streams Model. *Policy, Politics & Nursing Practice*, *3*(4), 358–366. doi:10.1177/152715402237970

Mahmud, S. (2007). Spaces for Participation in Health Systems in Rural Bangladesh: The Experience of Stakeholder Community Groups. In Spaces for Change? The Politics of Citizen Participation in New Democratic Arenas. London: Zed Books.

MIC. (2006). *Multi-indicator Cluster Survey, 2006, BBS, UNICEF*. Dhaka: GOB.

MICS. (2009). *Multi-indicator Cluster Survey, 2009, BBS, UNICEF*. Dhaka: GOB.

MoHFW. (2010). Final Draft of Health Policy. Dhaka: Ministry of Health and Family Welfare (MoHFW).

Nazneen, K. (2001). *Governance of the Healthcare Sector in Bangladesh*. Dhaka: University Press Limited.

Oberlander, J. (2003). *The Politics Of Health Reform: Why Do Bad Things Happen To Good Plans?* Health Affairs Web Exclusive. Retrieved 27 August 2009 from: http://content.healthaffairs.org/cgi/reprint/hlthaff.w3.391v1?maxtoshow=&hits=10&RESULTFORMAT=&fulltext=The+Politics+Of+Health+Reform%3A&searchid=1&FIRSTINDEX=0&resourcetype=HWCIT

Oliver, T. R., & Dowell, E. B. (1994). Interest groups and health reform: Lessons from California, *Health Affairs. Supplement*, *13*(2), 123–141.

Osman, F. A. (2004). *Policy Making in Bangladesh: A Study of the Health Policy Process*. Dhaka: A H Development Publishing House.

Osman, F. A. (2005). Implementation Constrained by a Lack of Policy Ownership: Evidence from Bangladesh. *The Asia Pacific Journal of Public Administration*, *27*(1), 19–36. doi:10.1080/23276665.2005.10779297

Osman, F. A. (2008). Health Policy, Programs and System in Bangladesh: Achievement and Challenges. *South Asian Survey*, *15*(2), 23–288. doi:10.1177/097152310801500206

Panday, P. K. (2001). The Role of Bureaucratic Elite in the Policy Making Process in Bangladesh., *Socialist Perspective: A Quarterly. Journal of Social Sciences*, *29*(1-2), 47–60.

Panday, P. K. (2008). Women's Political Participation in Bangladesh: Institutional Reforms, Actors and Outcomes. (Unpublished PhD thesis). City University of Hong Kong. Retrieved from http://dspace.cityu.edu.hk/handle/2031/5426

Pang, T., Sadana, R., Hanney, S., Bhutta, Z. A., Hyder, A. A., & Simon, J. (2003). Knowledge for better health - a conceptual framework and foundation for health research systems. *Bulletin of the World Health Organization*, *81*, 777–854. PMID:14758408

Perry, H. B. (1999). *Quest for a Healthy Bangladesh: A Vision for the Twenty-First Century*. Dhaka: University Press.

Perry, H. B. (2000). *Health for All in Bangladesh*. Dhaka: University Press.

Rabbani, G. (2009). Non-Governmental Actors are Coming Forward as Policy Actors: Example from Operational Framework for Pre-Primary Education. *Social Change*, *3*(2), 7–20.

Rahman, R. M. (2006). Human rights, health and the state in Bangladesh. *BMC International Health and Human Rights, 6*(4). Retrieved 22 May 2990 from http://www.biomedcentral.com/1472-698X/6/4

Reich, M. R. (1995). The Politics of Health Sector Reform in Developing Countries: Three Cases of Pharmaceutical Policy. *Health Policy (Amsterdam)*, *32*(3), 47–77.

Rhodes, R. A. W. (1997). *Understanding Governance: Policy Networks, Governance, Flexibility and Accountability*. Buckingham, UK: Open University Press.

Robinson, S. E., & Eller, W. S. (2010). Participation in Policy Streams: Testing the Separation of Problems and Solutions in Subnational Policy Systems. *Policy Studies Journal: the Journal of the Policy Studies Organization*, *38*(2), 199–216. doi:10.1111/j.1541-0072.2010.00358.x

Roper, W. L. (2007). Here We Go Again-Lessons On Health Reform Advances in science and clinical practice, not the political process, will continue to drive the pace of reform. *Health Affairs*, *26*(6), 1551–1552. doi:10.1377/hlthaff.26.6.1551 PMID:17978372

Schurmann, A. T., & Mahmud, S. (2009). Civil society, health, and social exclusion in Bangladesh. *Journal of Health, Population, and Nutrition*, *27*, 536–544. PMID:19761087

Shiffman, J., & Wu, Y. (2003, November). Norms in tension: Democracy and efficiency in Bangladeshi health and population sector reform. *Social Science & Medicine*, *57*(9), 1547–1557. doi:10.1016/S0277-9536(02)00547-6 PMID:12948566

Stout, K. E., & Stevens, B. (2000). The Case of the Failed Diversity Rule: A Multiple Streams Analysis. *Educational Evaluation and Policy Analysis*, *22*(4), 341–355. doi:10.3102/01623737022004341

Sundewall, J., Forsberg, B. C., & Tomson, G. (2006). Theory and practice—a case study of coordination and ownership in the Bangladesh health SWAp. *Health Research Policy and Systems*, *4*(5), 1–8. PMID:16704726

Talukder, M. N., Rob, U., & Mahabub, U A M. (2007). Lessons learned from health sector reform: A four-country comparison. *International Quarterly of Community Health Education*, *28*(2), 153–164. doi:10.2190/IQ.28.2.e PMID:19131306

The Daily Star. (29 April, 2004).

The Daily Star. (26 July 2008).

The Daily Star. (13 September, 2008).

The Daily Star. (23 September, 2008).

The Daily Star. (10 January, 2009).

The Daily Star. (1 November, 2009).

The Daily Star. (16 September, 2009).

The Daily Star. (05 June 2010).

The Daily Star. (10 March 2010).

UHS. (2006). *Urban Health Survey 2006*. Bangladesh: BBS.

Verschuere, B. (2009). The role of public agencies in the policy making process: Rhetoric versus reality. *Public Policy and Administration*, *24*(1), 22–46. doi:10.1177/0952076708097907

Walt, G., & Gilson, L. (1994). Reforming the health sector in developing countries: the central role of policy analysis. *Health Policy and Planning, 9*(4).

WB. (2005). *The Economics and Governance of Non Governmental Organizations (NGOs) in Bangladesh*. Poverty Reduction and Economic Management Sector Unit South Asia Region.

WHO/UNICEF/UNFPA. (1999). *Women-friendly health services Experiences in maternal care, Report of a WHO/UNICEF/UNFPA Workshop, Mexico City, 26-28 January*. Retrieved from http://www.unicef.org/health/files/womenfriendlyhealth-services.pdf

KEY TERMS AND DEFINITIONS

Agenda Setting: Policy actors deal with lots of policy problems during the stage of agenda setting. A specific problem takes place as an agenda item in the process when that problem is accepted as a real problem.

Caretaker Government: The caretaker government of Bangladesh is a form of government system in which the country is ruled by a selected government for an interim period during transition from one government to another, after the completion of the tenure of the former.

Interest Group Politics: Interest group politics mean politics among the core stakeholders who have specific interest.

Policy Process: Policy process refers to inter-linkage among problem identification, problem recognition, policy formulation, implementation and evaluation in a specific policy.

ENDNOTES

1 Policy process refers to inter-linkage among problem identification, problem recognition, policy formulation, implementation and evaluation in a specific policy.

[2] Interest group politics mean politics among the core stakeholders who have specific interest.

[3] Bangladesh is a South Asian country.

[4] Previous 'National health policies' of Bangladesh have covered a number of issues on health. Basically health policy is a package for providing the health services in Bangladesh.

[5] Here "public" means people who are not part of any organization or elite group.

[6] One of the major political parties of Bangladesh.

[7] The caretaker government of Bangladesh is a form of government system in which the country is ruled by a selected government for an interim period during transition from one government to another, after the completion of the tenure of the former.

[8] In the interim caretaker Government, advisors take the place of Ministers, but they are not Members of Parliament and are meant to be apolitical.

[9] In this study National Institute of Population Research and Training (NIPORT) Dhaka, MoHFW, Bangladesh ; Mitra and Associates, Dhaka, Bangladesh and Macro International, Calverton, Maryland USA were the key actors.

[10] In this study involved organizations were National Institute of Population Research and Training (NIPORT), MEASURE Evaluation, International Centre for Diarrhoeal Disease Research, Bangladesh (ICDDR,B), and Associates for Community and Population Research (ACPR).

[11] Bangladesh Bureau of Statistics, Planning Division, Ministry of Planning, Government of the People's Republic of Bangladesh, and UNICEF played dominate role in research agenda setting.

[12] James P. Grant School of Public Health, Center for Health Systems Studies, BRAC University, Bangladesh has taken necessary initiatives to conduct the study.

[13] Medical care before delivery.

[14] A wide range of policy actors who are directly or indirectly involved in particular policy.

[15] A professional body formatted by the BRAC University School of Public Health.

[16] One of the leading political parties of Bangladesh.

[17] Teacher-student relationship, working relationship and relationship from school or University.

Chapter 9

A Systematic Approach towards the Typology of Functions of National Health System:

Provision of Functional Model of National Health System

Mostafa Zamanian
University of Tehran, Iran

Zohreh Karimmian
University of Tehran, Iran

ABSTRACT

As one of the main national systems in any country, the health system has always been considered by governments. What distinguishes health system from other systems is that its purpose is directly related to the public health. Different countries adopt different structural patterns in this field but one can consider relatively common functions for a national health system which includes all functional aspects for this system. In recent years, attempts have been made for offering a comprehensive model in describing the functions. The OECD determined principles needed to offer an appropriate typology that should be independent of the names of health programs in different countries. In this chapter, it's tried to provide an overview of the proposed models for structures and functions of the health system and to propose a comprehensive model for it with an emphasis on theoretical aspects of public policy-making and binding functions in any national development system. This comprehensive model, provides the possibility to evaluate the success of a health system.

DOI: 10.4018/978-1-4666-9944-1.ch009

INTRODUCTION

The health system has always been considered by governments seriously. It is a priority in major development plans. Different countries adopt different structural patterns in the health field depending on their circumstances and macro-economic, political and social considerations. But aside from structural differences, one can consider relatively common functions for a national health system which includes all functional aspects for this key system. In recent years, attempts have been made for offering a systematic and comprehensive model in describing the functions of the national health system by competent communities, enterprises and experts in the field of health policy. These efforts were directed towards appropriate partitioning of the internal relationship in the health system and explaining the expected purpose(s) of these interactions. In addition, the remarkable point is that there are many factors outside the health system that affect people's health such as poverty, education, political and social infrastructure in a country. Since these factors are affected by external factors, health systems are known as open systems. Thus there are important implications for approaches to these systems from the perspective that they must affect health systems to produce better health outputs or more efficient and fair behaviors. The main functional elements of health systems can be defined at the global level. The Organization for Economic Cooperation and Development (OECD) determined principles needed to offer an appropriate typology. This classification should be based on the health system features and independent of the names of health programs in different countries. In this chapter, it's tried to provide an overview of the proposed models for structures and functions of the health systems and to propose a new and comprehensive model for the health system which provides the possibility to evaluate the success of a health system.

BACKGROUND

Various models of the health system can be divided into two sets: structural models and functional models. Next, a brief definition of each of these two types and an overview of the proposed models in each type will be provided.

The Structural Models of the Health System

Using various economic and health indicators, these models classify health systems in different countries. These indices are mainly based on the functions and control knobs raised in conceptual models of the health system. According to the OECD, the method for proposing a new classification for health systems consists of two stages. In the first stage, variables and indicators must be defined to highlight the differences in health systems. In the second stage, these variables must come together to extract meaningful groups based on the above three principles (OECD, 2004). Many attempts have been made in this regard, which will be explained next.

Roemer Model (Roemer, 1956)

Roemer analyzed health systems with a political-institutional approach. Using a historical analysis approach, he grouped health systems at that time. That study examined the relationship between a country's health policies and its economic and institutional status. He offered four groups for health services programs:

1. Free enterprises.
2. Social insurance.
3. Public assistance system.
4. Universal service.

As can be seen, this type of grouping is related to different methods of financing in countries to offer services to individuals.

Field Model (Field, 1973)

Field divided health systems into five groups. In general, this classification is based on the independence of health system personnel, ownership of medical facilities and financing method. The indicators selected by Field try to measure the health system integration.

Roemer and Axelrod Model (Roemer & Axelrod, 1977)

Roemer altered his previous classification and offered five groups for health systems in the world. These groups are as follows.

1. Free enterprise model.
2. Welfare state model.
3. Health system model in underdeveloped countries.
4. Health system model in developing countries.
5. Community-based model.

These groups are formed based on the key role of political and economic aspects in determining the health system status.

Terris et al. Model (Terris et al., 1977)

Then Terris et al. proposed two models: national health services (NHS) and social health insurance (SHI). In the NHS model, service providers are civil servants, services are offered at public hospitals, and the entire population receives free services. In the SHI model, service providers are independent enterprises which offer services according to contracts with the government. In fact, insurance is the health system foundation in these countries. However, the type of insurance coverage varies by country.

The WHO Model (Kleczkowski et al., 1984)

In the World Health Organization (WHO) report, Kleczkowski et al. introduced economic development level and economic approach as the main factors affecting the health system performance. Due to these two factors, health systems can be divided into nine groups:

- **Economic Development:** Various factors such as industrialization and urban population are effective in determining the development level of different countries. Based on these two factors, countries are divided into two groups: developed and developing. Since the developing countries group is so broad, the GDP index is used and this group is divided into two parts: transitional developing countries and poor ones.
- **Economic Approach:** It indicates the extent of government responsibility in offering services to people in the community. Based on the organizing method of the health system, three types of economic approach can be defined (table 1).
    - **Permissive:** This approach is based on the distribution of the health system responsibilities, and there is minimum social organization for offering governmental services.

Table 1. Typology of WHO

	Economic Approach		
Economic Development	**Permissive**	**Participatory**	**Social**
Developed	Model 1	Model 2	Model 3
Developing (Transitional)	Model 4	Model 5	Model 6
Developing (Poor)	Model 7	Model 8	Model 9

- **Participatory:** It aims to balance social and individual approaches for service delivery. In this approach, the government role is more organized than the previous one.
- **Social:** In this approach, health is the people's social right, and it is the most organized approach for offering governmental services.

Frenk and Donabedian Model (Frenk & Donabedian, 1987)

Frenk and Donabedian argued that relatively many indices can be used for classification of state intervention in the health system, including:

- Payment method to service providers.
- The level of administrative centralization.
- Percentage of public sectors in the health system.
- Tools used by the government to control service delivery.
- Scope of the covered population.
- Extent and broadness of the resulting benefits for covered persons.
- Principles for determining the eligibility of individuals to receive services.

Based on the type of government control over the health service production and the eligibility of individuals, Frenk and Donabedian proposed a typology for state interventions. The type of government control on the production of health services reflects the relationship between the government and service providers. Eligibility of individuals reflects the relationship between the government and real and potential consumers.

The OECD Model (OECD, 1987)

The OECD introduced a range of health systems based on three criteria: availability, financing method and the type of service providers. The classification considers two approaches (patient sovereignty and social justice) and proposes three basic models.

1. National Health Services (NHS).
2. Social Health Insurance (SHI).
3. Private Health Insurance (PHI).

The social justice approach is very important in countries with the NHS system. In these systems, coverage is universal and financing is done through taxes. They are also known as Beveridge systems. The SHI systems are formed by moving toward the patient sovereignty approach and maintaining the social justice approach. In these systems, coverage is almost universal and financing is through employer-based compulsory insurances. They are also known as Bismarck systems. The PHI systems are formed by focusing on the patient sovereignty approach and ignoring social justice. In these systems, people can be covered either by private insurers either personally or by the employer. They are also known as free-market systems. It is clear that in these systems there are many people who have no insurance coverage.

Navarro Model (Navarro, 1989)

By studying the evolution of health systems in different countries, Navarro introduced the class coalition as an independent variable which affects the health system type. According to this concept, he proposed three models (NHS, SHI, and liberal) for the health system.

Hollingsworth et al. Model (Hollingsworth et al., 1990)

Hollingsworth et al. focused on the degree of state intervention in the financing and production of other resources. Based on two indicators (the degree of concentration and management focus), they classified the British health system in a group with a high degree of concentration controlled by the public sector. The Swedish health system fell in a group with a low degree of concentration controlled by the public sector, and the US the health system fell in a group with a low degree of concentration controlled by the private sector.

Roemer Model (Roemer, 1991)

In his continued research, Roemer compared and classified health system structures in some countries by proposing a conceptual matrix. This classification, on one hand, is based on an estimate of the type of health system policies for social intervention in the health services markets and, on the other hand, on the economic level of countries which is defined by the Gross National Product (GNP). The first dimension of the matrix proposed by Roemer refers to the health system policies. The following four types of policies can be introduced in the health system:

1. Entrepreneurial and permissive.
2. Welfare-oriented.
3. Universal and comprehensive.
4. Socialist and centrally planned.

Economic dimension of this matrix includes: 1) industrialized countries, 2) transitional countries, 3) very poor nations and 4) oil-producing countries.

The OECD Model (OECD, 1992)

Based on the method of financing and reimbursement of costs to service providers, the OECD classified health systems into eight different groups (Table 2).

Model 1: It is the simplest model commonly used in the private sector. The patient pays the treatment costs out-of-pocket according to Fee-For-Service system.

Model 2: In this model, the patient pays his/her costs to the service providers both through taxes as well as out-of-pocket payment.

Model 3: In this model, the costs for the insured persons (who were insured on own volition by paying the insurance premium) are directly repaid to them by the private insurer. On the other hand, patients pay the remuneration of physicians and medical institutions with the Fee-For-Service system. In fact, there is no relationship between insurers and service providers.

Model 4: In this model, financing rests with public insurances based on taxes which its value is totally dependent on the income of individuals. There is no relationship between insurers and service providers. Patients pay the remuneration of physicians and medical institutions with the Fee-For-Service system.

Model 5: This model is based on contracts between insurers and service providers. Due to such contracts, part or all of the services is provided free of charge to patients. The payment type to service providers is based on Fee-For-Service and capitation.

Model 6: In this model, income tax is compulsory. Public enterprises (whether the government or insurers) make their payments to service providers based on Fee-For-Service or capitation. In this model, people are somewhat obligated for payment and the insurance coverage and services are usually universal.

Table 2. Typology of OECD

	Financing	
Reimbursement	**Private/Voluntary**	**Public/Compulsory**
Out-of-pocket payment	Model 1	Model 2
Out-of-pocket payment with insurance reimbursement	Model 3	Model 4
Contract with third party	Model 5	Model 6
Budget and Salary Payment by third party	Model 7	Model 8

Model 7: Users of this model argue that it can be helpful to recruit physicians, pay their salaries and acquire healthcare centers in the first and second service levels in a non-government manner. The main difference between this model and previous models is that insurers own healthcare centers at the first and second service levels.

Model 8: In this model, financing is through income tax, and payment to service providers is based on fixed salary and budget. Healthcare centers belong to the local government, the central government or public insurers. In fact, the government is totally responsible for service delivery, financing, planning, management and evaluation.

Hsiao Model (Hsiao, 1998)

According to Hsiao, factors affecting the health system performance include:

- System centralization versus decentralization.
- Ownership.
- Financing and service providing.
- Vertical integration of the organization.
- Integration of financing and service delivery.

Hsiao classified the health system in different countries based on different financing and service delivery patterns (Table 3).

Hsiao Model (Hsiao, 2003)

Hsiao proposed five models for health systems based on different approaches in financing, organization, payment and legislation in health services.

Table 3. Typology of Hsiao (1998)

<table>
<tr><th rowspan="2">Financing</th><th colspan="3">Public Income Direct Funds toward</th><th rowspan="2">National Health Insurance</th><th colspan="2">Social Insurance</th><th rowspan="2">Private Insurance</th><th rowspan="2">Out of Pocket Payment by Patient</th></tr>
<tr><th>Facilities</th><th>Service Group</th><th>Poor People</th><th>Direct Provision</th><th>Indirect Provision</th></tr>
<tr><td>State Provider</td><td>×</td><td>×</td><td>×</td><td>×</td><td>×</td><td>×</td><td>×</td><td>×</td></tr>
<tr><td>Non-State Provider</td><td></td><td></td><td>×</td><td>×</td><td></td><td>×</td><td>×</td><td>×</td></tr>
</table>

1. **National Health Services (NHS) Model:** In this model, people are covered based on their residency in the country. No independent fund is established for financing health services, but financing is through taxes and other public resources. Anyone who lives in that country enjoys health services as a citizenship right.
2. **National Health Insurance (NHI) Model:** It focuses on universal coverage and equal access to health services for all people. Thus, here the formation of the national health insurance fund is a basic principle in which the people and the government directly participate. The condition for using health services in these countries is membership in the concentrated health insurance fund. In this system, service providers are paid for services based on the Fee-For-Service system, and the insurer purchases services from public and private providers.
3. **Social Health Insurance (SHI) Model:** It has been adopted by many countries in the world. In this method, there are several funds and people join them arbitrarily or according to their job. Usually the type of services, tariffs and rates of individual participation are controlled by the government. In this model, individuals can choose among service providers. In these countries, civil institutions are deeply rooted, people are aware of their rights, and competitiveness is a condition for survival in the healthcare market.
4. **Voluntary Health Insurance (VHI) Model:** In this model, the capital needed for the health sector is supplied by individuals and the insurance premium paid by the employer. As a result, unemployed and poor people are not covered by any insurance. The government must attempt to finance the uninsured people.
5. **Medisave with Catastrophic Insurance (MCI) Model:** It is a new model compared to mentioned ones. It is based on personal responsibility of individuals for their health and their families, and the government is responsible for offering services to those in need and refractory patients.

The OECD Model (OECD, 2004)

The OECD altered and simplified its classification by removing combined modes of service delivery and financing. It examined and classified different financing methods based on two criteria (prepayment and risk pooling) and proposed four financing methods (table 4).

In summary, the OECD considered Contribution and taxes as a financing method, and the delivery procedure of dominant services as the representative of financing method. This way, it divided health systems into three groups (table 5).

Based on this classification, in the public integrated model, financing is made by the government, and services are offered in public health facilities.

Table 4. Financing method according to OECD

		Prepayment	
		Exist	**Not Exist**
Risk Pooling	Exist	Out of Pocket payment	Medical savings accounts
	Not Exist	Spontaneous charity	Health Insurance

Table 5. Typology of the OECD

		Provision of Services	
		Public	**Private**
Financing	Public	Public integrated model	Public contract model
	Private		Private insurance-provider model

Lee et al. Model (Lee et al., 2008)

Lee et al. studied classifications in the context of health systems and concluded that determinant factors in the characteristics of a country's health system can be summarized as follows:

- Level of social integration.
- Level of state intervention.
- Financing method.
- Service delivery procedure.

Using the above criteria, Lee et al. classified health systems into four groups. The definitions proposed for models are similar to those by Navarro (1989) and Xiao et al. (2003) (table 6).

Tanner Model (Tanner, 2008)

Tanner argued that there is no general model for the health system for all countries. He divided health systems into the following three groups, based on the unique historical, political, and national conditions.

1. **Single-Payer Health Systems:** The government pays the costs of health services for all citizens.
2. **Employment-Based Health Systems:** The employer is required to provide health insurance for its employees.

Table 6. Model of Lee et al. (2008)

	NHS Model	SHI Model	NHI Model	PHI Model
1- Social Value of Health System Constitution				
1-1- Basic Principle	Universalism	Corporatism	Universalism	Liberalism
1-2- population Coverage Principle	Citizens	Insured people	Citizens	Volunteers
1-3- Boundary of social solidarity	Nation	Groups of insured people	Nation	Volunteers and others
2- Main Structure of Service Provision				
2-1- Existence of private service providers	Limited: England: 96.0%* (1998)	Germany: Relatively Limited (2003) 53.1% Japan: Extensive (1998) 35.8%	Extensive, South Korea: 17.5% (2004) Taiwan: 33%	Extensive, USA: 33.7% (1995)
2-2- Strength of state regulation on private sector	Extensive, Strong, Detailed	Germany: Limited- Medium- General Japan: Extensive- Strong- Detailed	Extensive, Strong, Detailed	Limited
2-3- Availability of citizen to providers	Limited	Limited	Unlimited	Unlimited
3- State Intervention into Health System				
3-1- Proportion of public financing in total health system expenditure	England: 83% (2001)	Germany: 78.6% (2001) England: 81.7% (2001)	South Korea: 54.4% (2001) Taiwan: 64.4% (2001)	USA: 44.9% (2001)
3-2- Source of Financing	Tax	Germany: Social insurance contribution Japan: Tax and Social insurance contribution	Tax and Social insurance contribution	Tax and Premium
3-3- State administration of financing	Individual	Multiple	Individual	Multiple
4- Type of state intervention	Service Provider	Regulator	Conductor	Regulator at low level

3. **Managed Competition-Based Health Systems:** The private sector offers health services. But the government manages the desired market by extensive control and regulation.

Next, the following table summarizes aforementioned structural systems, and lists and evaluates countries that use each type (Table 7).

Table 7. Summary of structural health systems

Providers	Criteria of Classification	Classification	Examples
1. Roemer (1956)	Financing Method	Free Enterprises	
		Social Insurance	
		Public assistance system	
		Public Services	
2. Field (1973)	- Independence of personnel in health system - Ownership of health facilities - The Role of professional associations - Financing Method	Private	USA- Western Europe - Russia in 19th Century
		Pluralistic	USA in 20th Century
		National Health Insurance	Sweden- France- Canada- Japan in 20th Century
		National Health Services	England in 20th Century
		Social Health Services	Soviet Union in 20th Century
3. Romer (1977)	Political aspects Economic levels	Free enterprise model	
		Welfare State model	
		Health system model in underdeveloped countries	
		Health system model in developing countries	
		Community-based model	
4. Terris et al (1977)	Type of services delivery	National Health Services	Sweden- England
		Social Health Insurance	Canada- Denmark- Finland- Norway- France- Italy- New Zealand- Ireland- Israel
5. Terris (1978)	Type of services delivery	National Health Services	Sweden- England
		Social Health Insurance	Canada- Denmark- Finland- Norway- France- Italy- New Zealand- Ireland- Israel
		Public Assistance system	Most of Asian, African and Latin American countries
6. WHO (1984)	Level of economic development Economic Approach	Developed- Permissive	USA- Australia
		Developed- Participatory-	England- Norway
		Developed- Social	Russia- Hungry
		Developing (Transitional)- Permissive	Columbia- South Korea
		Developing (Transitional)- Participatory	Nigeria- Mexico
		Developing (Transitional)- Social	Cuba- China
		Developing (Poor)- Permissive	Philippine- Thailand
		Developing (Poor)- Participatory	Bangladesh- India
		Developing (Poor)- Social	Ethiopia- North Korea

continued on following page

Table 7. Continued

Providers	Criteria of Classification	Classification	Examples
7. Frenk and Donabedin (1987)	The form of state control over the production of medical services eligibility of the population	Concentrated ownership- Citizenship	Sweden- England- New Zealand
		Concentrated ownership- Contribution/ Privilege	Spain- Venezuela and India
		Concentrated ownership- Poverty	Non-Socialistic and developing countries
		Dispersed ownership- Contribution/ Privilege	Mexico
		Dispersed ownership- Poverty	USA- Non-Socialistic and developing countries
		Concentrated financing- Citizenship	Canada- France- New Zealand- England
		Concentrated financing- Contribution/ Privilege	Brazil- Lebanon
		Concentrated financing- Poverty	USA
		Dispersed financing- Citizenship	Germany- Austria- Swiss- Belgium- Japan- Netherland
		Dispersed financing- Contribution/ Privilege	Argentina- Netherland- USA
8. OECD (1987)	Accessibility (Coverage) Financing method Delivery of Services	National Health Services	England- Denmark
		Social Health Insurance	Germany- Austria
		Private Health Insurance	USA
9. Navarro (1989)	Class Coalition	National Health Services	
		Social Health Insurance	
		Liberal Model	
10. Hollingsworth et al (1990)	Degree of concentration Management focus	High degree of concentration and control by public sector	England
		Low degree of concentration and control by public sector	Sweden
		Low degree of concentration and control by private sector	USA
11. Roemer (1991)	Economic level Health system policies	Industrialized countries- Permissive	USA
		Industrialized countries- Welfare oriented	West Germany- Canada- Japan
		Industrialized countries- Universal	England- New Zealand- Norway
		Industrialized countries- Socialist	Soviet Union- Czechoslovakia
		Industrializing countries- Socialist	Thailand- Philippine- South Africa
		Industrializing countries- Welfare oriented	Brazil- Egypt- Malaysia
		Industrializing countries- Universal	Israel- Nicaragua
		Industrializing countries- Socialist	Cuba- North Korea
		Very poor countries- Permissive	Ghana- Bangladesh- Nepal
		Very poor countries- Welfare oriented	India- Burma
		Very poor countries- Universal	Sri lanka- Tanzania
		Very poor countries- Socialist	China- Vietnam
		Oil-producing countries- Welfare oriented	Libya- Gabon
		Oil-producing countries- Universal	Kuwait- Saudi Arabia

continued on following page

Table 7. Continued

Providers	Criteria of Classification	Classification	Examples
12. OECD (1992)	Reimbursement Financing method	Out of pocket payment- private	USA
		Out of pocket payment- public	
		Out of pocket payment with insurance reimbursement- Private	France- USA
		Out of pocket payment with insurance reimbursement- public	
		Contract with third party- private	France- Germany
		Contract with third party- public	Belgium- Canada- Germany- USA
		Budget and salary payment by third party- private	England- Italy- Germany
		Budget and salary payment by third party- public	Belgium- Canada- France
13. OECD (1994)	Financing method Type of service delivery	Contribution- Mixed	Belgium- France- Germany- Austria- Luxemburg - Japan
		Taxation- Public	Ireland- Spain- Denmark- Finland- Greece- Portugal- Norway- Sweden- Italy- England
		Taxation- Mixed	Australia- New Zealand
		Taxation- Private	Canada
		Mixed- Mixed	Turkey- South Korea
		Mixed- Private	Netherland- Mexico
		Private- Private	USA- Swiss
14. Hsiao (1998)	Financing method Type of service delivery		
15. Hsiao et al (2003)	Financing method Organization Payment Regulation	National Health Services model	England- Denmark- Greece- Italy- Poland- Hungry- Czech Republic
		National Health Insurance model	Canada- Finland- Norway- Spain- Souh Korea- Taiwan- Sweden
		Social Health Insurance model	Germany- Japan- Austria- Belgium- France- Netherland- Swiss
		Voluntary Health Insurance model	USA
		Medisave with catastrophic insurance model	Singapore
16. OECD (2004)	Financing method Type of service delivery	Public integrated model	Northern Europe Countries
		Public contract model	Japan- South Korea- European countries which are not in the Public integrated model
		Private insurance-provider model	Swiss- USA
17. Lee et al (2008)	Extent of social integration Level of state intervention Financing method Type of Service delivery	National Health Services model	England- Denmark- Greece- Italy- Poland- Hungry- Czech Republic
		Social Health Insurance model	Germany- Japan- Austria- Belgium- France- Netherland
		National Health Insurance model	Canada- Finland- Norway- Spain- South Korea- Taiwan- Sweden
		Private Health Insurance model	USA

continued on following page

Table 7. Continued

Providers	Criteria of Classification	Classification	Examples
18. Tanner (2008)	Financing method	Single-payer health systems	England
		Employment-based health systems	Germany
		Managed competition-based health systems	Swiss
19. Encyclopedia of Public Health	Financing method	Social Health Insurance system	Germany- France- Austria- Netherland- Japan
		Tax-based health system	Canada- Norway- Sweden- Finland- Australia- Italy- Spain- England
		Mixed health systems	

The following list includes all the used structural indicators. Each structural system can be explained based on these indicators.

1. **Financing Method:** In the financing process, proceeds received from primary and secondary sources are collected and accumulated in the common financial reserve fund and then allocated to the activities of service providers.
2. **Type of Service Delivery:** Service delivery can be considered as the most visible product of the health system and even some people confuse the service delivery system with the health system. Service delivery includes a wide range of activities. These activities can be classified with two different approaches: the first approach is based on the type of service providers and the second approach is based on the type of health services.
3. **The Basis for Political Philosophy:** Different countries have different political philosophies which are the basis for judgments on the performance of the health sector and other sectors. There are three approaches which determine political philosophy of countries in various fields: utilitarianism, liberalism, socialization.
4. **Type of State Intervention:** According to some experts in the health field, many health systems fail because states adopt wrong intervention methods and related tools. As a result, state intervention in the health system can be considered from two perspectives: type of intervention and level of intervention.
5. **Range of Covered Individuals:** The range of people covered by different services - which are offered by various service providers - can be divided into three groups: citizens, Contributors/Owners of privilege and the poor people.
6. **Economic Level:** Economic development is defined as grow along with increased manufacturing capacities including physical, human and social. In economic development, quantitative production growth will be achieved but

besides that, social institutions will transform, people's attitudes will change, the utilization capacity of existing resources will increase continuously and dynamically, and a new innovation will be made every day.

7. **Integration Level of the Health System:** Currently, many governments are changing to improve the quality and quantity of service delivery and reduce cost. In this respect, decentralization is one of the basic approaches to achieve this important goal. From the perspective of centralization level, governments can be divided into two categories: centralized and decentralized.

The Functional Models of the Health System

As shown in Figure 1, each functional model describes this meta-system by describing the functions, intermediate goals and ultimate goals. In other words, according to these models, a health system should fulfill the ultimate goal by realizing some functions of the intermediate goals path (figure 1).

Next, the main functional models in health systems are explained.

Londonio and Frenk Model (Londoño & Frenk, 1997)

According to this model, health systems must perform four basic roles to meet the population's needs. Two roles, i.e. financing and provision of services, are conventional functions performed by any health system. The other two roles are often implicitly satisfied or are not met at all. These neglected functions are modulation (a wider concept of regulation, including laying down fair rules and transparency) and articulation. Articulation refers to organization and management of a series of exchanges between the population's members and financing service providers so that resources can flow in the production and consumption of services. Table 8 shows the functions and sub-functions of the health system in this model (table 8).

Figure 1. Functional model of the health system

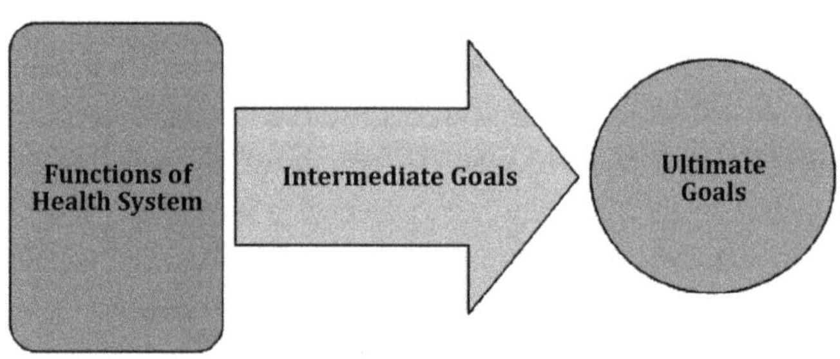

Table 8. Functions and sub-functions of the health system in the Londonio and Frenk model

Function	Sub-Function
Modulation	- Health System Development - Coordination - Financing Design - Regulatory - Customer Support
Financing	- Revenue Collection - Fund Pooling - Service Purchasing
Provision of Health Services	- Personal health services - Public health services
Articulation	- Articulating the relationships between people and service providers - Articulating the relationships between financing agencies and service providers

Commonwealth Fund Model (Davis et al., 2007)

The Commonwealth Fund was established in July 2005 in order to determine the characteristics of a health system with optimal performance. The output of this fund is supposed to be used as the base model in reforming the American health system. The studies conducted by this fund can be considered as an independent model in health system. According to this model, the ultimate goal of health system is to achieve healthy, productive and long lives. A high-performance health system is designed to achieve the following four intermediate goals:

1. Safe and high-quality care.
2. Access to care for all people.
3. Efficient and high-valued care.
4. Enhancement of system capacity.

These intermediate goals support achieving the mentioned ultimate goals.

Table 9 shows the functions and sub-functions of the health system according to this model.

Mills and Ranson Model (Mills & Ranson, 2001)

Mills and Ranson used Roemer's definition (1991) for modeling the health system. Accordingly, the health system is defined as the combination of resources, organization, financing and management which cooperate in offering healthcare services.

Table 9. Functions and sub-functions of the health system in the Commonwealth Fund model

Function	Sub-Function
Modulation	- Capacity building for evaluation/ Information - Policymaking and Planning - Control of social participation and system responsiveness - Creating the ability of accountability - Regulatory
Financing	- Revenue Collection - Aggregation and allocation of financial resources - Purchasing and Payment by provider
Provision of Health Services	---
Resource Generation	- Human resource management - Pharmaceutical material management

Table 10. Functions and sub-functions of the health system in Mills and Ranson model

Functions	Sub-Functions
Regulation	- Regulation of market entry and exit - Paying the remuneration of service providers - Quality control and service distribution - Control of standards
Financing	- Tax - Premium - Out of pocket payment
Provision of Services	---
Resource allocation	---

In this model, the health system elements are: management, provision of services, organization, plans, resource generation and economic support.

Table 10 shows the functions and sub-functions of the health system according to this model.

The World Health Organization Model (WHO, 2000)

The WHO (established on April 7, 1948) is a UN specialized agency which operates as a coordinating authority in the field of international public health. Its mission is to improve the situation of all the people in the world. The WHO explores the challenges and problems of the health sector in an annual report. These reports are published by subject and include important theoretical headings and practical challenges relevant to that subject. The 2000 WHO Report dedicated to the health

Figure 2. Functional model of the WHO for the health system

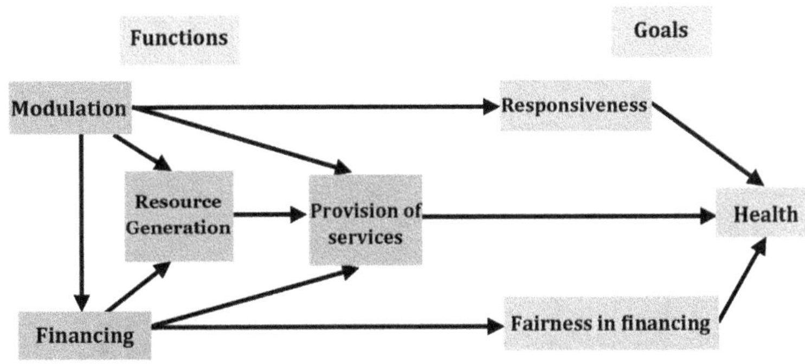

Table 11. Functions and sub-functions of the health system in the WHO model (2000)

Functions	Sub-Functions
Modulation/ Forward looking	Presented above
Financing	- Revenue Collection - Fund pooling - Strategic purchasing
Provision of Services	- Personal health services - Public health services

system. It has been the reference for many projects and researchers in this field. The report first defines the health system and determines its boundaries, and then examines its ultimate goals, intermediate outputs and functions. The following figure gives an overview of the ultimate goals and functions of the health system in this model (Figure 2).

Table 11 shows the functions and sub-functions of the health system according to this model.

The World Bank Model (World Bank, 2007)

In 2007, the World Bank published a report and in its first volume, very briefly described the theoretical framework of the health system used in this project. Based on this report and search in other available documents in the World Bank, a health system model was extracted. Next, this model will be explained. The following figure shows an overview of the health system in this model (figure 3).

Table 12 shows the functions and sub-functions of the health system according to this model.

Figure 3. The World Bank model for the health system

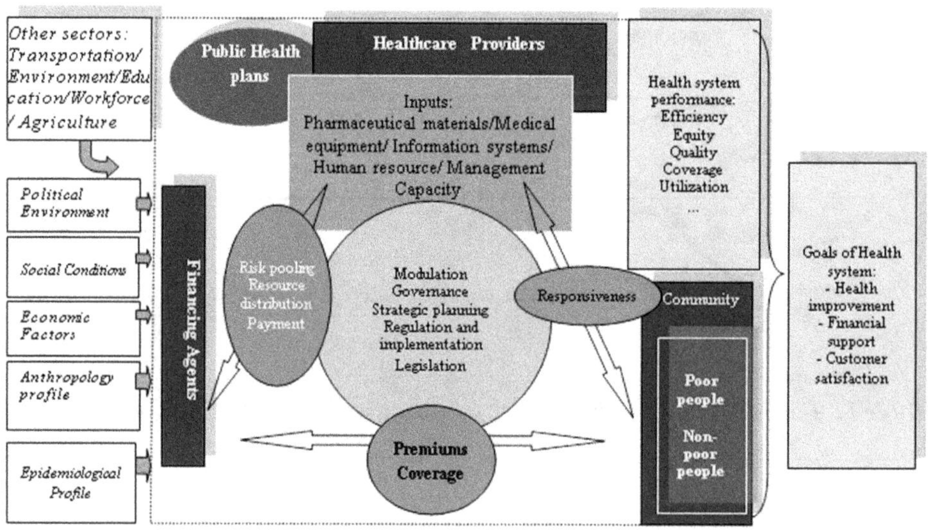

Table 12. Functions and sub-functions of the health system in the World Bank model

Functions	Sub-Functions
Modulation/ Forward looking	- Governance - Strategic Planning - Regulation and Implementation - Legislation
Financing	- Financial resources collection - Risk redistribution - Strategic Purchasing
Provision of services	---
Resource management	---

The USAID Model (USAID, 2009)

The United States Agency for International Development (USAID) is the United States federal government agency which claims to help develop the world, especially low-income countries (mostly African countries). It conducts theoretical analyses and implements projects in different areas of these countries.

This model adopted the WHO (2000) definition of the health system, that is, the health system consists of "all enterprises, institutions and resources allocated to producing health actions."

Like the WHO model, functions of this model include (Table 13):

Table 13. Functions and sub-functions of the health system in the USAID model

Functions	Sub-Functions
Modulation	- Capacity building for evaluation/ Information - Policymaking and Planning - Control of social participation and system responsiveness - Creating the ability of accountability - Regulatory
Financing	- Revenue Collection - Aggregation and allocation of financial resources - Purchasing and Payment by provider
Provision of Services	---
Resource management	- Human resource management - Pharmaceutical materials management

Table 14. Functions and sub-functions of the health system in the WHO model (2007)

Functions	Sub-Functions
Leadership/ Governance	- Governance - Strategic Planning - Regulation and implementation - legislation
Financing	- Financial resources collection - Risk redistribution - Strategic Purchasing
Provision of Services	---
Healthcare Workforce	---
Information systems management	---
Medical equipment, Vaccines and technologies management	---

The WHO Model (WHO, 2007)

The WHO (2007) published an article entitled "Strengthening the Health Systems to Improve Health Outputs, the WHO Framework for Action" and proposed a conceptual model for the health system. According to this report, the health system consists of all enterprises, people and actions and its primary goal is to develop, restore or maintain health.

To achieve their goals, all health systems must perform some basic functions, regardless of how they are organized.

Table 14 shows the functions and sub-functions of the health system in this model.

The Proposed Functional Model

After analyzing various functional models for the health system, it is time to propose an integrated model which contains the strengths of those models and covers their shortcomings. This model is shown in Figure 5. Its important elements are as follows:

Inputs of the Health System

- **Effects of Non-Health Sectors:** A problem facing any health system is how to interact with other sectors such as transportation, environment, education, and energy. These are known as inter-sectoral issues in the literature.
- **Political Environment:** The political environment is another input for the health system. It affects the health system performance with tools such as legislation and budgeting. Moreover, some characteristics of the health system such as responsiveness, efficiency, and transparency are partly influenced by the macro-political environment.
- **Social Conditions:** This component affects the health system by affecting factors such as people's participation, demands, and life style.
- **Economic Conditions:** Economic conditions of each country provide the health system with important limitations and opportunities. For example, in countries with high per capita income, the possibility for universal coverage of individuals and reducing financial risks for health is much higher than low-income countries.
- **Geographical Conditions:** Another input to the health system is geographical conditions which affects its priorities and performance. Access to the full basket of food, common diseases, essential vaccines for prevention, and so on are largely dependent on the geographical conditions of countries.
- **Epidemiological Conditions:** By influencing the pattern of disease spread and priorities in the prevention of communicable diseases, epidemiological conditions are an important input for the health system.

Ultimate Goals

Hsiao suggests that we must clarify, at the systematic level, that what final outputs are important to the community and distinguish them from intermediate outputs. It is true that intermediate outputs are important and affect the ultimate output but they are just temporary results.

According to the functional model of the health system, the following ultimate goals can be considered for the health system.

- **Health Level Improvement:** Good health has an intrinsic value to people. Moreover, a certain level of health services is necessary for the protection of life and treatment of severe morbidities. Thus, the maximization of health level can be considered as one of the most important goals for the health system.
- **Health Distribution Improvement:** Not only the improvement of health level is considered as one of the main goals but also equality in its distribution is an important goal for the health system.
- **Protection against Financial and Social Risks:** In some references, "affordability" is considered as a policy objective of the health system. One of the characteristics of healthcare is the uncertainty of high treatment costs. Therefore, the affordability goal in some countries has been set as the ultimate goal of achieving adequate coverage of financial risks for citizens.
- **Public Satisfaction:** It is clear that public satisfaction is the ultimate goal for political leaders and policy makers in democratic societies. Even the leaders of authoritarian governments must satisfy the public in the long term. Blendon et al. (1990) concluded that public dissatisfaction with the health system performance contributes to political pressures for the health system reform: dissatisfaction with the status quo is largely related to the common belief that the healthcare system needs fundamental change and restructuring.

Intermediate Goals

Often, intermediate outputs are confused with ultimate goals. Targeting improved access, quality and/or performance is important in health policies but it has derivative importance versus the ultimate goal of the health system. We would like to achieve higher technical quality in health services because it has a positive effect on health status. Improved service quality in health services is desirable as long as it has a positive impact on patient satisfaction and health outputs. The maximization of efficiency allocation allows improving health status and risk coverage under budget constraints. Finally, the success of a nation in achieving these intermediate outputs should be evaluated based on their contribution to ultimate outputs.

According to this model, the intermediate goals are inherently among intermediate/process outputs of the health system. These goals are:

- **Efficiency:** A system is efficient when it produces and offers appropriate services (considering goals) in an appropriate manner. Such a definition leads to two specific concepts for efficiency: technical efficiency and allocative efficiency.

- **Safety:** The provided care is safe when it is delivered in a way that leads to greater reliability for the cared processes and minimal medical errors.
- **Access:** In some cases, access simply means whether services are offered in a particular area or not. Here, the point is the physical availability which can be measured by the distribution of available inputs (beds, physicians or patients) compared with the general population. The second concept is a definition which better reflects the meaning of this word: effective availability means that how easy people can receive care services? The difference between physical availability and effective availability is due to the fact that several barriers (such as cost, travel time, poor and low quality services) may limit individuals to use facilities that are physically available.
- **Quality:** "Quality" can be meaningful only in the quantity of provided care for a patient. The second basic meaning of "quality" which is used by health professionals refers to clinical quality. This sense includes both the skills of care providers (e.g. surgical skills) and the accuracy of diagnostic and therapeutic decisions.
- **Coverage:** Countries always struggle to increase the range of benefits whose citizens deserve (programs, interventions, goods and services). For this purpose, they provide access to goods and services for broader population groups and finally, for all citizens. Ultimately, they attempt to protect their citizens against inappropriate financial and social consequences of using healthcare.

Functions of the Health System

The health system functions in this model include modulation, provision of service, financing, human resource management, medical equipment and drugs management, and information and knowledge management. Each of these functions and their lower levels sub-functions are as follows:

- **Modulation:** After reviewing the modulation in different models in previous sections, one can mention the following sub-functions to cover all aspects of the health sector and avoid parallelism and overlap in different sub-sections as much as possible. Since modulation is an input for other functions of the health system, there may be overlap between some sub-functions in some areas and other sub-functions in the health system. This is due to the management- and policy-based nature of modulation. These sub-functions are as follows:
    - **Policy Making:** Based on the systemic view to health and the system definition (as a set of various elements and their interrelations to achieve a single goal), all elements and their relationships should pursue a single

goal so that the activities within the system are directed towards general goals. Thus, the first sub-function in modulation is policy-making so that the position of elements and activities within the system are clarified, and they can go towards the specified goals with greater strength. Perhaps this sub-function is the most important and crucial element in modulation. Weakness and inefficiency in policy-making has high impacts on the whole system which cannot be compensated with considerable spending and it is just a waste of resources. On the other hand, the strength and intelligence of this element is very effective in the system effectiveness and efficiency and accelerating the achievement of the system goals.

- **Intelligence:** According to the literature of Intelligent systems (Graham Mann; and Luoma and Leppänen, 2007), it can be said that these systems have the following characteristics:
  - Ability to extract and store knowledge.
  - The human-like logical process.
  - Learning from experience.
  - Access to solutions in a way similar to natural evolution processes.
  - Ability to monitor the status of the entire system.
  - Getting feedback from the system performance and inputs.
  - Ability to modify the system.
  - Ability to monitor and adapt to the changing environment.
- **Creating Cooperation and Solidarity:** Creating cooperation and solidarity can be performed at two levels:

- Management of inter-sectoral collaboration (the health system and other sectors).
- Management of intra-sectoral collaboration (elements of the health system).
  - **Regulation:** In a clear understanding, regulation refers to the use of coercive power by the government for imposing limitations on organizations and individuals. Regulation tools may include laws, decrees, orders, instructions, administrative rules and guidelines issued by governments and non-government bodies such as the self-regulated organizations, to which the regulation power is delegated by governments. Regulation is not the use of incentives or encouragement (i.e., indoctrination) for affecting individual and organizational behavior. An effective regulation requires good design along with governmental ability in the application and implementation of regulation. Many failures may occur in the setting up and operation of regulations. If there is no regulation in the first place, serious regulation failures may worsen the situation. A key regulation failure occurs when a regulatory agency is

captured by the regulated organizations (i.e., organizations that are supposed to be regulated by the agency) and it advocates the interests of capturing groups instead of developing public interests. The study of L. J. White (2000) was used to explain the regulation. He divided the regulation into three types: economic regulation, information regulation and health/safety/environmental (HSE) regulation.

- **Accountability:** Accountability is often defined as the obligation of an individual or organization to account for its responsibilities (Audit Bureau of Trinidad and Tobago, 2003). At the organizational level, accountability refers to a process in which an organization is committed to balance between the needs of its stakeholders and decision processes and activities, and match its outputs with its commitments (Global Accountability Report, 2003). Edwards and Holmes interpreted accountability as "means by which individuals and organizations report to their superior authorities" (Edwards and Holmes). They believe that effective accountability needs clear expression of goals (whether based on special rules or the realization of preset performance levels), transparency of decisions and relationships, honest reporting on the use of resources and achievements, an inspection process by regulatory authorities in order to determine the satisfaction level of results and mechanisms to encourage and punish those in charge. Accountability comes in two basic types: accountability of officials to superiors in the hierarchical organizational structure (horizontal accountability), and public accountability of officials to the people (vertical accountability). One important result of accountability is "responsible leadership." Responsible leadership along with accountability to the people increases public trust which is the essence of survival and prosperity of any nation (Audit Bureau of Trinidad and Tobago, 2003). Accountability can also be divided into two other types: functional (or short-term) and strategic (or long-term). Functional accountability is measured simpler and is related to the efficient and effective use of resources and the immediate effects of their usage. Strategic accountability is related to the long-term effects and considers the organization's success in achieving long-term goals (Conradi, 1998).
- **System Design:** Based on the organizational architecture studies (Kaufmann, 200), the following cycle can be considered for system design (Figure 4).
- **Performance Evaluation:** The purpose of performance evaluation is the assessment, evaluation and judgment on the performance of various elements of the health sector according to rules and regulations,

and effectiveness, efficiency, economical and ethical criteria in order to improve the quality of services.

- **Provision of Services:** This is the most visible function of the health system which includes demand management, determining the service package, supply management, provision of service, infrastructure and support.
- **Financing:** As mentioned earlier, financing is one of the most important determinants of the health system performance in terms of equity, efficiency and quality. It includes resource mobilization, allocation and distribution at all levels (national and local) and the payment method to service providers. This function refers to "methods used to mobilize resources that support public health plans, provide access to basic health services and form the health service delivery systems" (Shiber and Akiko, 1997). The details of each sub-function are as follows:
    - **Revenue Collection:** Revenue collection refers to mobilize funds from primary (households and firms) and secondary sources (the government and charity institutions). Financial resources can be collected through eight basic mechanisms: out-of-pocket, optional insurance rated based on income, optional insurance rated based on risk, compulsory insurance, general taxes, allocated tax, financial assistance of non-governmental enterprises and agencies, and the sale of public assets.
    - **Risk Pooling:** The second important aspect of financing is to accumulate capital from individuals or households (the pool members) and manage it in such a way that all participants are protected against the risk of paying cost diseases out-of-pocket. Financing based on both taxes and health insurance includes integration. Note that customers' fee-for-service does not include resource integration.
    - **Purchasing Health Services:** Health services are purchased by public or private agencies which spend money directly for providing or purchasing services for their stakeholders. In many cases, the buyers of health services are the agency that integrates financial resources such as the Ministry of Health, social security agencies, regional health boards, insurers, individuals or households (who pay out of pocket when consuming services). For good performance of the health system, financing agencies should produce good amount of revenue, efficiently integrate the risk, provide appropriate incentives for providers, and allocate resources to efficient, effective and fair interventions and services. Figure 5 shows how financing works (figure 5).
- **Human Resource Management (HRM):** Given the importance of human development and the introduction of human as the development axe, which is obvious in the UN Millennium Development Program, HRM is very impor-

tant in developing economic and social systems. Of course, HR is not equally important in different sectors. Considering the importance of the human dimension of development in recent years, many countries put emphasis on human capital in their development plans. Clearly, the human capital aspects have a special place in the health system. HRM has serious structural and performance weaknesses in the health sector of many developing countries, and structural decentralization is one of the main problems of their health systems. HR is one of the most important resources in the health service delivery system because it is responsible for using health technologies in the management and provision of services in order to promote health. On the other hand, personnel expenses usually account for 60 to 80 percent of total current expenditures in the health sector. Thus, emphasis on qualitative and quantitative development of human resources will improve efficiency, prevent waste of national resources and, ultimately, enhance social capital. According to HRM definitions, general functions include supply management, organization management and maintenance management.

- **Medical Equipment and Drugs Management:** A health system should guarantee access to medical equipment and drugs through high-quality, safe, efficient and economical technologies.
- **Information and Knowledge Management:** This function is initially divided into two sub-functions: knowledge management and information management. Each one can contain lower level sub-functions.

The necessity of knowledge management in the health system refers to the important role of knowledge in the fulfillment of its goals. It can be argued that almost all the health, education, research, monitoring, and managerial activities in the health system rely heavily on complex knowledge and information. According to global statistics, a physician typically allocates one third of his/her time to information analysis and knowledge promotion. However, the realization of expected outcomes of a national health system (such as lower costs, reduced medical errors, increased quality of care, and increased collaboration and innovation in the health sector) is largely dependent on the use of knowledge management systems in the healthcare sector.

That is why today transition from data-driven decisions to knowledge-based decisions in the form of evidence-based public health (EBPH) is considered in the health systems of developing and developed countries (table 15 and figure 6).

Figure 4. Organizational architecture cycle (Kaufmann, 2000)

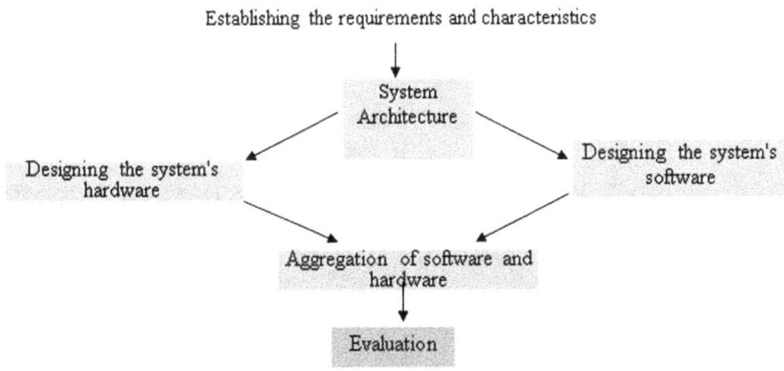

Figure 5. Financing process

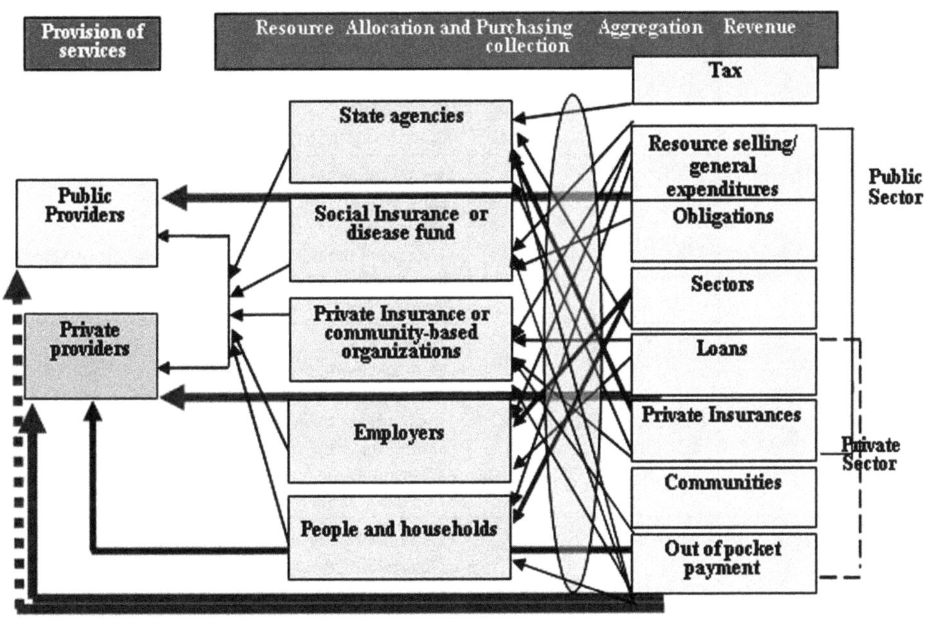

FUTURE RESEARCH DIRECTIONS

As presented, the model tries to provide a comprehensive view on the performance of the health system, independent of the type of the structural model. Hence, it can be invoked as a basis model in the evaluation of health systems. In other words, in addition to conventional patterns in the evaluation of health systems which are currently used and focused primarily on indicators of health in the community, the

Table 15. Functions and sub-functions of the proposed model

Functions	Level 1 Sub-Function	Level 2 Sub-Function
Modulation	Policymaking	- Strategy Formulation - Establishing the goals, directions and service prioritizing - Defining the role of health system players
	Intelligence	- Forward looking and monitoring the overall system status - Understanding the environment and its changes - Learning and experience accumulation - Obtain new suggestions and ideas - Modifying the plans, policies, mechanisms and structure of health system
	Collaboration and alliance	- Intersectoral collaboration (health system and other sectors) - Coalition building (elements of health system)
	Regulation	- Economic regulation - Information regulation - Health/ Safety/ Environmental regulation
	Responsiveness	- Creating transparency - Contribution - Addressing litigations
	System Design	- Establishing the requirements and characteristics of health system - Designing the health system hardware (Structures) - Designing the health system software (processes, plans, job description and so on) - Aggregation of hardware and software
	Performance Evaluation	- Determining the evaluation criteria - Data and evidence collection - Documentation and analysis of data and evidences - Recognizing the pros and cons of health system - Determining the prioritized changes and interventions - Propose making evidence-based changes
Financing	Revenue collection	- Determining the sources of revenue - Determining the sourcing mechanisms - Determining the agents - Determining the collection mechanisms of financial sources

above model can be used to evaluate the national and regional health management system analytically. Obviously, based on the functional classification proposed in this model, the strengths and weaknesses of different patterns of health system can be assessed. The causal analysis of functions and sub-functions of the proposed model would be useful in providing health system reform policy.

Figure 6. An overview of the proposed model of health system

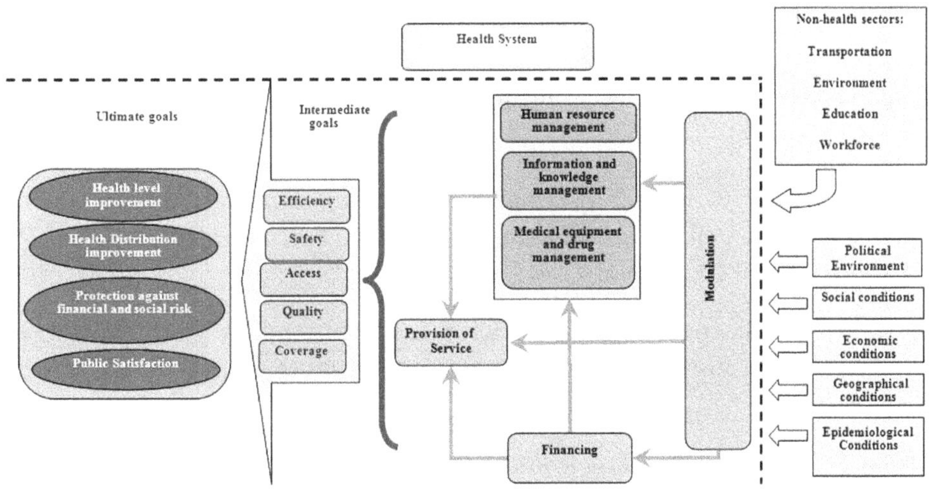

CONCLUSION

The comprehensive deployment of the health system requires different tools. Each tool is a ring in the intertwined chain of this system. At the end, a coherent and targeted network is formed which in its entirety realizes its main mission: providing and ensuring the public health.

This chapter presented a comprehensive overview of structural models in the national health systems in the world. Then, the national health system was reviewed and analyzed functionally from different perspectives. Finally, a comprehensive functional model was proposed.

With a holistic view to the health system, the proposed model fills the gaps in the previous models and improves the literature on the functional field of health system. This model also breaks different functions into sub-functions and provides a more accurate picture of the functional scope of health system. Thus, the model can be used in order to evaluate the performance of a health system.

REFERENCES

Davis, K., Schoen, C., Schoenbaum, S. C., & Doty, M. M. (2007, May). *Mirror, Mirror on the Wall: An International Update on the Comparative Performance of American Health Care, The Commonwealth Fund*. Retrieved from http://www.commonwealthfund.org/

Field, H. H. (1973). Environmental Design Implications of a Changing Health Care System. In Environment and Cognition (pp. 127-157). New York: Seminar Press.

Frenk, J., & Donabedian, A. (1987). State intervention in medical care: types, trends and variables. *Health Policy and Planning*, *2*(1), 17–31. doi:10.1093/heapol/2.1.17 PMID:10282125

Hollingsworth, J. R., Hage, J., & Hanneman, R. (1990). *State intervention in medical care: consequences for Britain, France, Sweden, and the United States, 1890-1970*. Chicago: Cornell Univ Press.

Hsiao, W. (1998). *Health care financing in developing nations.* Paper prepared for the World Bank Institute Flagship Course on Integrated Health Care Financing Approaches.

Hsiao, W. C. (2003). *What is a health system? Why should we care.* Harvard School of Public Health, working paper, 33.

Kleczkowski, B. M., Roemer, M. I., & Werff, A. V. D. (1984). *National health systems and their reorientation towards health for all: guidelines for policy-making*. Academic Press.

Lee, S. Y., Chun, C. B., Lee, Y. G., & Seo, N. K. (2008). The National Health Insurance system as one type of new typology: The case of South Korea and Taiwan. *Health Policy (Amsterdam)*, *85*(1), 105–113.

Londoño, J. L., & Frenk, J. (1997). Structured pluralism: Towards an innovative model for health system reform in Latin America. *Health Policy (Amsterdam)*, *41*(1), 1–36. doi:10.1016/S0168-8510(97)00010-9 PMID:10169060

Mills, A. J., & Ranson, M. K. (2001). *The design of health systems. International Public Health.* Gaithersburg, MD: Aspen Publishers.

Navarro, V. (1989). Why some countries have national health insurance, others have national health services, and the US has neither. *Social Science & Medicine*, *28*(9), 887–898. doi:10.1016/0277-9536(89)90313-4 PMID:2652327

OECD. (1987). *The Reform of Health Care: A Comparative Analysis of Seven OECD Countries*. OECD.

OECD. (1992). *The Reform of Health Care: A Comparative Analysis of Seven OECD Countries*. OECD.

OECD. (2004). *The Reform of Health Care: A Comparative Analysis of Seven OECD Countries*. Paris: Organisation for Economic Co-operation and Development.

OECD. (2004). The Reform of Health Care: A Comparative Analysis of Seven OECD Countries. Paris: Organisation for Economic Co-operation and Development.

Roemer, M. I. (1956). *Medical Care in Relation to Public Health: A Study of Relationships Between Preventive and Curative Health Services Throughout the World.* World Health Organization.

Roemer, M. I. (1991). Health care costs and financing in world perspective. *The Yale Journal of Biology and Medicine, 64*(5), 435. PMID:1814057

Roemer, M. I., & Axelrod, S. J. (1977). A National Health Service and Social Security. *American Journal of Public Health, 67*(5), 462–465. doi:10.2105/AJPH.67.5.462 PMID:324295

Tanner, M. (2008). The grass is not always greener: A look at national health care systems around the world. *Cato Policy Analysis Paper,* (613).

Terris, M., Cornely, P. B., Daniels, H. C., & Kerr, L. E. (1977). The case for a national health service. *American Journal of Public Health, 67*(12), 1183–1185. doi:10.2105/AJPH.67.12.1183 PMID:596502

USAID. (2009). *Sustaining health gains –Building systems*. Washington, DC: United States Agency for International Development.

WHO. (2000). *World Health Report 2000 – Health systems: improving performance*. Geneva: WHO Press.

WHO. (2007). *Everybody's business. Strengthening health systems to improve health outcomes: WHO's framework for action*. WHO.

World Bank. (2007). *Healthy development: the World Bank strategy for health, nutrition and population results*. Washington, DC: The World Bank.

ADDITIONAL READING

Kohn, L. T., Corrigan, J. M., & Donaldson, M. S. (Eds.). (2000). *To err is human: building a Safer Health System* (Vol. 6). National Academies Press.

KEY TERMS AND DEFINITIONS

Health: Complete physical, mental and social relaxation, not merely the absence of disease and disability (WHO, 2000).

Health System: The health system includes all activities whose main goal is to preserve, enhance or restore the health (WHO, 2000).

Healthcare: Healthcare includes providing services and implementing prevention, treatment, and rehabilitation plans in various aspects of health (Encyclopedia of Public Health).

Public Health: Public health is the science and art of preventing diseases, increasing life expectancy and raising the general level of human health through applying individual, collective and institutional methods and strategies in society (Winslow, 1920).

Chapter 10
On-Site Clinics:
A New Model of Health Coverage in Local Government

Robert Yehl
Valdosta State University, USA

Mary Eleanor Wickersham
College of Coastal Georgia, USA

Virginia B. Sizemore
Valdosta State University, USA

ABSTRACT

With the continued rising cost of health insurance and the fiscal constraints as a result of the 2007-09 economic recession requiring local governments in the U.S. to make cuts in employees, services, and benefits, it appears that on-site health clinics are one method of reducing, or at least, slowing health care costs. This chapter analyzes the use and benefits of such clinics for local government managers that is a new, but potentially effective method of both controlling costs and improving employee health.

CHANGING TIMES CALL FOR NEW IDEAS

A hallmark of the U.S. healthcare system for the last 70 years has been employer-sponsored health coverage. Growing out of the need to provide benefits as a means of remaining competitive in both hiring and retaining employees, employers

DOI: 10.4018/978-1-4666-9944-1.ch010

often offered coverage with low deductibles, co-pays and low-cost prescriptions. Historically speaking, federal, state, and local governments were initially slow to respond to this influx of health insurance benefits that permeated U.S. industry in the post-World War II society. Although some of the larger municipal governments began offering coverage to employees in the 1950s, it wasn't until the passage of the Federal Employees Health Benefits Program in 1960 that federal employees saw direct participation by their employers. By the end of the decade most state and local government employees had followed suit. Once implemented the benefit package for public employees often served as a key recruitment tool, since public sector pay seldom matched private sector wages (Cox, 2011, p. 2; Falk, 2012, p. 8; Kaiser Family Foundation, 2012).

As cautious as they were in providing employer-sponsored health care, governments have been equally slow to address the rapid escalation in health costs over the last two decades. They have preferred to absorb rising costs while the private sector increasingly shifted these costs to employees. (Kavanaugh, p. 2, 2011; Claxton, Rae, Panchal, Damico, Lundy, Bostick, Kenward, & Whitmore, 2012). Saddled with high cost plans and low deductibles, governmental agencies throughout the country watched their health costs soar, a trend escalated by this so-called "Cadillac coverage," insurance that costs as much as 20 percent more in the public than in the private sector (Barro, pp. 2-5, 2011). Adding to the rise in costs were the mandates included in the 2010 Patient Protection and Affordable Care Act that require preventive coverage with no co-pays, coverage of employees' children up to age 26, and prohibitions on coverage limits for essential services. These and other requirements have further increased costs to both fully-insured and self-insured health plans. Such high-cost, low-deductible, and rich benefit plans take up an increasingly higher share of governmental budgets at a time when, in many areas, local government revenue is declining (Gross, Huh, Sylvester, & Zahradnik, 2012). One report estimates that health benefits offered by state and local governments reflect more than five percent of annual expenditures (Barro, p. 1).

The economic recession that began in 2007 forced local governments, in particular, to make reductions-in-force and cuts in services and benefits. A number of these governmental units came face-to-face with the fact that continued health care benefits to which government employees were accustomed were no longer sustainable. The growing public expectation for effective and efficient government that operates like the private sector, rising costs of health care, and reduced revenue became a triple threat to local governments. One approach that appears to be gaining in popularity in getting a handle on health costs has been the implementation of on- or near-site health care clinics, perhaps best described as a modern version of the "company doctor."

On-site clinics are not a new phenomenon — there has been widespread interest and successful use of these clinics in the private sector for decades. However, local governments have slowly realized that direct provision of primary care can contain costs in five key ways: by moving away from the standard fee-for-service model of private care; by making less-costly primary care services more accessible and affordable; through direct contracting for labs and generic drugs; by taking advantage of the potential for prompt identification of worksite specific issues for "real time epidemiology" (Nash, 2005, p. 24); and by establishing patient-centered medical homes that foster disease management and promote wellness activities. These direct savings may be multiplied through improved quality of care that results in enhanced employee productivity and reduced absenteeism.

There are currently over 90,000 local governments in the United States. Estimates vary on the number of these governmental units providing clinics, however, a survey of 1,500 municipal and county governments with populations of more than 10,000 indicated nine percent of these local governments were providing on-site clinics with an additional 12 percent considering implementation (ICMA, 2011).

This chapter analyzes the trend for clinic implementation as a potentially effective model for lowering cost, improving access, and enhancing the quality of health care coverage.

WHY WORKSITE CLINICS HOLD THE PROMISE OF SAVINGS

Moving away from the fee-for-service model of care. On-site clinics are, to a great degree, a rejection of health care as is currently practiced in most community settings. These clinics constitute what Chase describes as a "disruptive model of care" (2011). Worksite clinics that operate on a cost-plus or contract fee basis remove incentives inherent in the fee-for-service reimbursement model to "do more, bill more" (Chase, 2011). Savings may also be achieved by removing much of the cost of the claims payment function. Chase estimates that the cost of the "insurance bureaucracy tax" is as much as "40 percent" (2012). Clinic provider Novia executive Bill Crimmons reports:

Generally speaking, the savings are significant. . . . Most family practice doctors in private practice must charge about $500 to $600 per hour in billable charges to earn $100 an hour. In our clinics, we're running at $289 an hour, with only three visits per hour and the doctor still earns $100 an hour. That's roughly 50 percent savings (Byrne, 2009, p. 4).

Direct contracts for labs and generic drugs. Further savings may be derived through contracted services for labs and other diagnostic services and bulk purchase of generics. Generic drugs can often be purchased less expensively by a clinic than through group health plans, which may garner financial benefit on top of premiums through charging more for pharmaceuticals when the insurer owns the mail order pharmacy or the pharmacy benefits manager program.

Making primary care accessible and affordable. By refocusing on primary care in the worksite clinic in lieu of specialty care in the community, savings can be achieved. "[P]rimary care physicians achieve better generic (that is, not disease-specific) outcomes than do specialists at much lower costs, even though specialists may achieve better 'quality' of care in their particular area of competence" (Starfield, Shi, Grover, & Macinko, 2005, p. W5-102). Bias built into current payment systems in the U.S. has resulted in higher reimbursement for specialists than for primary care (Sandy, Bodenheimer, Pawlson, & Starfield, 2009; Yurk, Christensen, & Wright, 2008), costs that are multiplied when employees seek out specialists first in lieu of primary care. Nash (2005, p. 67) describes shifting health clinics toward primary care as the "low-hanging fruit" in achieving savings. Chase puts it even more directly: "more primary care = healthier population = less money spent" (2011).

Immediate access, short-wait times, and no or very low co-pays may foster increased use of primary care at the worksite clinic. Port St. Lucie, Florida city employees, for example, are allowed to stay on the clock during visits because their clinic operates so efficiently that employees are seldom away from work for more than one hour (Balona, 2009). Employees are also attracted to the "one-stop shopping aspect" that is available in some larger clinics, where ancillary services, including medication dispensaries, are on site. A 2009 study comparing chronic medication compliance between community and worksite clinics found that medication compliance at on-site clinics was almost ten percent higher than in community settings. Improving medication compliance "can significantly lower overall healthcare costs . . . [and] improve the lives of chronically ill patients" (Sherman, Frazee, Fabius, Broome, Manfred, & Davis, 2009, pp. 53, 57).

Occupational health. Occupational health within the worksite clinic may also provide opportunities for savings. Some researchers believe that "[i]n-house medical personnel . . . have a better understanding of the interaction between an employee's health, his or her ability to perform the job, and the culture of the company" (Pachman, Stempien, Milles, & O'Neill, 1996, p. 1048). Awareness of job duties may help with return-to-work or limited-duty assignments that keep experienced workers on the job and may help reduce turnover and expensive workers' compensation claims.

Worksite clinics as medical homes. Local governments increase the potential for savings and improved quality when they create an "environment where financing and provision of services are integrated," and where "primary care providers serve as 'gatekeepers', an important role in controlling cost, utilization, and the rational allocation of resources" (Shi, 1995, p. 428). Access to claims data from within and outside the clinic, the use of predictive analytics, and population health data can guide health plan changes and incentives that control costs, while electronic health records and case management can foster improved care and outcomes (Nash, 2005). With the advent of electronic medical records (EMRs) it is now easier for this information to be shared. Sanford and Lake Mary, Florida operate joint clinic facilities that are open on alternate days. Even if employees need to visit a clinic the next day for a follow-up visit the medical staff have instant access to their medical files. At QuadMed, an early implementer of worksite clinics in the private sector, when population statistics indicated that "obesity was a major contributing factor to healthcare spending" (McCarthy & Klein, 2010, p. 5), the company adjusted its benefit program to encourage participation in wellness-focused weight-loss and diabetes management programs. Population health data tracking also provides a means for establishing accountability for clinic staff and vendors and allows the organization to set internal and external goals that can drive performance.

Care within a medical home offers "the ability to change practice patterns, such as drug prescribing, ordering of tests and procedures, and specialist referrals, along with the potential for early diagnosis and treatment to avoid ED [emergency department] visits, hospitalizations and other costly downstream complications" (Tu, Boukos, & Cohen, 2010, p. 4). Provider familiarity with the patient also allows for identification of patterns that may indicate a new health risk to the individual patient, reducing expensive redundancies in care; encouraging compliance and wellness, and reducing "potentially adverse effects of medical interventions" (Starfield, Shi, & Macinko, 2005, p. 487). Some companies integrate the company's wellness program with a clinical focus on predominate but treatable chronic diseases such as obesity, smoking, diabetes, and hypertension. (McCarthy & Klein, 2010, p. 1). Worksite clinics as medical homes may also reduce costly "defensive medicine" that results from the lack of any longitudinal doctor-patient relationship of trust that is a foundation of primary care.

CHALLENGES TO WORKSITE CLINIC SUCCESS

Local governments considering worksite clinics face challenges in start-up including: approval for capital for an office location and medical equipment; cost of promotional efforts for employees; and, if a vendor contract is in place, minimum revenue agreements for some initial period. Governments may also experience push-back from local providers and institutions that see worksite clinics as competitors. Byrne suggests that "[m]any worksite clinics must employ independent physicians rather than navigate accusations of scavenging business and conflict of interest" (2009, p. 2). Local governments in smaller communities should consider the potential of negative economic outcomes that could result if their worksite clinics "have a detrimental effect on the viability of other community physician practices, in which the patient mix would shift toward a greater proportion of those covered by Medicare and Medicaid, which tend to pay lower rates than commercially insured patients" (McCarthy & Klein, 2010, p. 10).

Employers must ensure arms-length handling of individual medical records to foster employee trust (Towers-Watson, 2012). Long-established "corporate practice of medicine" prohibitions set out by the American Medical Association warn physicians to avoid situations in which the "physicians' judgment may be influenced by a business' motivation to reduce costs and maximize profits" (Gorman & Miller 2011, p. 487).

Worksite clinics are also subject to compliance programs, Health Insurance Portability and Accountability Act (HIPAA) regulations, state medical board and nursing guidelines for licensure, staffing, and oversight, workers' compensation laws, pharmacy board dispensary rules, federal Occupational Safety and Health Administration (OSHA) and other safety regulations, public building mandates for access and egress, patient referral laws, laboratory regulations, and health inspections (Gorman & Miller, 2011; Oliphant & Murray, 2012; Savely, Hamilton, Degani, Weinberg, & Muraca, 2011). Oliphant and Murray (2012, p. 65) warn employers that such clinics may "implicate employee benefits laws," which may include risk of losing "grandfathered" plans that are an option under the 2010 Patient Protection and Affordable Care Act.

COST-EFFECTIVENESS OF WORKSITE CLINICS

Anecdotal data from local governments provide strong evidence of the overall effectiveness of government worksite health clinics (see case studies), but proving return on investment to elected officials may be another matter entirely. Cost savings, says Executive Director of the National Association of Worksite Health Centers Larry Boress, "are often the hardest to quantify." Lack of quantitative data and any national benchmarks for calculating return on investment (ROI) (Sherman & Fabius, 2012, p. 394) make it difficult to determine return on employer investment in a worksite clinic. The fact that employees use both community and clinic providers, the presence of normal, episodic spikes in health care costs due to a few employees with serious health problems (referred to as "shock" claims), and lack of comparative data from the past limit ability to pinpoint the sources of savings.

Table 1. Worksite clinic successes

Organization	Success	Source
Pitney Bowes	For each dollar spent on clinics, the company has "achieved savings of $1 in care costs" and "another $1 in increased productivity."	Chordes 2009, 75
Syngenta Crop Protection	Clinic "provides employee health care services two to three time more cost-effective than do off-site health care clinics."	Chenoweth and Garrett 2006, 84
CareHere (Clinic Vendor)	Helped their clients decrease the health care costs growth trend by half.	Mooradian 2008
CHC Meridian (Clinic Vendor)	50 percent decrease in hospital admission rate, 42 percent reduction in hospital outpatient services; and 32 percent reduction in overall costs.	Levy 2007, 52
Take Care Health (Clinic Vendor)	Reports "a $2 - $4 return on investment for every dollar spent" by clients.	Chordas 2009, 75
Briggs and Stratton	Cut emergency and urgent care visits by half; stabilized health care costs.	Moore 2011, 17

The longer history of worksite clinics in the private sector has resulted in some data that further supports cost savings to the employer. Table 1 provides published reports of savings that could be replicated in public sector clinics. Employee participation is critical and may take time and incentives to build a sustainable clinic. A national survey of larger private companies found that only 25 percent of employees used worksite clinics that were available to them (Hewitt, 2008, p. 14), although some organizations report much higher participation. Higher participation can reduce the costs of managing outside claims and improve ROI.

Despite the fact that local government clinics often cite cost reduction as the primary reason for operating their clinics, "more than half either don't know (39 percent) or don't track (14 percent) ROI" (Towers-Watson, 2012, pp. 1, 4). This Towers-Watson data is confirmed in a smaller survey conducted by the authors with 40 local government-sponsored worksite clinics across the U.S. Only 16 of 40 survey respondents could offer hard data on ROI, but ten of the 16 had demonstrated mean savings of $1,269 per employee.

Government managers should be forewarned that per-employee health costs may rise in the first year or two of operations. This is a common but generally short-lived

Figure 1. Percentage of respondents reporting sources of cost savings after clinic implementation (n = 27)

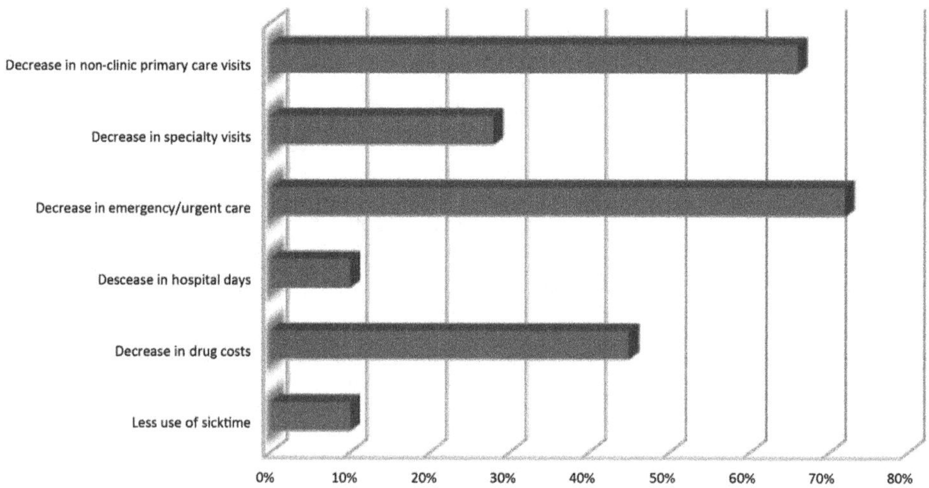

occurrence at new clinics due to pent-up demand from patients seeking care due to the more affordable costs of co-payments and medications. Industry reports of ROI for worksite clinics range from one to four years, depending on the initial capital investment in office space (Canadian Medical Association Journal, 2011; Liddick, 2005; Moore, 2011), though respondents to the authors' survey reported return on initial investment in only 1.8 years.

Through Internet searches, news and industry reports of government operated worksite clinics, and contact with clinic management providers for lists of governments with whom they contract, the authors surveyed approximately 100 local government clinic operations in 20 states. Forty responses were received and Figure 1 illustrates sources of savings identified by these respondents. Notable are savings through decreased use of expensive urgent and emergency care, most likely the result of convenient and affordable employee and dependent access to primary care. Even a 10 percent reduction in hospital days and sick time can have a significant cost savings effect.

Direct savings may also be achieved through ancillary contracts and onsite services. In the author's survey, just over half of the clinics surveyed operate a dispensary and most clinics limit pharmaceutical choices to generics only. Of 17 respondents who keep such data, 82 percent reported that their drugs purchased for the dispensary cost less than drugs purchased through the health plan. These cost savings also accrue to employees, while improving medication compliance and, there-

Figure 2. Clinic effectiveness (n = 37)

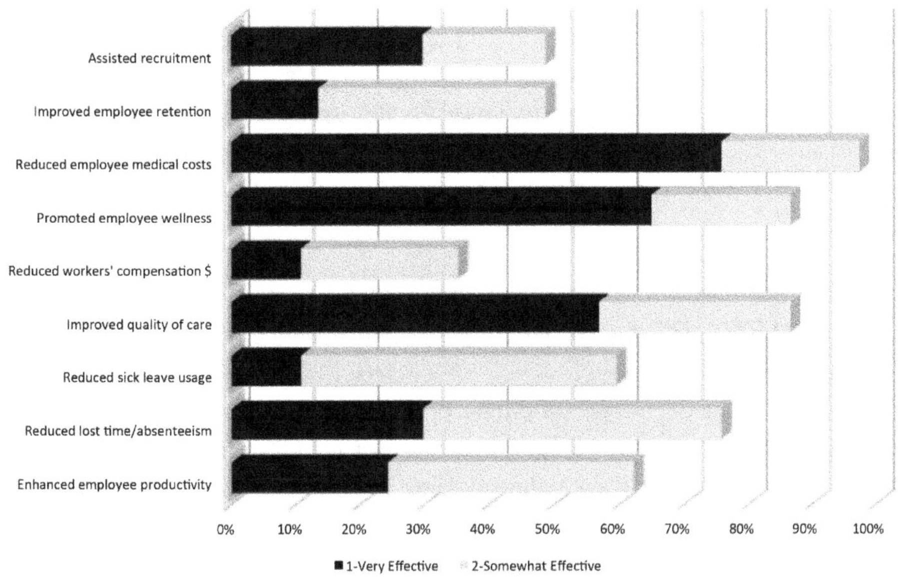

fore, outcomes. Employees also appreciate the benefit of $0 co-payments available at the vast majority of worksite clinics.

Some cost-savings are less easily measured or may promote employee lifestyle changes that will provide other direct and indirect long-term savings. Figure 2 illustrates the views of survey respondents on cost-effectiveness of their clinics. Of primary importance is the clinics' and employers' team approach to improved employee wellness, an effort that should produce longer-term savings. About half of governments responding to the authors' survey are investing in wellness activities such as smoking cessation, weight management, chronic disease management, wellness services, laboratory services including drug testing and immunizations. Nutrition, pharmacy, and urgent care services are offered at over 40 percent of surveyed locations.

Data from the private sector indicate potential for additional savings when benefit plans are altered to encourage employees to use the clinic as a medical home, where the focus is on primary care and management of costly chronic disease, which accounts for over 75 percent of U.S. health care spending (Centers for Disease Control and Prevention, 2009, p. 1). Sherman and Fabius point out that "a favorable shift in the population health risk profile can be viewed as a leading indicator of future health care utilization and costs" (2012, p. 398). Though results may not be immediately quantifiable, such linkage may have the long-term benefit of providing both hard and soft cost savings (LaPenna, 2010, pp. 71-79). Chenoweth and Garret (2006) note, however, that the final decision on keeping an intervention should not be based solely on financial costs. There are benefits—employee morale, better labor-management relations, and improved employee health—that cannot be readily quantified or may be long-term. Tracking and trending population outcomes measures such as health risk assessments, sick leave and urgent care usage, hospital days, and specialist visits can provide additional information about clinic effectiveness.

CLINICS IN THE REAL WORLD

So what has been the experience of clinics operating at the local government level? Two communities in the state of Georgia were studied to help answer this question: Camden County and the city of Valdosta. Both have taken different approaches to clinic development, but officials in these communities believe the clinics have been sufficiently successful to foster commitment to ongoing operations.

Camden County, Georgia

Slow and steady. That's the approach to growth adopted by Camden County's government-operated Living Well Onsite Health Clinic. "I don't want to say that we didn't know where we were going when we started, but at every step we began to realize greater possibilities for this clinic," says Camden County Budget and Finance Director Mike Fender.

Those "possibilities" have astonished elected officials and have drawn in two of Camden County's city governments and the Public Service Authority, with the county's remaining city considering joining the clinic. "This whole process was triggered by the fact that our costs were out of control," says Fender. "We are a self-insured plan, and our stop-loss policies had gone from $60,000 to $700,000, with exclusions for our costliest patients. We knew we had to do something to reverse the trend."

Reverse the trend they have. For the past five years, the county has seen no increases in its medical costs, despite the fact that they have added services, including an Employee Assistance Program with substantial mental health benefits that begins in 2014. The reasons for the savings are numerous, but in general they relate to better management of chronic disease and a focus on wellness, increased use of the Living Well Clinic in lieu of the emergency room, and better compliance due to generic medications onsite and at a local grocery, where some medications are free as a loss leader for the sale of other medications and groceries.

Mary T. Smith, the county's insurance consultant, explains that the county's initiation into the provision of health care was nothing more than what amounted to a "company nurse," a registered nurse on staff to distribute bandages for scrapes and minor cuts and over-the-county pain medications and to assist with some employee training. "When we saw the amount of money going for chronic diseases," explains Smith, "we realized the potential for cost savings through more intensive disease management."

Nearly all worksite clinics are run by vendors or outside providers, effectively creating a natural wall between the employer and the employees' records. In starting its own clinic with county employees, Camden County had the bigger challenge of earning the trust of employees. "Employee trust was key, if people were going to participate. Some were afraid that they might lose their jobs due to poor health status. We had lots of work to do to prove to them that this about *their* health and *their* plan." The clinic and its employees are, of course, subject to HIPAA regulations, and any data that goes to the county is aggregated to protect privacy. The ability to pass on the cost savings from the clinic helps reinforce the direct benefits to employees, says Smith, many of whom were not seeing a doctor on a regular basis, due to cost, prior to the clinic's opening.

The clinic is forbidden by law from treating its employees' workers compensation injuries, but awareness of and analysis of the injuries by clinic staff has helped in prevention of injury, according to Fender. "We have a community panel of physicians for workers' compensation," he says, "but our clinic staff can look at the claims and see where we might make changes to reduce the chance of an injury. The clinic administrator serves on the safety committee for the county and helps with recommendations for changing processes to reduce accidents and injuries, a sort of "real-time epidemiology" (Nash, 2005, p. 24) that has the potential to reduce injury and costs.

That initial "company nurse" has grown into a full-blown doctor's office with a physician on site four days a week, two nurse practitioners, several RNs, and one medical assistant, all employees of the county. Living Well has not attempted to become a "medical home" for its employees at this point, according to clinic administrator Dawn Haney, who explains that the clinic serves primarily as a place to seek urgent care needs, to conduct case management, to coordinate wellness activities and teaching, and to dispense low-cost generic drugs. "We do have a few patients who visit here exclusively because of their health problems," she says, "but in almost all cases, we work with physicians in the community." The clinic has not ruled out serving as the "medical home" for employees at some future date because of the potential for additional savings. Research has shown that local governments increase the potential for savings and improved quality when they create an "environment where financing and provision of services are integrated," and where "primary care providers serve as 'gatekeepers', an important role in controlling cost, utilization, and the rational allocation of resources" (Shi, 1995, p. 428).

"One of the challenges for local governments," explains Fender, "is that they run the risk of offending their citizens if they appear to be competing with local providers. We have made every effort to avoid that conflict." Researchers have noted push-back from local physicians who believe the clinic is "skimming the cream," the county's fully insured patients, and leaving them with public payers with low reimbursements (McCarthy & Klein, 2010, p. 10). "To prove the point, we give significant 'wellness points' to our employees when they have a physical with their community-based primary care providers. Those points, along with other activities, can reduce employees' premiums up to 20 percent."

The "wellness points" program is a newer addition to the program. Originally established to create incentives for employees to take charge of their own health, the clinic worked with the administrative services organization to give points for completion of a Health Risk Assessment and getting the annual physical, among other options. "We're working now to move to an outcomes-based rewards system," explains Smith. "It's tricky. We will have a health care attorney to help sure that we stay within the bounds of the law, but we will have options for 'wellness points' for all employees that reduce the premium for making progress toward individual goals and participating in wellness activities like exercise. The county's Public Service Authority operates a wellness center, so this gives us an avenue to not only give discounts for participation but to track attendance, which earns points."

The clinic uses an electronic medical record (EMR), which helps the providers and RN case managers assure that medicines dispensed at the clinic do not conflict with community-based prescriptions. Case managers also monitor patient biometrics and conduct intensive disease management for those with chronic diseases, charting progress through the EMR.

Administrator Dawn Haney also tracks visits at the clinic and compares the costs of those visits to the cost of a community visit to determine savings. "Return on investment is hard to quantify in an exact manner, because we are often talking about avoided costs," says Smith, "but we know that we are seeing significant savings when a patient brings her child with an earache here, rather than going to the emergency room. Even our regular non-urgent visits provide savings, because we do not have the overhead costs of filing claims." Some experts estimate that just avoiding claims filing can save as much as 40 percent (Chase, 2012). Haney reports that savings on visits range from $72 to $172, depending on the level of care, when compared to community-based reimbursement.

The major proof of success, says Fender, lies in the county's budget: no increases in costs for the county for over five years. One of the cities that has joined the clinic came in with a 144 percent medical loss ratio. After the first year, with the clinic's help, they had cut the loss to 55 percent. "As the new cities have come on," Fender explains, "we are setting up a sort of natural experiment. The county allows covered employees and dependents and non-covered employees and dependents to use the clinic, though we hope the non-covered employees will begin to see the value of participation in the health plan because of the added health resources they can access. One city allows covered employees and dependents, but not non-covered employees, and the other city allows covered employees only. It will be interesting to compare savings a couple of years down the road. I suspect that we will find that expanded use brings greater savings."

Employees are also winners, according to Haney. Their premiums have remained stable or gone down, thanks to wellness points, and if they use the clinic, they do not have to take time off to visit the doctor. "I think this program has really been a real morale builder," agrees Fender. "The employees appreciate what we are doing in working with them to improve their health and save money for everyone."

Going it alone is not always the easiest route. "We have grown into this," says Fender, "and we are still working to improve the clinic operations, but we believe this is preferable to using a vendor. We have seen a lot of places that started clinics, but dropped them because they couldn't see a return on investment. It's also hard to justify the big outlay for a full-service clinic, when it is not a proven commodity and it takes time to get employees invested. We've taken the slower route, and it's worked for us. Our record demonstrates that."

Valdosta, Georgia

Like Camden County, the city of Valdosta, Georgia was also experiencing a jump in health care costs. Although self-insured, the city had experienced three years of near- and double-digit increases in claims expenses. The city took action on two fronts. First, the city initiated several plan changes for its 570 employees including increasing deductibles and co-pays, and establishing a tiered-system for prescription drugs. Additionally, the city began assessing a health insurance premium of $27.50 per pay period for employee-only coverage (family coverage already required a premium contribution); tobacco users pay an additional $25.00 per pay period. Aware of the relationship between health coverage and recruiting and retention of quality employees, City Manager Larry Hanson explains that the city began looking at alternatives to control the unsustainable increases, while limiting costs to employees and establishing a mechanism for improving employee health. When the city began planning for the clinic they were hoping to partner with Lowndes County to share in initial set-up costs. However, at the last moment the county decided not to pursue the clinic and the city decided to proceed on their own and the clinic opened April, 2011. According to Hanson, the city has not regretted that decision.

The city selected CareHere to manage and operate their clinic through a RFP process. CareHere, which is based in Nashville, Tennessee currently manages over 160 health and wellness centers of which about one third are with local governments and school districts. Hanson said that the city liked the approach taken by CareHere in partnering with them to select the clinic's doctor and other medical staff. While initially rolling out the clinic with limited hours, it is now open 4 and a half days a week and is operating at 98 percent capacity. To increase capacity and respond to employee requests, the city is now considering extending hours by adding Saturday service. The city was able to use an existing property and renovating the building to clinical standards cost about $30,000 in capital expenditures. The city also spends about $30,000 annually on supplies, including generic medications that are dispensed at the clinic. "It is less expensive for us to purchase these medications and give them away rather than have employees use pharmacy services," said Hanson. The clinic is staffed by a physician, physician's assistant, and nurse on a staggered basis.

The city and CareHere made a concerted effort to educate employees about the clinic and services and it appears to have paid off in two ways. One, Hanson says, is that many employees are using the clinic as "their first choice for health care." Operating the clinic as a "medical home" has the potential for significant cost savings. While comparable marketplace office visits and services cost $82.91, CareHere provides the service for $56.56. CareHere estimates that for every dollar invested by the city in the clinic, $1.30 is returned in savings. Two, while there is no evidence that the clinic has reduced health care expenditures to date, it appears to have slowed the rate of increase in claims costs to a manageable level. The clinic costs the city about $400,000 a year to staff and actual claims increased by only $30,000 or less than one percent from FY2012 to FY2013 as shown in Figure 3. A slow down in double digit claims increases will have a definite impact on future health care expenditures by the city.

There are a number of intangible benefits as well. Employees can easily schedule appointments on line and can usually get an appointment within 24 hours. Appointments are scheduled in 20-minute increments so that staff is not overloaded with patients at any one time and most people are in and out of the clinic within 30 minutes.

"Because the clinic scheduling is so efficient and employees spend so little time there it is not necessary for employees to go off the clock and burn sick leave," Hanson noted.

The city also contracts for a flat rate for all lab tests with a third party at a fraction of the cost of the same tests at local doctors' offices, where costs are higher due to mark-up on lab fees to pay for lab staff, interpretation of results, and a profit margin.

Of course the primary way to reduce health care expenditures is to have healthier employees. The city is encouraging employees to be pro-active with their health.

Figure 3. Claims history FY2005-FY2013
Source: City of Valdosta Comprehensive Annual Financial Reports

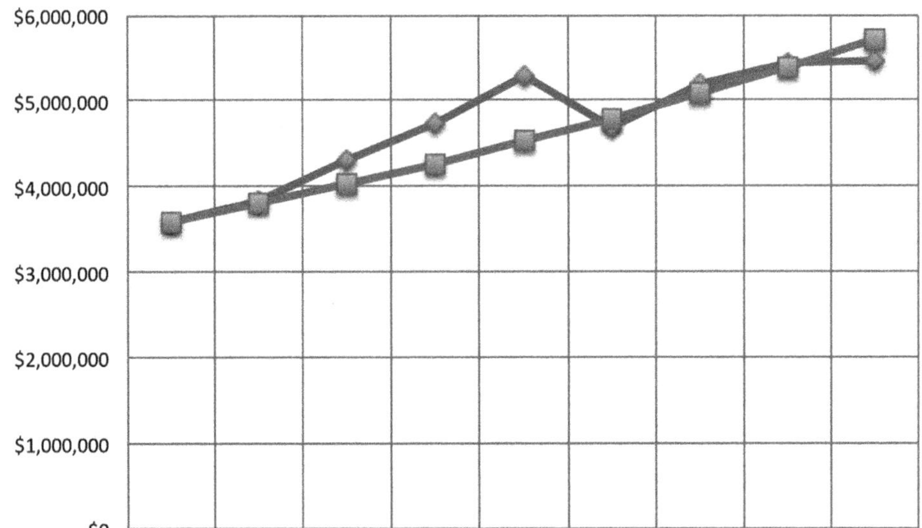

	FY05	FY06	FY07	FY08	FY09	FY10	FY11	FY12	FY13
Actual	$3,584,226	$3,826,749	$4,302,967	$4,727,383	$5,298,332	$4,677,586	$5,179,010	$5,443,831	$5,473,208
Projected	$3,584,226	$3,799,280	$4,027,236	$4,268,871	$4,525,003	$4,796,503	$5,084,293	$5,389,351	$5,712,712

CareHere sponsors annual health fairs and conducts health risk assessments (HRA) to raise awareness among employees of chronic, but treatable diseases such as hypertension, high cholesterol, obesity, and diabetes. About 43 percent of employees have completed a HRA. By charging tobacco users with a higher premium the city is also providing a financial incentive in order to change a poor health habit. Healthier employees will have a long-term impact on both expenditures and lost time due to illness.

Surveys of those using the clinic show very favorable opinions about the facility. First, virtually all of the respondents would recommend the clinic to a family member or co-worker (n=63) and about 98 percent believe that it is a valuable feature of their health plan. As for time spent in the waiting room, 86 percent of those surveyed had wait times of 10 minutes or less for a scheduled appointment; 60 percent of these respondents had wait times of five minutes or less.

Even though the city offers a generous health insurance plan by comparable standards, the cost of physician co-pays and medications keep health care out of reach by many employees. A 2012 survey by the Commonwealth Fund found that even low and moderate income families had some difficulty affording health care because of the cost-sharing requirements compared to their income. Over half of those underinsured surveyed (51 percent) had financial difficulties receiving health care (xi, xii). This is supported by the Valdosta employee survey as 48 percent identified "no co-pays" as the main reason for choosing the clinic. Comments on clinic surveys provide further anecdotal evidence that doctor co-pays and prescription drugs were deterrents for some employees in seeking health care prior to the clinic's opening.

While it is too early to quantify the financial impact on the city's clinic on overall health care costs, the city manager believes that in the short term the clinic is "keeping health care affordable" for the city. The city appears to have subscribed to many of the "best practices" of clinics identified earlier that should, in the long term, create healthier and consequently more productive employees.

CONCLUSION

While direct savings on health care costs for employers and employers are primary drivers for governmental decisions to open worksite health clinics, it is likely that savings have been derived from the new model of health as much as from better control over costs of care. Easy access to care, low or no co-payments and deductibles, a relationship with a primary care physician within a medical home, and onsite occupational care are "best practice" components of clinics that may contribute to improved health and cost-savings. Once implemented, clinics appear to have a high level of satisfaction.

While the authors' survey data demonstrated no statistically significant relationships in clinic implementation and direct savings in health care expenditures to date, the operation of local government clinics is still in an early stage of development. Just as in the private sector, the prospect for savings and improved health over the long-term appear real.

Dependence on data from a clinic vendor is an inadequate means of determining financial success (Sherman & Fabius, 2012), so local governments must be cautious when using such data in determining whether or not to open a clinic. While there is no uniform tool for measuring cost savings, the simple use of per-employee total costs (with a comparison of community versus clinic costs), population health monitoring in key areas, and measures of employee productivity and satisfaction can provide a preliminary means of benchmarking among worksite clinics. Another alternative is comparing growth trends in health care costs prior to the clinic opening with national trends and actual performance of the clinic, though adequate time must be allotted to account for pent-up demand that may increase costs in the first year of operations. At a time when efficiency and effectiveness are essential expectations of governments, measuring performance of clinics provides an opportunity to demonstrate good fiscal and human resources management, while enhancing employee productivity through better management of health care. While additional research and a broader development of clinics are needed, it can be argued that on-site clinics have a potential to meet these expectations. The authors suggest that employers consider services that reduce lost time from the workplace, encourage a holistic approach that not only includes basic primary care but wellness and healthy lifestyles, disease management, dispensary services, and easy access.

It is estimated that for clinics to be financially successful about 500 employees are required. It is possible that even small government entities can benefit by partnering with neighboring communities, school districts, or other multi-employer operations. Once implemented, a fiduciary responsibility is created on the part of elected and appointed officials and the clinic needs on-going assessment and evaluation. Because of the fishbowl that is local government, employers should not over-promise savings but look at the clinic as an additional tool that promotes employee health, retains staff, and can reduce health care expenditures for the long-term.

REFERENCES

Anonymous. (2011). The doctor is in – at your workplace. *Canadian Medical Association Journal, 183*(13), E983.

Balona, D.-M. (2009). Health-care clinics for government workers may save time, money. *Orlando Sentinel*. Retrieved from http://www.orlandosentinel.com/news/orl-loc-lid-clincs031509,0,7551669.story

Barro, J. (2011). *Cadillac coverage: the high cost of public employee health benefits*. Civic Report No. 65. Center for State and Local Leadership. Manhattan Institute. Retrieved from manhattan-institute.org/csll

Byrne, R. (2009). *Worksite health clinics put new focus on employee health*. HealthLeaders InterStudy's Ohio, Kentucky, and Indiana Health Plan Analysis 10:1, 1-5. Retrieved from: http://www.noviacareclinics.com/assets/uploads /IKO_Worksite-Health_09.pdf

Centers for Disease Control and Prevention. (2009). *The power of prevention: chronic disease . . . the public health challenge of the 21st century*. National Center for Chronic Disease and Health Promotion. Retrieved from: http://www.cdc.gov/chronicdisease/pdf/2009-power-of-prevention.pdf

Chase, D. (2011). Employers solving healthcare crisis one on-site clinic at a time. *Insurance Thought Leadership*. Retrieved from http://www.insurancethoughtleadership.com/index.php/site/healthcare/employers-solving-healthcare-crisis-one-onsite-clinic-at-a-time/#axzz1x1a44iPx

Chase, D. (2012). Marcus Welby is dead – long live Marcus Welby. *Insurance Thought Leadership*. Retrieved from http://www.insurancethoughtleadership.com/index.php/site/authors/69#axzz1x1a44iPx

Chenoweth, D. H., & Garrett, J. (2006). Cost-effectiveness analysis of a worksite clinic. *AAOHN Journal, 54*(2), 84–89. PMID:16509183

Chordas, Lori. (2009). On-the-spot care. *Best's Review,* (May), 74-75.

Claxton, G., Rae, M., Panchal, N., Damico, A., Lundy, J., Bostick, N., . . . Whitmore, H. (2012). *Employee health benefits 2012 annual survey*. Kaiser Family Foundation, Health Research & Educational Trust, and NORC. Retrieved from http://ehbs.kff.org/pdf/2012/8345.pdf

Collins, S. R., Robertson, R., Garber, T., & Doty, M. M. (2013). *Insuring the Future: Current Trends in Health Coverage and the Effects of Implementing the Affordable Care Act*. New York: The Commonwealth Fund.

Cox, W. (2011). Out of sync: Government and private employee compensation in Illinois. Illinois Policy Institute.

Falk, J. (2012). *Comparing the compensation of federal and private-sector employees*. Congressional Budget Office.

Gorman, K., & Miller, R. (2011). Managing the risks of on-site health centers. *AAOHN Journal, 59*(11), 483–490. doi:10.3928/08910162-20111017-02 PMID:22017191

Gross, L., Huh, K., Sylvester, A., & Zahradnik, R. (2012). *The local squeeze: falling revenues and growing demand for services challenge cities, counties, and school districts*. The Pew Charitable Trust. Retrieved from: http://www.pewstates.org/uploadedFiles/PCS_Assets/2012/Pew_Local_Squeeze(1).pdf

Hewitt Associates. (2008). *Wellness and beyond: employees examine ways to improve employee health and productivity and reduce costs*. Retrieved from: http://www.aon.com/attachments/thought-leadership/Wellness_and_Beyond.pdf

International City-County Management Association. (2011). *Local government employee Insurance Program*. Accessed at: https://icma.org/Documents/Document/Document/303133.Washington

Kaiser Family Foundation. (2012). *Premiums, cost-sharing and coverage at public, private and non-profit employers: a view from the 2012 employer health benefit survey*. Retrieved from: http://www.kff.org/insurance/ snapshot/chcm112012oth.cfm

Kavanaugh, S. (2011). *Containing health care costs: proven strategies for success in the public sector*. Government Finance Officers Association and Colonial Life.

LaPenna, A. M. (2010). Workplace Clinics and employer managed healthcare: a catalyst for cost savings and improved productivity. Boca Raton, FL: CRC Press.

Liddick, Betty. (2005). Sick over health care costs, companies get some relief with on-site medical centers. *Workforce Management, 84*(5), 82.

McCarthy, D., & Klein, S. (2010). *QuadMed: transforming employer-Sponsored health care through workplace primary care and wellness programs*. The Commonwealth Fund. Retrieved from: http://www.commonwealthfund.org/~/media/Files/Publications/Casepercent20Study/2010/Jul/Triplepercent20Aimpercent20v2/1424_McCarthy_QuadMed_triple_aim_case_study_v2.pdf

Mooradian, D. (2008). Jobsite health clinics open doors to savings. *HealthLeaders InterStudy – Tennessee Health Plan Analysis, 20*(4), 1-4.

Moore, A. V. (2011). The doctor is in – at the workplace. *Benefits Magazine,* (December), 14-19.

Nash, J. L. (2005). *Making the business case for integrated health and wellness*. Academic Press.

Office of the National Coordinator for Health Information Technology. (n.d.). *Benefits of EHRs: improved diagnostics and patient outcomes*. Retrieved from http://www.healthit.gov/providers-professionals/improved-diagnostics-patient-outcomes

Oliphant, L. T., & Murray, C. C. (2012). Fit for an on-site clinic. *HRMagazine*, *57*, 1, 61, 63, 65.

Pachman, J. S., Stempien, D., Milles, S. S., & O'Neill, F. N. (1996). The hidden savings of a corporate on-site medical center. *Journal of Occupational and Environmental Medicine*, *83*(10), 1047–1048. PMID:8899583

Sandy, L. G., Bodenheimer, T., Pawlson, L. G., & Starfield, B. (2009). The political economy of U.S. primary care. *Health Affairs*, *28*(4), 1136–1144. doi:10.1377/hlthaff.28.4.1136 PMID:19597213

Savely, S., Hamilton, W., Degani, F., Weinberg, A., & Muraca, P. (2011). A survey of environmental safety at 20 medical clinics. *Journal of Environmental Health, 73*(6), 86–94. PMID:21306100

Sherman, B. W., & Fabius, R. J. (2012). Quantifying the value of worksite clinic nonoccupational health care services. *Journal of Occupational and Environmental Medicine, 54*(4), 394–403. doi:10.1097/JOM.0b013e31824b2157 PMID:22418274

Sherman, B. W., Frazee, S. G., Fabius, R. J., Broome, R., Manfred, J. R., & Davis, J. (2009). Impact of workplace health services on adherence to chronic medications. *The American Journal of Managed Care, 15*(7), 53–59. PMID:19589007

Shi, L. (1995). Balancing primary versus specialty care. *Journal of the Royal Society of Medicine, 88*, 428–432. PMID:7562823

Starfield, B., Shi, L., Grover, A., & Macinko, J. (2005). The effects of specialist supply on populations' health: Assessing the evidence. *Health Affairs*. Retrieved from http://content.healthaffairs.org/content/early/2005/03/15/hlthaff.w5.97.full.pdf

Starfield, B., Shi, L., & Macinko, J. (2005). Contribution of primary care to health systems and health. *The Milbank Quarterly, 83*(3), 457–502. doi:10.1111/j.1468-0009.2005.00409.x PMID:16202000

Towers-Watson. (2012). *2012 Onsite health center survey report*. Retrieved from: http://www.towerswatson.com/assets/pdf/7705/Realizing-the-Potential-of-Onsite-Health-Centers.pdf

Tu, H. T., Boukus, E., & Cohen, G. (2010). *Workplace clinics: a sign of Growing employer interest in wellness.* Center for Studying Health System Change Research Brief.

Yurk, M. J., Christensen, K., & Wright, E. (2008). *Overuse of specialty care increases costs in Indiana*. Center for Health Policy.

Chapter 11
Bridging the Gaps with Nonprofits: The Intersection of Institutions, Interests, and the Health Policy Process

Laura Caccioppoli
Villanova University, USA

ABSTRACT

This chapter will examine how nonprofits are both bridging the gaps left behind from health policy, and are at the intersection of institutions, interests, and the policy process. Using cultural competency as a theoretical lens, the chapter will make use of the current literature, demographic trends, and other qualitative and quantitative data to situate three case studies. As the Affordable Care Act, and other health policies tout themselves as solutions to gaps in health care services for minorities, this chapter offers an overview and evaluation of these policies as well as an explanation of the role nonprofits have in filling necessary service delivery and advocacy.

INTRODUCTION

In 2010, President Barack Obama signed the Affordable Care Act into law with the stated goal of "ensuring all Americans have access to quality, affordable health care" (Affordable Care Act, 2010). Indeed, the pulse of American health care was not good.

DOI: 10.4018/978-1-4666-9944-1.ch011

The law, which helps more people attain health insurance coverage, and prevents insurance companies from denying those with preexisting conditions, still contains gaps that minorities, who are most vulnerable, fall through. It is a well-documented fact that those with lower socioeconomic status; ethnic, racial and other minorities are often those at the highest risk for developing non-communicable diseases (Cesare et al., 2013). Even when all other variables are held constant (insurance, status, income, socioeconomic status, etc.) racial minorities are still "less likely to be given appropriate cardiac medications or to undergo bypass surgery, and are less likely to receive kidney dialysis or transplants. By contrast, they are more likely to receive less desirable procedures, such as lower limb amputations for diabetes and other conditions" (Smedley, Stith, & Nelson, 2003). This gap in healthcare for racial and ethnic minorities does not just pertain to more technical procedures – it is also found in more common procedures.

The gaps that exist are neither limited to any particular minority group, nor are they limited to any type of care. There are other health disparities that exist, for a sample, consider the Minnesota Department of Health and Human Services (DHS), who conducted a survey to measure the gaps that exist just in their long-term care facilities. The state found that there was a lack of adequate affordable housing, lack of universally designed houses and/or apartments, and a lack of beds for those with dementia. Moreover, when looking through the lens of cultural competency, those surveyed felt they were unprepared to handle the United States' changing demographics; for example, immigrant needs and the needs of those in the Lesbian, Gay, Bisexual, and Transgender (LGBT community) to name a few (Myott, 2010).

The role of nonprofits then is mission critical to providing quality culturally competent service delivery, advocating for health policy changes. The need for nonprofits has been recognized and nonprofits have responded, in fact healthcare represents 57% of nonprofit workers and the sector has shown tremendous growth despite the recession (Lambert, 2013). In terms of providing service delivery, quality nonprofits can be a cost effective alternative to state run institutions. Indeed many states, including Connecticut, have called for expanding the use of nonprofits in order to help lower costs (Commission on Nonprofit Health and Human Services, 2011). Moreover, nonprofits can serve more niche-based consumers such as those with Multiple Sclerosis (MS). The National Multiple Sclerosis Society (NMSS) helps provide education on the disease, and can help offset the cost of medications, and provide other valuable services to both the person with MS and their support system (National Multiple Sclerosis Society, 2014). Additionally, nonprofits, such as the NMSS, organize supporters, to help provide the political clout needed to make real policy changes. Lastly, nonprofits can also act as patient advocates, ensuring that patients are able to achieve culturally competent health care services – by providing translators, or even helping to get patients to the clinic.

This chapter will analyze where current policies are falling short, where nonprofits are able to step in, and how nonprofits can help drive policy changes. While there is a clear need for nonprofits, there are already nonprofits that are beginning to tackle this challenge. If we are to learn from the precedent of these nonprofits and utilize the aspects that are working, it is necessary to examine some nonprofits that are successful in providing quality, competent service delivery, as well as advocacy.

As the Affordable Care Act, and other health policies tout themselves as solutions to gaps in health care services for minorities, this chapter offers an overview of the role nonprofits should have in filling necessary service delivery and advocacy.

BACKGROUND

In order to understand the role that nonprofits can play in filling the gaps left behind by the Affordable Care Act (ACA), it is important to know the following: how do we understand health care in America, what is the nature of the gaps in health care, who are the key players / process, and what are nonprofits? Answering these questions provides the foundation needed to discuss the issues, controversies and problems more fully.

How Do We Understand Health Care in America?

Public health and health policy experts have been trying to quantify, qualify, and rate health care systems for many years. Generally speaking, there are a few ways one can tackle this task. First, a country can be ranked on how much money is spent on health care as a proportion of its gross domestic product. The Organisation for Economic and Cooperative Development (OECD)'s *Health at a Glance*, report from 2013 shows that the United States ranks first in this category, at 17.7 percent.

While measuring health as an expenditure of GDP is helpful in understanding how much a country is spending on medical care, it is not useful in determining the quality of health care received for the amount of money spent (table 1). Fortunately, the World Health Organization (WHO) performed a study to more accurately measure the performance of health systems. The WHO's assessment and ranking of health systems was based upon the following four criteria: overall health regarding level attained and distribution, responsiveness of the health system, efficiency, and quality. The study measures the level of health care, responsiveness, and efficiency against the overall expenditures on health care. For more information regarding the methodology of the study, please refer to the WHO's report: *Measuring Overall Health System Performance for 191 Countries.*

Table 1. Health expenditure as a percentage of GDP, 2011

United States	17.7
Netherlands	11.9
France	11.6
Germany	11.3
Canada	11.2
Switzerland	11.0
Denmark	10.9

The report may look familiar to those who have studied public health or health policy, as it is one of the more commonly cited studies, especially because it transformed the way Americans view their own health care. Even though the United States spends the most on health care as a percentage of GDP, and indeed, per capita, they rank at 37th out of 191 countries on the WHO's rating scale. Ranking in first was France, followed by Italy, and San Marino. Germany came in at 25. The United States, however, came in just behind Costa Rica, and just before Cuba (Tandon, A et al., 2000)

Some may argue that the ranking system devised by the World Health Organization is unfair, in that it does not consider how the people of a country feel about their access to health care, and treatment. Indeed, measuring a patient's overall satisfaction regarding health care can be incredibly useful in terms of determining how well a country is doing at providing care. Considering that the United States and its capitalist ethos places much weight in consumer satisfaction, it does seem logical to compare patient satisfaction, which is precisely what the Harvard School of Public Health did in its 2001 study "The Public Versus the World Health Organization" (Blendon, 2001). In this examination, the Harvard School of Public Health relied on national opinion surveys to help illuminate the perception of patients in fifteen European countries, the United States and Canada. In this ranking, the United States fared somewhat better, but not much. Ranking the highest were the Danes, where 91 percent of Danes said they were "very" or "fairly" satisfied with their health care. Finland came in at 81 percent, France at 65 percent, and only 40 percent of Americans stated that they were satisfied with their health care (Blendon, 2001).

Indeed, it is clear that the United States health care system is not performing as well as it could. Moreover, reviewing the WHO ranking suggests that the United States does not rank well in terms of equity, distribution of health care, or fairness in financing. It is in these aforementioned categories that the true gaps in health care exist. The nature of these gaps can both help explain why the United States ranks where it does in terms of health care, and can also provide insights into the ways that nonprofits can bridge these gaps.

The Nature of the Gaps

While more specific issues regarding minorities' lack of access to healthcare will be more fully addressed later in the chapter, it is necessary to understand some terminology to discuss the gaps in health care. Additionally, it is necessary to understand the nature of these gaps. There are two important key terms to know when discussing health care and those who are disadvantaged. The first is *equality*, which Patel & Rushefsky define as "treat[ing] people who are in the same situation the same way, or treat[ing] people in different situations differently (p.190)." Put more simply, when a health care system is *equal*, there is no discrimination on the basis of race, sexual orientation, religion, age, etc. Then there is *equity*, which Patel & Rushefsky note adds a social justice aspect to health care. *Equity* can be understood providing what is necessary in order for people to overcome disadvantages. What does this look like in the health care system? Consider Patient A, a forty year old woman who has multiple sclerosis and is having an exacerbation that requires her to travel to Philadelphia to receive an intravenous steroid treatment twice a month. Each treatment takes approximately three hours. She lives in the suburbs of Philadelphia, and has insurance through her employer, and she speaks English. Now consider Patient B, a forty year old Latina woman who lives in a less affluent area of Philadelphia, on the border of the suburbs. She too is experiencing a multiple sclerosis exacerbation and the same intravenous steroid treatment as Patient A. Patient B also has employer based health insurance. She does not speak English, and does not have a car. Equality of health care would suggest that both Patient A and Patient B should receive the treatments they need, and Patient B should not be turned away on the basis of her race. Equity would suggest that Patient B would also need translated materials in order to better understand her condition, prognosis, and health. Patient B would probably also need some sort of transportation to the clinic.

The reality is that there is discrimination in the United States health care system (Berk & Schur 1998). There is discrimination amongst who is able to obtain health insurance, versus who is not. There is also discrimination on the type of insurance a person can receive. Those who work at a larger firm may be able to receive better health insurance than those who do not. Additionally, a person who has a higher income may be able to afford insurance that covers a wider range of procedures (Jecker, 1993; Enthoven, 2003). In terms of insurance coverage, those who are living below the poverty line are often eligible for Medicaid, but those who are living just barely above the poverty line are not able to receive government assistance. In fact, those who are living in poverty, are much more likely to have no insurance (Collins et al. 2004; Hoffman, Carbaugh, & Cook 2004). Those who are younger, minorities, noncitizens, or foreign-born individuals are also likely to be uninsured (Hoffman, Carbaugh, & Cook 2004).

In terms of type of insurance, there is also inequality within the United States health care system. For those who have good insurance plans, receiving treatment and utilizing preventative medicine to reduce the risk of getting sick is easy. For those who are under insured, or on government programs such as Medicaid, acquiring quality services is often more difficult (Hoffman et al. 2001; Broyles, Narine, & Brandt 2002; Fairbrother et al. 2003; Committee on the Consequences of Uninsurance 2002). Indeed, the problem is compounded for those who are most vulnerable in society, such as children.

Even though in 2012 Medicaid or the Children's Health Insurance Program (CHIP) covered about 44 million children, there are still about 7.2 million children who remain uninsured. Additionally, the difference in terms of quality of treatment between Medicaid and private insurance is stark (Childrens Defense Fund, 2012).

Byrd and Clayton (2003) also note that disparities in health care among low-income and minorities are not a new phenomenon, but rather part of the history of the United States.

Regarding equity, there are several gaps that exist in the United States health care system. The barriers that affect equitable health care are many and varied. There are the obvious factors: lack of health insurance, and cost-sharing provisions. Then there are the factors that are not as easily identified: lack of transportation, lack of childcare, lack of health care providers in a certain region, and language barriers (Stoddard, St. Peter, & Newacheck 1994). Put another way, for many there are competing demands: clothing, food, and shelter may take precedent over health care, especially when income is tight (Long, 2003).

Voters in the United States have come to the consensus that the United States is not providing the best health care for the best value. The most recent presidential candidates have also emphasized the view that the health care system needs to be changed. President Barack Obama has certainly made headway with his signature piece of legislation, the Patient Protection and Affordable Care Act (ACA). While the ACA has attempted to address the equality of health care, namely, trying to expand insurance so that all people have access to health care, the Congressional Budget Office still estimates that 23 million people will still be without health insurance by 2019. The ACA also does not go far enough in ensuring that all persons are treated equally. According to a report by the Associated Press, insurance companies are maneuvering around the ACA. An example is insurance companies changing their policies so as to require those with chronic illness to pay a greater portion of their costs associated with their chronic illness. This amounts to discrimination against those complicated, long-term diseases (Politico, 2014). Additionally, the law does little to help address the bigger problem of equity of health care.

Political Arena

Key Actors

To understand what more can be done, it is necessary to understand the political environment in which this is all occurring. Health care and policy are created, and implemented within a myriad of institutions, and political actors. There is the public sector, which includes, government (local, state, and federal). Next, there is the private sector, which includes health care providers, professionals and purchasers (people needing these services and insurance companies). Often, people forget about the third sector, or nonprofit sector, which includes many of the same actors (purchasers, providers) as the private sector. The third sector will be discussed more at length later in the chapter.

The way in which actors partake in the formulation of policy, can be understood as the policy cycle. This cycle, as described by Baumgartner & Jones, includes agenda setting, policy formulation, budgeting, implementation, evaluation, and modification or termination of policy (2008). Actors participate at each stage of the policy cycle in order to advocate for its own interests – this often results in policy that is messy (Baumgartner, & Jones, 2008; Patel & Rushefsky, 2006).

Institutions

The United States turns to its Constitution to determine the legitimacy of a policy, and indeed, help in formulating policy. The Constitution devised a government with three branches so that not one branch would have too much power. The result of this arrangement was that the Executive, Legislative (composed of a House of Representatives and a Senate), and Judicial branches had a separation of power and a means by which they could check and balance the power of the other branches. The set-up of these somewhat coequal branches of government sharing power leads to a political environment that creates competition. As a result, if there is one party in control of the Executive branch, and a different part in control of the Legislative branch, gridlock may occur. Moreover, the fierce competition for preeminence in policy arenas can make it difficult to formulate consistent, comprehensive policies, especially in the area of health policy (Baumgartner & Jones, 2008). Equally important, policies must hold up to the spirit and values of the United States Constitution, or face the chopping block of the Supreme Court. It is clear then, that the creation of policy in the United States is highly dependent upon the constitutional environment of the health policy process.

The political environment is also focused on the Congress. Congress is the legislative body, in other words, Congress is who produces policy. Congress itself is a highly decentralized body. Several committees and subcommittees exist in both the House of Representatives and the Senate. It is in these committees that questions are asked, solutions are examined, and policies get proposed before being voted on by the chamber as a whole (Oleszek 2014).

If a bill gets through committee and is actually brought to a vote, there are still barriers to passage. Congress is currently experiencing unprecedented polarization in Congress, which makes even more difficult for members to agree on any bill, let alone a bill as controversial as health reform.

Politics

With all the partisanship, and incentives to represent interests, it is certainly difficult to enact any substantial policy changes. There are a few theories as to how policies are actually passed and implemented. The theory of *incrementalism* suggests that policy makers prefer policies that change small aspects of an existing bill instead of comprehensive change. A policymaker may choose these smaller incremental changes as a way to reduce the potential fall out of a negative impact, or other politically risky consequence. The cost of this type of decision-making can be the lack of new or creative ways to solve problems (Rosenbaum, 1985). Consensus or coalition building is often key in incrementalism. The process by which conflicting interests and values come together is tricky. Logrolling (trading votes) is a common tactic, so too is pork-barrel politics (directing government projects to a legislator's home district). These types of coalitions and trades can result in a policy that looks drastically different from its original form.

Herbert Simon, an American political scientist, sums up the theory as "satisficing." In other words, Congress seeks to "satisfy" certain interests with a solution that "suffices," or meets some minimum acceptable level.

Perhaps the most intuitive and certainly the most dramatized political aspect of policy making is the electoral cycle. In this view, policy decisions are calculated based on potential electoral consequences. No doubt, this mentality is especially true around elections. In short, Patel & Rushefsky describe this policymaking process as "drive by the need to produce short-term tangible benefits."

Nonprofits

Lastly, it is important to know a little about what nonprofits are. Nonprofits are exactly that, institutions that do not earn a profit. Nonprofits may, however, have an operating surplus, but the extra earnings are reinvested into the organization in order to support future programs or services. This is uniquely different from the private sector, where profits are dispersed to shareholders. The nonprofit sector is also different from the public sector, that of the government, which is why nonprofits are sometimes referred to as the *third sector*.

In order to better understand the difference between the private sector, the public sector, and the third sector, let us examine the services they provide. The private sector is the marketplace. In the market place, producers create goods and supply them to a consumer, who wants the goods – as long as the consumer can pay the price, they get the good. Indeed, the market regulates prices for services, because the producers who are seeking to make a profit, can only charge as much as a consumer is willing to spend for an item, or risk another competitor providing the good at a lower cost.

According to Sargeant & Sheng (2010), the public sector varies from the private sector in that the public sector provides services that are important to society, but that do not generate enough profit to make it worthwhile for an individual to create and maintain the service. These institutions are provided for and funded by the government.

There are of course those services that do not enjoy popular support and thus taxpayers (who are also voters) are not willing to fund. As a result, only some fundamental human needs can be provided for through the public sector. This creates a gap where there are important human needs that need to be met, but are not being provided for by either the private or public sector. That is where nonprofits step in. Nonprofits operate by collecting money from government institutions (in the form of grants, and in the case of 501(c)3 organizations tax exemptions), corporations, and individuals and then putting that money towards services and programs that are not currently being tended to by either the market or government. For the purposes of this chapter, only 501(c)3 organizations will be considered.

A 501(c)3 is a specific type of tax exempt nonprofit organization. Those nonprofits who designated as 501(c)3 organizations by the Internal Revenue Service (IRS) are often called "charitable organizations" or "public charities." The IRS sets strict rules on organizations that receive tax-exempt status. First, the organization must benefit the public interest, and not private shareholders. Additionally, net earnings must be reinvested into the nonprofit itself, to help provide more programs and services. Lastly, and perhaps most importantly, 501(c)3 organizations are restricted in the amount of legislative activities they participate in (IRS.gov). It is important to remember that 501(c)3s are allowed to participate in advocacy and legislative activities; they *are not* allowed to spend a majority of their time or money focused on this activities. Examples of 501(c3) organizations are: churches, hospitals, colleges & universities (IRS).

In sum, through understanding how the United States health care system is viewed, the nature of the gaps that exist, the environment in which health policy is created, and what nonprofits are, it is possible to delve into the issues, problems, and controversies surrounding health care, and the role that nonprofits have in solving these problems.

BRIDGING THE GAPS

Issues

The goal of the Affordable Care Act (ACA) was to provide quality, affordable health care to all Americans. Even with this new law, there are still many gaps that exist in the current health care system. Moreover, the gaps that exist are affecting the most disadvantaged citizens, minorities. The ACA focuses its efforts on equality of health care, specifically on the issue of insurance. The issue of equity in health care is currently not addressed and is a main reason why the ACA leaves many chasms for the most disadvantaged members of society to fall into.

Let's expand on each of these issues more broadly. First, we will consider some of the gaps that exist, next an examination of what the ACA actually accomplished, followed by the means by which the ACA set out to provide quality affordable health care, and lastly an examination of the principles of equality and equity within the ACA.

Minorities and those in low-income groups generally do not have the same access to health care as their white and/or wealthier counterparts (Byrd and Clayton, 2003). This has been a historical trend in American health care, but it is important to remember that this is not true for every single person who is a minority or living in poverty. Complicating the issue is the fact that in general, minority groups have a host of other disadvantages: lower education level, higher crime rates, and high unemployment rates. Not only can all these factors influence health, it is also likely that these rates have more to do with poverty than they do race (Committee on the Consequences of Uninsurance, 2002).

According to the Bureau of the Census 2004, minorities are more likely to be uninsured than non-minorities. For example, 19.5 percent of African Americans were uninsured as compared to 11.1 percent of non-Hispanic whites. Moreover 18.7 percent of Asians and a staggering 32.7 percent of Hispanics were uninsured in 2003.

In addition to being uninsured, age-adjusted death rates are higher for minorities than whites. The lack of access to health care begins before birth as minorities often have less access to prenatal care (National Center for Health

Statistics 2004). Related to prenatal care is the issue of birth weight, and premature birth; according to a 2003 Agency for Health Care Research and Quality study, minorities have higher rates of low-birth weight and premature births. Low birth weight, and premature birth are also risk factors for infant mortality, so it is no surprise that minorities also have higher rates of infant mortality. The same study also shows that access to health care does not improve after birth – minorities are also less likely to receive all their vaccinations. Additionally, the study also found that for minority women, the statistics are even more daunting. For example, the study found that minority women are less likely to screenings (such as pap smears or mammograms), and that minorities with breast cancer are "less likely to receive surgery and more likely to receive no treatment than whites" (Patel & Rushefsky, 2006).

An additional problem for minorities, in particular Blacks, is chronic illness. Unlike their white counterparts, Blacks often go longer without diagnosis and without treatment – this has the obvious consequence of increase mortality rates. Generally speaking, the earlier a person is diagnosed and can start treatment, the more effective that treatment is. More alarming is that even after a treatment has begun, Blacks often receive less aggressive interventions than their white counterparts (U.S. Department of Health and Human Services, 1991).

While the U.S. Department of Health and Human Services "Health Status of Minorities and Low-Income Groups" report may seem out of date, being printed in 1991, but unfortunately, the findings still hold true. Even when all other variables are held constant (insurance status, income, socioeconomic status, etc.) racial minorities are still "less likely to be given appropriate cardiac medications or to undergo bypass surgery, and are less likely to receive kidney dialysis or transplants. By contrast, they are more likely to receive less desirable procedures, such as lower limb amputations for diabetes and other conditions" (Smedley, Stith, & Nelson, 2003).

Indeed, a study as recent as 2013 has also concluded that minorities are still facing barriers to health care and health inequities. According to Cesare, et. al, those of low socioeconomic status, or those who live in impoverished communities "have a higher risk of dying from non-communicable diseases (NCDs) than do more advantaged groups and communities." The authors even suggest ways to combat NCDs in these communities; they include strategies that may seem odd, considering they suggest early childhood development programs (and other improvements to education, as well as employment changes, instead of strictly medical tactics. The authors note that improving education, and removing barriers to secure employment will help begin to remove some of the educational and financial barriers to health care. Moreover, the authors argue for universal insurance to help further reduce these financial burdens.

Given that the ACA seeks to remedy many of these barriers to accessing quality affordable health care, what can be said about President Obama's attempt to solve these problems through the ACA? The Democrats and Congress did make a noble effort to expand health insurance. The logic was that through expanding health insurance, more people would have the access needed to acquire medical services, but what did the ACA really do?

The entire reform is itself some 400,000 words, and to fully explain the law itself would be a book in itself. For the purposes of this chapter, painting with broad strokes will suffice. Put simply, the ACA did three things. First, it expanded health care coverage. It also put some regulations on the insurance companies. Third, it changed taxes in order to provide funding.

In terms of expanding coverage, the Congressional Budget Office (CBO) estimates that about 32 million more people will health insurance of some form or another by 2019. None of this coverage will come from a public option, that is, government insurance program. The pubic option, which was talked about when the administration was pushing health reform, did not make the final bill. Instead, the expansion comes in several ways. Part of the expanded coverage comes from lowering eligibility standards for Medicaid. The main way that Medicaid expansion worked was through making those without children eligible for coverage. Overall, the CBO estimates that some 16 million additional people will be covered through Medicaid.

As an important side note, for the first five years of Medicaid expansion, the federal government will foot the bill. This is different from the usual way Medicaid is paid for, which is a split between the federal government and the state (Reid, 2010).

The new law also plans to increase the number of people with health insurance through insurance exchanges. These exchanges, run by either the state or the federal government, will provide five levels of coverage: "bronze," "silver," "gold," "platinum," and "catastrophic." The various plans are meant to give those in looking for insurance, a choice insurance options to meet their needs (Reid, 2010).

For those who were unable to afford insurance, the exchanges help provide a range of coverage options that may fit a person's budget. If however one is still unable to afford coverage, the government offers tax credits that are meant to help offset the cost of insurance. In addition to setting up exchanges, the ACA also helps provide coverage through employer based insurance programs.

Those companies that have more than forty-nine people on payroll are required to provide an insurance plan to employees. Like those looking to buy insurance, but need help offsetting the costs, the federal government offers tax credits to small employers to help them provide insurance.

In terms of regulating insurance companies, the ACA made it illegal to deny insurance to someone with a preexisting condition. In order to accommodate taking on a higher risk pool, those with preexisting conditions, the ACA required that everyone buy insurance under what is known as the individual mandate. It is no surprise that healthy individuals may not feel the need to purchase insurance, even if it is mandated. There is a penalty for not purchasing insurance, though the penalty may not be enough to dissuade people from dodging the mandate. The penalties ramp up, so the penalty for not having coverage in 2014 is one-percent of yearly household income or $95 per person for the year ($47.50 per child under 18 years of age) – whichever is higher. The penalty in 2015 will be 2% of yearly household income, or $325 per person for the year ($162.50 per child under 18), whichever is higher. In 2016, the cost of the penalty will be 2.5% of income or $695 per person. After 2016, the cost is adjusted for inflation (healthcare.gov).

A portion of the new health care law was designed to fund the law itself. The Congressional Budget Office (CBO) put the cost of the reform at around $940 billion for the first ten years. This is no pocket change, and thus Congress had to create new taxes and fees in order to fund the policy. Some of the ways the ACA is funded are: a new Medicare tax (earning more than $200,000 per year) can except the tax paid on Medicare to be raised to about 3.8 percent. The law also taxes pharmaceutical companies, health insurance companies, and medical device manufacturers. Additionally, the law will be funded through the abovementioned penalties.

From the strategies the ACA employs to bring about this quality, affordable health care, it is clear that Congress was focusing on the issue of *equality* of health care. By changing the way people obtain insurance, and the eligibility requirements for government run programs such as Medicaid, the law sought to give more people the opportunity to receive health care despite the ability to pay for medical care. The notion that everyone should be able to obtain health care regardless of age, gender, income, etc. is the key principle of equality we discussed earlier. The question remains, did the ACA meet this goal? The answer is not so clear.

While the many more people will have health insurance thanks to the new law, the CBO predicted that 23 million Americans would still be uninsured in 2019. Other countries, such as the United States' neighbor to the north, Canada, provide universal coverage to every citizen. Similarly, most other developed countries provide similar equality of coverage (Reid, 2010).

Despite the campaigning of the health reform law taking a social justice tone, the ACA did little to solve the inequities in the health care system. As noted above, minorities and in particular racial minorities, still receive less adequate medical care and treatment than whites. Indeed, Brown et al., Cesare et al., and Gornick et al., noted that insurance is not enough. Gornick et al.: state that race and income have substantial effects on mortality and use of services among Medicare beneficiaries. Providing health insurance is not enough to ensure that the program is equitable for all beneficiaries. This is especially important because Medicare provides universal coverage to all those 65 years or older, so the study can highlight the inequalities and inequities within the health care system by holding type of insurance coverage constant. Additionally, to ensure that there is equal *and* equitable treatment, other barriers besides insurance must be addressed. Areas such as patient and provider communication, health literacy, language barriers, culture, social support, and transportation must be addressed (Brown, Ettner, & Piette, 2004).

CONTROVERSIES

There are several controversies surrounding the ACA in particular, and health reform more broadly. As previously mentioned, there are many key players in health care reform: the insurance industry, the government (state, local, federal), patients, doctors, pharmaceutical manufacturers, and medical device companies, to name a few. Each of these actors has specific, and often competing interests. In order to reconcile these competing interests, logrolling, pork barreling, and satisficing occurs. Accordingly, the ACA went through many iterations before coming to its final form, for example, the proposed public option for insurance was struck out of final version of the ACA.

President Obama's health reform also faced a Congress that was deeply divided. The Democrats in Congress pushed through the reform on sheer will alone. In fact, not one Republican, House or Senate, signed the final copy of the ACA (Devins, 2012). There is also a lack of buy-in from the states – Kaiser Health News notes that there are only 36 states participating in the health exchanges. Additionally, according to Congressional records, the Republicans in Congress have tried to repeal or change the ACA over fifty times. Furthermore, according to the Pew Research Center, Congress is more polarized than ever, and so are the people who elected them.

At the heart of the controversy is a not a battle of whether or not people should receive health care, but rather, it is a battle of ideology. The Democrats believe that government has a responsibility to provide health care for the people, and that government should play a crucial role in helping the American people attain quality, affordable health care. The Republicans, however, believe that while Americans should have access to quality, affordable health care, they often believe that the federal government does not have a role to play.

With both the government and voters becoming ever more polarized, and fundamental disagreements about the role of government in health care reform, the question remains: how do we solve the problems in health care with a plan that brings both sides of the aisle together?

PROBLEMS

The problems in solving health care are tightly tied to the controversies of health reform. No doubt partisan polarization only exacerbated the tensions between the actors in health care policymaking. In addition to the controversies that exist, there are a few other key problems that are causing our health care system to fail. First, health care in the United States is very expensive. As we noted, the United States already spends the most on health care. The cost of medical procedures, hospital stays, and prescription drugs all cost more in the United States than they do in other countries like France or Canada (Reid, 2010). Moreover, doctors in the United States pay more for medical school than their counterparts overseas. So too, U.S. doctors pay more in malpractice insurance.

Then there are the insurance companies. Insurance companies in the United States are generally for-profit companies, that is, they exist to make money. Reid, 2010 points out that the language health insurance companies use highlights the mentality of the industry: "the money paid to doctors, hospitals, and pharmacies for treatment of insured patients is referred to as a 'medical loss'" (p.37). The insurance companies see paying for treatments as cutting into the overall profit of the company. No other developed country views insurance and payment for services in this way.

While the ACA does cap administrative costs for private insurers at around 15 to 20 percent, it is still high when compared to British and Canadian insurance companies who only spend about five percent on administrative costs (Reid, 2010). United State health insurance companies may also deny claims, which is no doubt helpful for insurance companies looking to make a profit. While the ACA does make changes, both denying coverage for preexisting conditions, and the practice of rescission, and putting caps on payments, are no longer allowed, insurance companies are still allowed to deny claims. Lastly, the United States still links insurance to employment, so if a person loses her job, she loses her coverage.

Another problem for health insurance companies, and the heath care system in general is that there are still barriers for minorities. Even with the ACA, a lack of cultural competency pervades the American health care system (Caccioppoli, 2014). Without insurance companies and health care providers addressing issues of culture, the United States will continue to provide services that are unequal and inequitable.

SOLUTIONS AND RECOMMENDATIONS

The potential solution to the United States' health care ailments must be one that is founded on the principles of equality *and* equity. As the literature has shown, equality without equity maintains the current gaps in the health care system while giving the illusion of a more just health care system. Next, the solution must acknowledge the key actors and engage in the policymaking process. Lastly, the solution must acknowledge the tumultuous state of American politics.

While it would be very bold indeed to say that this chapter has *the* solution, there is reason to believe that nonprofits will be a critical element in the solution.

A key component to solving these problems is the use of nonprofits, specifically, 501(c)3s. It may seem strange, however nonprofits have the potential to address equality of health care, issues of equity, and engage in all levels of policymaking and implementation. Furthermore, nonprofits are able to skirt around much of the controversy, making them more likely to be embraced by both Democrats and Republicans.

To begin, nonprofits have been a fabric of the American identity and an alternative to government since the nation's founding. French political philosopher Alexis de Toucqueville noted the importance of associations (which are nonprofits), during his visit to America in the 1830s:

Americans of all ages, all conditions, and all dispositions constantly form associations. They have not only commercial and manufacturing companies, in which all take part, but associations of a thousand other kinds, religious, moral serious, futile, general or restricted, enormous or diminutive. The Americans make associations to give entertainments, to found seminaries, to build inns, to construct churches, to diffuse books, to send missionaries to the antipodes; in this manner they found hospitals, prisons, and schools. If it is proposed to inculcate some truth or foster some feeling by the encouragement of a great example, they form a society. Wherever at the head of some new undertaking you see the government in France, or a man of rank in England, in the United States you will be sure to find an association. (Tocqueville, [1835] 1945, II p.106)

In his travels through the new, young republic of the United States in the 1830s, Tocqueville found that associations, or nonprofits, were responsible for stepping in where the government or private interests did not. All members of the society utilized associations of one form or another, and indeed care for people with disabilities, education, and healing were provided for through these associations.

Politics and Cost

Regarding partisan polarization, both Democrats and Republicans can get behind the use of nonprofits. For Democrats, the key issue is providing quality, affordable health care. Many Democrats feel that the private sector is unable to bring costs down to a level where all persons are able to participate in the health care system. Nonprofit organizations have the potential to drastically reduce costs because the emphasis is not on making profits. For Republicans, there is no sacrificing of principles. Rather than government stepping in to ensure health care, nonprofits will assume the role, which means there is no threat of government encroachment. Some more conservative individuals may try to argue that nonprofits will kill the market element, which is another fundamental value of republicans. This is simply not true. When examining other developed countries that utilize nonprofits as a cost effective measure, such as Germany, insurance companies are private nonprofit agencies (Reid, 2010). These nonprofit agencies are still able to compete for customers, by offering additional services, or selling supplemental insurance packages etc. Additionally, it does not mean that there are not some health care professionals that operate for-profit businesses. While the market may look different, there are still the common principles and elements that will remain unchanged even with the implementation of nonprofits.

Furthermore, the United States already attempted to utilize the private sector to help reduce health care costs. The managed care revolution, private sectors competing for government contracts, and H.M.O.s, did not end up reducing overall health care costs (Berenson, 2008). It is also true that other countries have had success in utilizing nonprofits to help manage costs and provide more equitable access to health care services. Whether looking at Canada, Germany, France, or Britain – or looking East to Japan, one thing is clear, these countries are spending less money and providing better quality health care to more of its citizens; and the care is distributed more justly (OECD; WHO; Reid, 2010). In fact, some states have already seen that nonprofits can be a viable solution to improving health care. A 2011 bipartisan report from the Connecticut Commission on Nonprofit Health and Human Services has recommended and advocated for the use of nonprofits to help reduce health care costs and to better provide for Connecticut's most vulnerable populations. The report also notes that nonprofits are also better than the government at providing these services, which are not provided for by the private.

Equity

What about the issue of equity?

Earlier, it was noted that one of the biggest inequities in the United States' health system is the lack of physicians and health care services in low-income communities. The main reason for this was that it is not necessarily the most profitable for physicians to accept Medicaid, or to serve in less affluent areas. The result is that the most vulnerable members of society, even with insurance, often go without necessary health care and treatments. Unlike for-profit ventures, nonprofits do not look to make profits to pass on to shareholders. Nonprofits can utilize fee-for-service methods to both sustain themselves, and attempt to build extra earnings that can be utilized to help offset the costs for those who cannot pay.

Moreover, nonprofits have the potential to provide unique culturally competent health care services to specific populations. The rollout of the ACA notably failed at engaging one of the fastest growing demographics in the United States, the Latino community (Caccioppoli, 2014). Without a culturally competent campaign to get Latinos health insurance coverage, the federal government missed a huge opportunity to provide health insurance to a group that might otherwise not be able to afford coverage. As previously mentioned, there is clear racial and ethnic discrimination going on in the American health care system, such as minorities receiving less adequate, or aggressive treatments for the same ailments as whites. Culturally competent care is critical if equitable care is to be provided.

Culturally competent care, and equitable treatment does not necessarily need to take place at the hospital or insurance level, although, they certainly should. Nonprofits can also occupy a specific niche. Consider the National Multiple Sclerosis Society (NMSS), a nonprofit dedicated to eliminating multiple sclerosis, through research and advocacy. The NMSS also works to provide services for all those affected by multiple sclerosis, including family members, caregivers, etc. The NMSS and organizations like it provide a valuable alternative resource for health care users. The NMSS helps provide services like funding for research. It also unites those affected by multiple sclerosis – leading to innovative solutions such as members of the society donating their old walkers or wheelchairs (that they can no longer use due to progression of the disease, or the death of a loved one), so that a person who could not afford the item will still have access to a necessary assistive device.

Surplus is only one aspect of calculating the performance of a nonprofit, they also consider fulfillment of their mission statement. As a result, a nonprofit with a mission to provide quality health care to low-income African American women in Northeast Philadelphia, may have more of an incentive to create a transport service that helps women get to and from appointments. Since any surplus earned by the nonprofit has to be reinvested into the organization, nonprofits also have the opportunity to expand and improve upon existing programs.

Perhaps most importantly, nonprofits (especially high impact nonprofits) also engage in advocacy. Crutchfield and Grant, note in their updated 2012 book, *Forces for Good*, that nonprofits mobilize members and provide the political clout needed to make real social changes, particularly through advocacy. The more nonprofits advocate, the better they can serve. The authors go on to note that if nonprofits are to be successful in both their advocacy and service delivery, they must act in ways that are bipartisan, as that is the only way they will gain the necessary support for their endeavors. The ability for nonprofits to advocate means that the constituents they serve will be well represented in Congress. Moreover, it means that all people including the most vulnerable will have a seat at the policymaking table. For racial minorities, or those with chronic illness, having a seat at the table will mean that policies will be designed with their needs in mind – and overtime, more culturally competent service delivery will provided.

FUTURE RESEARCH DIRECTIONS

Research on minorities and healthcare typically focuses on the problems, not the solutions. Likewise, most of the research regarding health care reform focuses on the failings of the private and public sector, and not on the potential of the third sector. Public health and epidemiological studies have repeatedly shown that addressing issues of equity, such as health literacy, education, transportation, etc. has a real impact on the overall health of a community. Knowing that nonprofits have already begun to address these issues indicates that increased support and partnership with local or state governments can provide insights into the ways in which nonprofits can truly improve American health care. Until more nonprofits begin to collaborate with state and local governments, it will be necessary to explore the way other countries utilize nonprofits.

CONCLUSION

The United States health care system is currently facing many ailments. From skyrocketing costs, to a lack of return on the spending, the health care system is in crisis. The Patient Protection and Affordable Care Act, President Obama's signature legislation, begins to address some of the issues of equality in the health care system, but does not provide the truly comprehensive health reform it touted. For minorities, access to quality, affordable healthcare is still difficult. Doctors often have a small presence, if any, in low-income neighborhoods. Women, and racial minorities face discrimination in the system even with health insurance; for those without coverage, the situation is even worse. To complicate matters, the political environment in which healthcare policy is made is complicated to say the least. With numerous actors and interests, creating and passing comprehensive health care reform is difficult. Furthermore, partisan polarization in the United States Congress is at an all time high. With representatives and senators voting along their party's ideological lines, only a truly bipartisan solution will survive.

Nonprofits have the potential to be this solution. Unlike the private sector, which failed at its chance to improve health care, the nonprofit sector does not seek to fill the pockets of shareholders. This allows nonprofits to focus on providing quality care and fulfilling its mission. Unlike the private sector, nonprofits have no incentive to deny claims, or discriminate against those insured. Moreover, nonprofits are able to perform these services at significantly lower costs than the private sector – as evidenced by other countries, and innovative solutions from the state of Connecticut.

In addition to reducing overall health costs and providing a more equal health care system, nonprofits have the potential to address the issue of equity. Nonprofits use surplus money to expand programs, and experiment with new ways to provide better services to their constituents. Furthermore, nonprofits mobilize their constituents to help them engage in the policymaking process.

REFERENCES

Affordable Care Act. (2010). Retrieved October 14, 2014, from http://hhs.gov/healthcare/rights/law/index.html

Baumgartner, F. R., & Jones, B. D. (2008). *Agendas and Instability in American Politics*. Chicago: University of Chicago Press.

Berenson, R. (2008). Health Affairs. *Medicare Advantage Plans at a Crossroads-Yet Again.* Retrieved October 14, 2014, from http://content.healthaffairs.org/content/28/1/w29.full

Berk, M. L., & Schur, C. L. (1998). Access to care how much difference does medicaid make. *Health Affairs*, *17*(3), 169–180. doi:10.1377/hlthaff.17.3.169 PMID:9637973

Blendon, R. (2001). The public versus the world health organization. *Health Affairs*, 18. PMID:11585157

Broyles, R. W., Lutchmie, N., & Brandt, E. N. Jr. (2002). The temporarily and chronically uninsured: Does their use of primary care differ? *Journal of Health Care for the Poor and Underserved*, *13*(1), 95–111. doi:10.1353/hpu.2010.0159 PMID:11836917

Caccioppoli, L. (2014). Cultural competency and the rollout of the affordable care act. *PA Times Online.* Retrieved October 14, 2014, from: http://patimes.org/cultural-competency-rollout-affordable-care-act/

Census. (2004). *Health Insurance.* Retrieved October 14, 2014, from http://www.census.gov/hhes/www/hlthins/hlthins.html

Cesare, M. D., Marmot, M. G., Blakely, T., Asaria, P., Khang, Y., & Ezzati, M. (2013). Inequalities in non-communicable diseases and effective responses. *Lancet, 381*(9866), 585–597. doi:10.1016/S0140-6736(12)61851-0 PMID:23410608

Childrens Defense Fund. (2012). *Uninsured children.* Retrieved October 14, 2014, from http://www.childrensdefense.org/policy-priorities/children-health/uninsured-children/

Collins, S. R., Davids, K., Doty, M., & Ho, A. (2004). *Wages, benefits, and workers' health.* New York: The Commonwealth Fund. Congressional Budget Office. Cost estimates for health care legislation. Congressional Budget Office. Retrieved October 14, 2014 from http://www.cbo.gov/publications/collections

Commission on Nonprofit Health and Human Services. (2011). *State of Connecticut.* Retrieved October 14, 2014, from http://ct.gov/opm/lib/opm/finance/hhs_commission/final_report_comission_on_nonprofit_health_and_human_services.pdf

Committee on the Consequences of Uninsurance. (2002). *Institute of Medicine. Care Without Coverage: Too Little, Too Late.* Washington, DC: National Academy Press.

Crutchfield, L. R., & Grant, H. M. (2008). *Forces For Good: the six practices of high-impact nonprofits.* San Francisco: Jossey-Bass.

de Tocqueville, A. (1945). *Democracy in America* (Vol. 2). (H. Reeve, Trans.). New York: Random House. (orig. publ. 1835)

Devins, N. (2012). Party polarization and judicial review: Lessons learned from the affordable care act. *Northwestern University Law Review, 106*(4), 1821–1848. Retrieved from http://www.law.northwestern.edu/depts/legalpub/lawreview/v106/n4/1821/LR106n4Devins.pdf

Enthoven, A. (2003). Employment-based health insurance is failing: Now what? *Health Affairs.* doi:10.1377/hlthaff.w3.237 PMID:14527258

Fairbrother, G., Gusmano, M. K., Park, H. L., & Scheinmann, R. (2003). Care for the uninsured in general internists' private offices. *Health Affairs, 22*(6), 217–264. doi:10.1377/hlthaff.22.6.217 PMID:14649449

Galewitz, P. (n.d.). *Most states to rely on federal website for 2015 enrollment*. Kaiser Health News. Retrieved October 14, 2014, from http://www.kaiserhealthnews.org/stories/2014/april/24/two-states-likely-to-set-up-own-exchange-for-2015.aspx

Gornick, M. E., Eggers, P. W., Reilly, T. W., Mentnech, R. M., Fitterman, L. K., Kucken, L. E., & Vladeck, B. C. (1996). Effects of race and income on mortality and use of services among medicare. *The New England Journal of Medicine*, *335*(11), 791–799. doi:10.1056/NEJM199609123351106 PMID:8703185

HealthCare.gov. (2014). Fees you pay if you don't have health insurance coverage. *HealthCare.gov*. Retrieved October 12, 2014, from http://www.healthcare.gov/fees-exemptions/fee-for-not-being-covered/

Hoffman, C., Carbaugh, A., & Cook, A. (2004). *Health insurance coverage in america: 2003 data update*. Washington, DC: Kaiser Commission on Medicaid and the Uninsured.

Hoffman, C., Schoen, C., Rowland, D., & Davis, K. (2001). Gaps in health coverage among worker-age americans and the consequences. *Journal of Health Care for the Poor and Underserved*, *12*(3), 272–289. doi:10.1353/hpu.2010.0739 PMID:11475546

IRS.gov. (2014). Exemption requirements – 501(c)3 organizations. *IRS.gov*. Retrieved October 14, 2014, from http://www.irs.gov/charities-&-non-profits/charitabale-organizations/exemption-requirements-section-501%28c%29%283%29-Organizations

Jecker, N. (1993). Can an employer-based health insurance system be just? *Journal of Health Care Politics. Policy and Law*, *18*(3), 657–673.

Krause, E. A. (1977). *Power and illness: the political sociology of health and medical care*. New York: Elsevier.

Lambert, J. (2013, December 10). *NPQ. Infographic: what is driving nonprofit sector's growth?* Retrieved October 13, 2014, from https://nonprofitquarterly.org/policysocial-context/23359-infographic-what-is-driving-nonprofit-sectors-growth.html

Long, S. K. (2003). *Hardship among the uninsured: choosing among food, housing and health insurance. New Federalism*. Washington, DC: The Urban Institute.

Myott, S. (2010). 2009 *County Long-Term Care Gaps Analysis Survey*. Department of Human Services Continuing Care Administration. Retrieved October 14, 2014, from http://dhs.state.mn.us/main/groups/aging/documents/pub/dhs16_153750.pdf

National Center for Health Statistics. (2004). *Health United States 2004*. Hyattsville, MD: Centers for Disease Control and Prevention, U.S. Department of Health and Human Services.

National Multiple Sclerosis Society. (2014). *Home*. Retrieved October 12, 2014, from http://www.nationalmssociety.org/

OECD. (2013). *Health at a Glance 2013*. Retrieved October 14, 2014 from http://oecd.org/els/health-systems/health-at-a-glance-2013.pdf

Oleszek, W. J. (2014). *Congressional Procedures and the Policy Process*. Washington: Congressional Quarterly Press.

Patel, K., & Rushefsky, M. E. (1995). *Health Care Politics and Policy in America*. Armonk, NY: M.E. Sharpe.

Pew Research Center. (2013). *Partisan polarization in congress and among public is greater than ever*. Retrieved October 14, 2014, from http://www.pewresearch.org/fact-tank/2013/07/17/partisan-polarization-in-congress-and-among-public-is-greater-than-ever/

Politico. (2014). *Protecting the sick? Not so easy*. Retrieved October 14, 2014, from http://www.politico.com/story/2014/08/insurance-discrimination-obamacare-110095.html

Porter, E. (2013). Health care and profits, a poor mix. *The New York Times*. Retrieved October 14, 2014, from http://www.nytimes.com/2013/01/09/business/health-care-and-pursuit-of-profit-make-a-poor-mix.html?pagewanted=all&_r=0

Reid, T. R. (2010). *The Healing of America: a global quest for better, cheaper, fairer health care*. New York: Penguin Press.

Rosenbaum, W.A. (1985). *Environmental Politics and Policy*. Washington, DC: CQ Press.

Sargeant, A., & Shang, J. (2010). *Fundraising Principles and Practice*. San Francisco: Jossey-Bass.

Smedley, B. D., Stith, A. Y., & Nelson, A. R. (2003). *Racial and Ethnic Disparities in Healthcare: a Background and History. In Unequal Treatment: Confronting Racial and Ethnic Disparities in Health Care* (pp. 455–527). Washington, DC: National Academy Press.

Smedley, B. D., Stith, A. Y., & Nelson, A. R. (2003). *Unequal Treatment Confronting Racial and Ethnic Disparities in Health Care*. Washington, DC: National Academies Press.

Stoddard, J., St. Peter, R., & Newacheck, P. (1994). Health insurance status and ambulatory care for children. *The New England Journal of Medicine, 330*(20), 1421–1425. doi:10.1056/NEJM199405193302006 PMID:8159197

Tandon, A., Murray, C. J. L., & Evans, D. (2000). *Measuring overall health system performance for 191 countries*. World Health Organization.

U.S. Department of Health and Human Services. (1991). *Health Status of Minorities and Low Income Groups* (3rd ed.). Washington, DC: U.S. Government Printing Office.

Watson, S. (1994). Minority access and health reform: A civil right to health care. *The Journal of Law, Medicine & Ethics, 22*(2), 127–137. doi:10.1111/j.1748-720X.1994.tb01285.x PMID:7921079

KEY TERMS AND DEFINITIONS

Advocacy: The process by which a group of people acts and engages the political process to create change.

Affordable Care Act: President Barack Obama's signature health care law, signed in 2010 and sought to provide Americans with quality, affordable health care.

Communicable: To be transmitted from one to another, especially regarding disease.

Cultural Competency: A theory and practice that focuses on addressing, acknowledging, and appreciating cultural diversity.

Equality: The act of treating people the same.

Equity: Related to equality but adds the social justice element of providing those with disadvantages the opportunities needed to overcome those disadvantages.

Nonprofit: An Internal Revenue Service designation for an organization that does not seek profit, but rather, reinvests earnings back into the organization.

Chapter 12
Redesigning the Organizational Structure to Reach Efficiency:
The Case of Ministry of Health and Medical Education of Iran

Mohammad Arabi
University of Allameh, Iran

ABSTRACT

The structure of an organization requires partial modification or even total redesigning due to the changes in missions, strategies, policies and objectives once environmental and technological changes take place. This evolutionary redesign and implementation of its plan can have the maximum effectiveness and efficiency when all aspects and components of a coherent structure are considered carefully. This research has considered redesigning the structure of the Ministry and outlines the methodology and undertaken activities in order to evolve the structure of the central department of Ministry to prove how a re-design in organizational structure followed by policy coherence can maximize the output in healthcare sector.

INTRODUCTION

Any organization requires effective and efficient leadership along with necessary requirements such as various sources in order to achieve its mission, objectives and vision. This is the main bottleneck of organizations when they are going to bring fundamental changes. From the perspective of organizational change and develop-

DOI: 10.4018/978-1-4666-9944-1.ch012

ment and related issues, the following aspects can be considered as dimensions and the main components of a comprehensive transformation of the organization:

1. Change in objectives, goals, strategies and policies.
2. Developments in science and organizational technology.
3. Development of human resources and skills, capabilities and competencies.
4. The transformation of the structures, systems and organizational systems and processes
5. Change in organizational culture.
6. And change in knowledge, attitude and style of management and leadership of managers (especially leaders and senior managers of an organization).

The last case is more important than others which is in fact a major stimulus to fulfill them.In fact, the senior managers are the ones who prepare this way to transform other pillars with having deep knowledge, competence and courage (Thurow, 1999) in the basic decision-makings and by creating necessary administrative and technical infrastructure. In the meantime, organizational structure with all its dimensions and its key components (Scott & Davis, 2005) is one of the most important tools in the hands of managers and many managerial techniques and tools can be formed based on its framework. It can even be said that it clarifies the structure, the total outline of the systems, processes, organizational relationships and responsibilities and ways of doing things.

Organizational structure in its simplest definition is the division of duties and coordination between personnel of the organization and it shows the framework of relationships governing occupations, systems and organizational processes and human resource (including individuals and groups) who try to achieve the specified goals (Scott,2005;Galbraith,1977).The structure of an organization (such as the Ministry of Health and Medical Education) requires partial revision or even total redesigning due to the changes in missions, strategies, policies and objectives once environmental and technological changes take place. This evolutionary redesign and implementation of its plan can have the maximum effectiveness and efficiency when all aspects and components of a coherent structure are considered carefully, and these components are as follows:

- Chart of organizational units (including the original chart and detailed ones).
- Duties of units (up to the lowest level of responsibility centers such as the offices, departments and units).
- Occupational structure (list of jobs and positions, job descriptions, job characteristics and qualifying conditions).
- Decision-making structure (structure assemblies, councils, committees and community centers of, decision-making, policy-making and authority).

This research outlines the methodology and undertaken activities and main results of this project in the structure of central department of Ministry. Firstly, the model and macro methodology of redesigning the structure of Ministry has been explained. Then, various main components of this model are clarified. Last but not least, the results are briefly explained in three main stages.

BACKGROUND

According to the conditions and requirements set forth by the Department of Development and Resources Management of Ministry of Health and Medical Education of Iran in 2008, the research project of "redesigning the organizational structure" was defined and its implementation began in July the same year. This project considered redesigning the structure of the Ministry in three levels of headquarters, the headquarters of universities of Medical Sciences and Health Services (as provincial branches of health Ministry and regional organizations) and the hospitals with Board of Trustees all as a single and coherent unit including the basic dimensions of an organizational structure. In order to redesign and implement the process in a scientific way, compatible with the native conditions of Ministry and current requirements of country, following entries are considered:

- Complete and accurate understanding of the situation (package 1 of questions that was sent to every units and various departments of universities and hospitals, then collected and analyzed).
- Analysis of content and structural dimensions, and also optimal architecture design variables (package 2 of questions that was completed by experts and professionals in different structural levels and was analyzed in a software system).
- Review of whole structural history of Ministry and its changes over time.
- All related laws and regulations.
- Detailed mission of Ministry (the intersection of the approximately one thousand fields of mission and offering service with more than 60 roles of strategic management and operations management).
- Investigation of the perspectives and goals and orientations and micro /macro policies of Ministry and Healthcare system in Iran.
- Benchmarking and comparative study (4 countries comprehensively;140 countries in the field of food and drug; more than 16 standards and 20 top hospitals in the field of hospital structure).
- The opinions of previous experts and managers of Ministry.
- Study of the existing problems and bottlenecks.

In the context of an integrated methodology and based on the natural models (Scott,2005)with regards to defining strategies, this structure has been applied and after designing the macro architectural structures of the Ministry of Health, detailed designing of structure in various levels has been took place. In order to provide necessary contexts to operationalize the designed structures, as well as reviewing all aspects, two subjects of " comprehensive design and definition of all dimensions of organizational structure" and also " the definition of very large and intensive interacted process with various components of Ministry(such as managers and experts of departments, universities and hospitals) are considered as two main bottlenecks that their absence is obvious in many structural processes in Iran and also definition of transition plan and settlement of structure has been included in second phase as an innovative activity to provide required conditions to execute design dimensions more and better.

This research has been conducted via three phases: In the first stage (input stage), the basic studies that were considered as input of redesigning the structure, are briefly introduced. In the second stage (processing and analysis stage), first the principles and policies adopted by the Board of Studies as input to the design principles are outlined, and two fundamental views/ approaches of designing the structure are described to the headquarters of the Ministry (the process and mission views). Then four processing elements as determining and effective basic on design outputs are explained. These four elements are:

1. Architecture of Ministry structure.
2. Models and frameworks of determining systems.
3. Organizational standards.
4. A model to determine the independent agencies of Ministry.

Finally, in the third stage (output stage); structural scenarios designed for central department of the Ministry of Health and Medical Education are presented and briefly described.

MODEL AND MACRO METHODOLOGY TO REDESIGN THE STRUCTURE

Based on what was noted in the introduction, we can now look at the model and macro methodology of project (figure 1). This model has been changed at first and in several stages of the project to meet the needs of the design group.

In Figure 1, the green color shows components of input stage; brown shows the components of processing and analysis stage and blue shows the output stage.

Figure 1. Model and methodology of structural reform

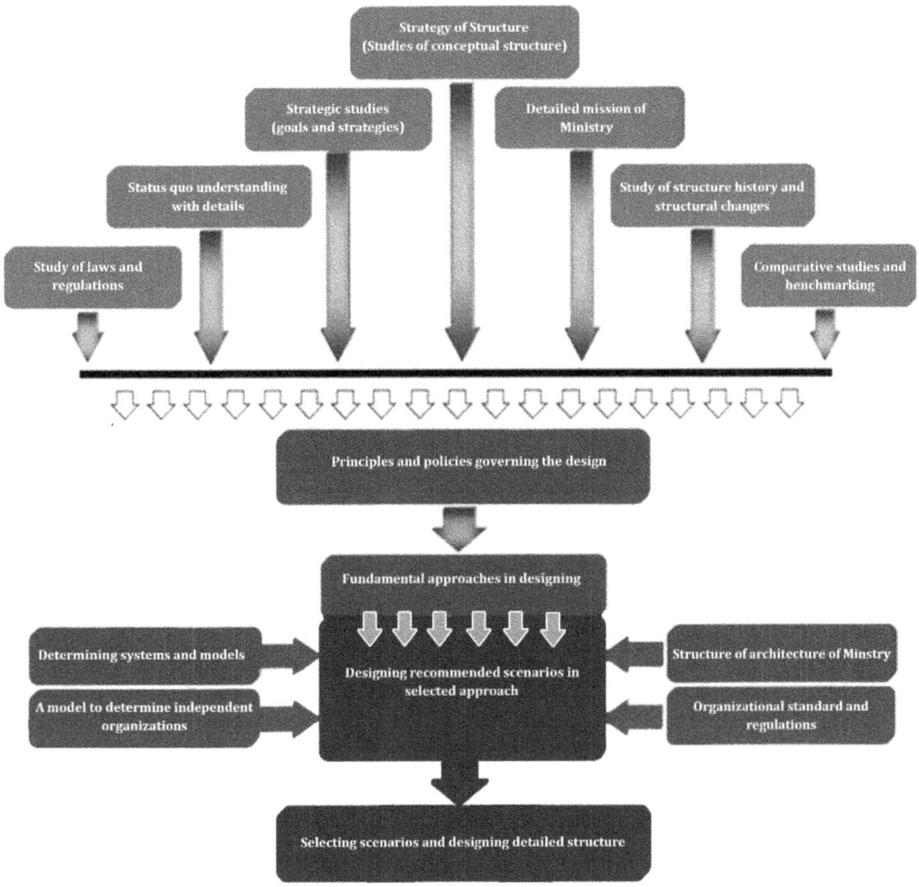

Stage I: Input

In order to extract and determine the orientation of the structure and the principles and policies that governing the design, seven major activities were planned and implemented. In this section of the paper, it is necessary to provide a brief description of these activities and their achievements. Remarkably, each of these seven activities has its own separate and detailed report and detailed methodology and among them, the activity of "determining structure strategy" or "study of conceptual structure" will be discussed a little more detailed than the rest of them.

1. Status Quo Understanding

In any action of designing or re designing or making changes in a phenomenon or an entity, the necessity of understanding the phenomenon / entity in question is obvious. In issues of organization and management, depending on which area of expertise, designing or redesigning or making changes take place; the stage of recognition takes titles such as "need assessment/need analysis", "Pathology", "Status quo understanding" or " AS-IS recognition". Status quo understanding of the structure of central department of Ministry of Health took place with the aim of understanding the existing organizational units as well as missions and duties, the available occupations and positions, both internal and external stakeholders, a list of upper hand terms, regulations and guidelines of the activities listed, list of systems used, customers and clients for every departments within the organization and also considering comments and issues and structural problems of various departments; and the following basic steps were taken:

- Designing and developing package one in four groups appropriate to the various departments (a total of 110 booklets), including:
  - **Package One-A:** Special for vice-principals (each package contains two booklets).
  - **Package One-B:** Special for vice-presidents of minister (student / coordination / Parliament) (each package contains three booklets).
  - **Package One-C:** Special for main units (centers / offices / main departments) (each package contains two booklets).
  - **Package One-D:** Special for affiliate organizations (each package contains a booklet).
- Sending packages and continued follow-up for completing them.
- Receiving and analyzing 350 completed booklets (one booklets for every organizational unit).
- Designing software system (using Excel) in order to enter related information from package one of various departments to this system and summarizing and integrating them.
- Study and analysis of information contained in the completed packages separately based on every offices and departments in headquarters and deputies.
- Holding expert meetings with more than 90% of organizational units at all levels, with the aim of:
  - Identifying current and desired tasks.
  - Knowing the volume of tasks.
  - Identifying structural problems.
  - receiving comments and suggestions.

2. Study of Laws and Regulations

In this area, collection, review and analysis of all laws, regulations and upper-hand documents related to organizational structure of organizations and ministries as well as the special rules of the Ministry of Health and Medical Education have been considered in the agenda. These laws and documents included the following major items:

- Parliament resolutions, with emphasis on:
    - Law of the Fourth Economic, Social and Cultural.
    - Development plan.
    - Civil Service Management Code.
- The approvals of the Council of Ministers, with emphasis on the administrative reform.
- Directives of Vice Presidency of Human Capital and Management Development(formerly management organization).
- The approvals of the Supreme Council with emphasis on the Supreme Council of Cultural Revolutionary and the Administrative Supreme Council.

The results included compiling a comprehensive report on the laws and regulations related to the Health Ministry structure at three levels of headquarters (central departments), universities and selected hospitals and the report of this level includes a good summation and integration of mentioned laws and regulations. For example, Civil Service Management Code has been studied as one of the most important inputs of this project. Chapter IV of this Code is in relation to the organizational structure of the administrative systems. Of important issues in this Code are:

- Article 29, paragraph (c); vertical levels at the national and provincial executive agencies, including the highest-ranking executive, is determined as follows:
    - Ministries and government institutions, maximum at 4 levels
    - Provincial units, maximum at 3 levels
- Article 29, paragraph (d); Each of the ministries that are governed by the Vice President, can expect a maximum of five deputies in their organizational structure and appropriate to the size and diversity of tasks and the number of organizational positions. Each deputy can have a maximum of 5 heads, deans, directors or similar titles.
- Article 35- All executive agencies are required to offer their proposal of organizational structure reform under the provisions of this chapter within one year.

Here there are two examples presented (figure 2 and figure 3), taken from the summation of laws and regulations and principles in order to redesign the structure of the Ministry of Health.

Figure 2. The rules and principles to redesign the structure of the Ministry of Health, part A

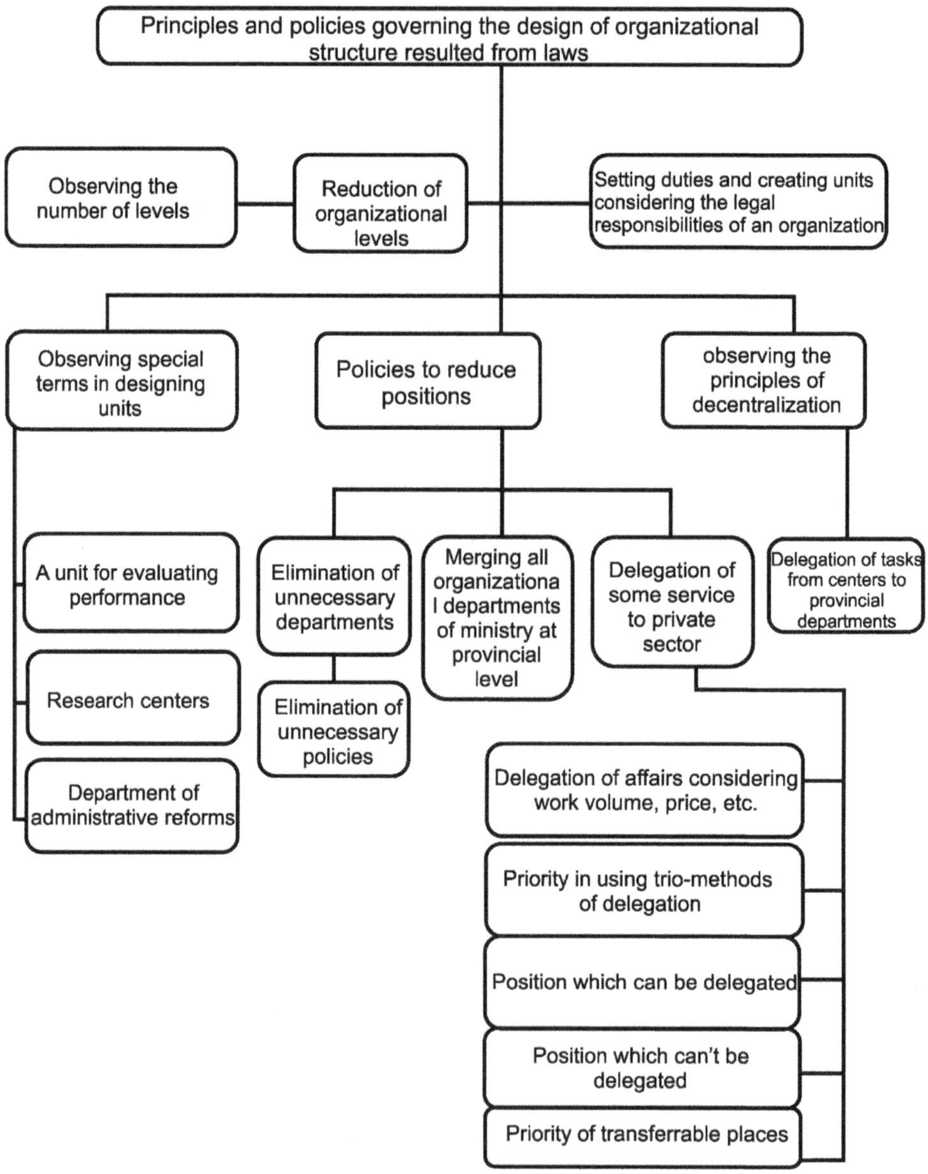

3. Study of the History of Ministry Structure and Structural Changes

Activities conducted in the following areas: Collection, review and analysis of existing documentation in the field of structural changes and redesigning the structure of the Ministry, including mergers, liquidations, abstraction, and creation of responsibility centers in:

- Headquarters of Ministry.
- Provincial departments of Ministry.
- Affiliated organizations of Ministry.

Since the establishment of the medical department so far and with the aim of pathology and evaluating the results of structural changes as well as holding required meeting with experts or those involved in the structural changes of the past. Results are drafting history of the organizational structure of the Ministry of Health that includes a good summation of structural changes and the professional activities that took place on reform of the ministry in the past. Examples of these trends have been presented in the form of some charts below (figure 4, figure 5 and figure 6).

4. Designing and Developing a Detailed Mission of Ministry of Health and Medical Education

Activities carried out in this heading are as the following:

- Extracting mission areas in detail and based on value chain analysis.
- Extracting roles playable by the various components of Ministry, in three headings:
    - The roles of "strategic management" in detail and differentiation (23 roles).
    - The roles of "operations management" in detail and differentiation (23 roles).
    - The roles of "operation and performance" in detail and differentiation (17 roles).
- Developing a separate mission for headquarters of Ministry and the headquarters of the Medical Sciences Universities.
- Extraction of the responsibilities due to roles that are defined based on played or non-played by various components of Ministry.
- Developing a detailed mission Matrix resulted from mission areas of Ministry with operational and managerial roles.

Figure 3. The rules and principles shall be used to redesign the structure of the Ministry of Health, part B

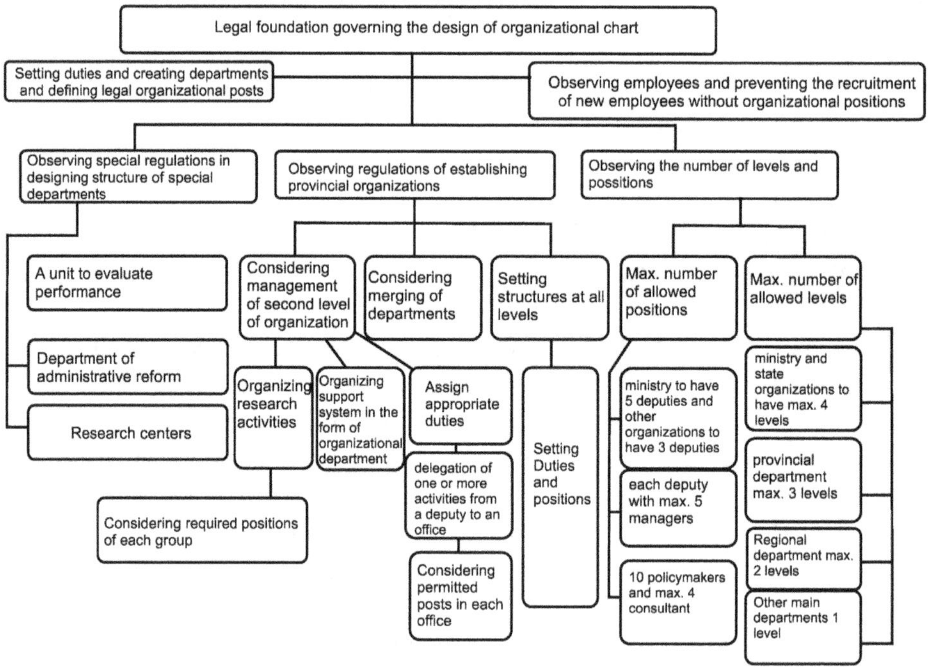

Figure 4. Trend of changes in health departments since 1926 until today

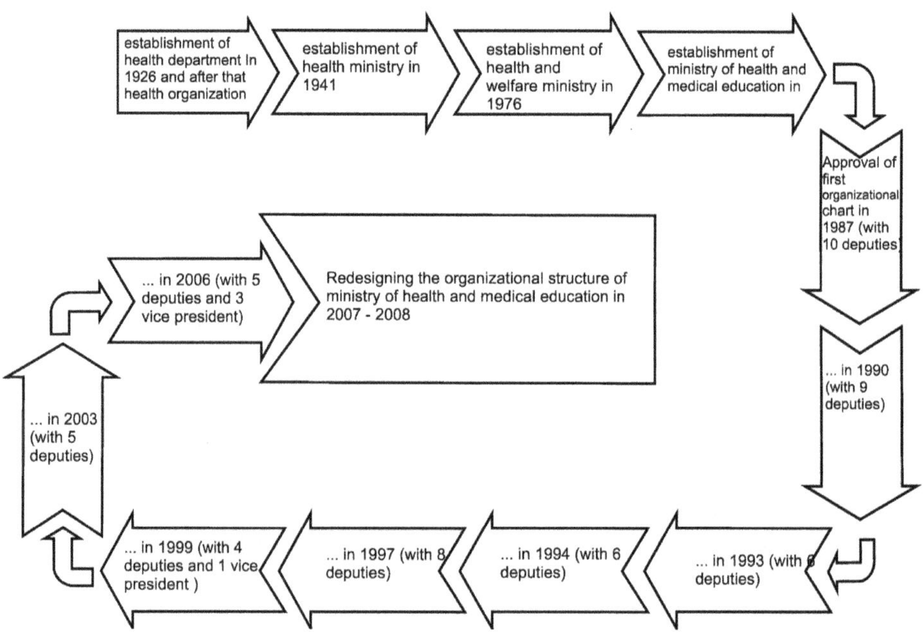

Figure 5. Evolution of health and medical education field in Iran since the establishment of regional health organizations until 2007

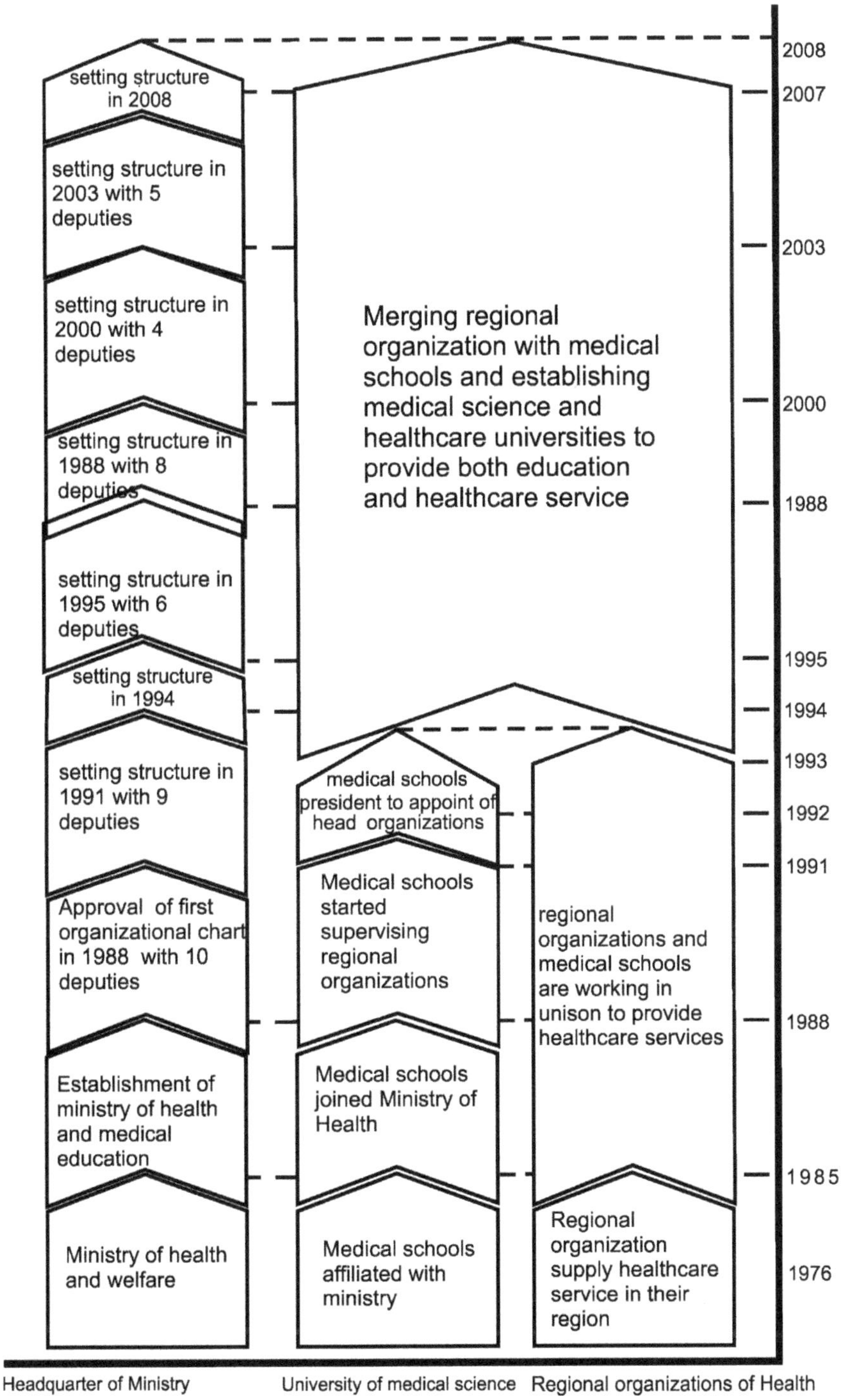

Figure 6. Evolution in deputies of headquarter of health and medical education Ministry in organizational charts approved during 1988-2008

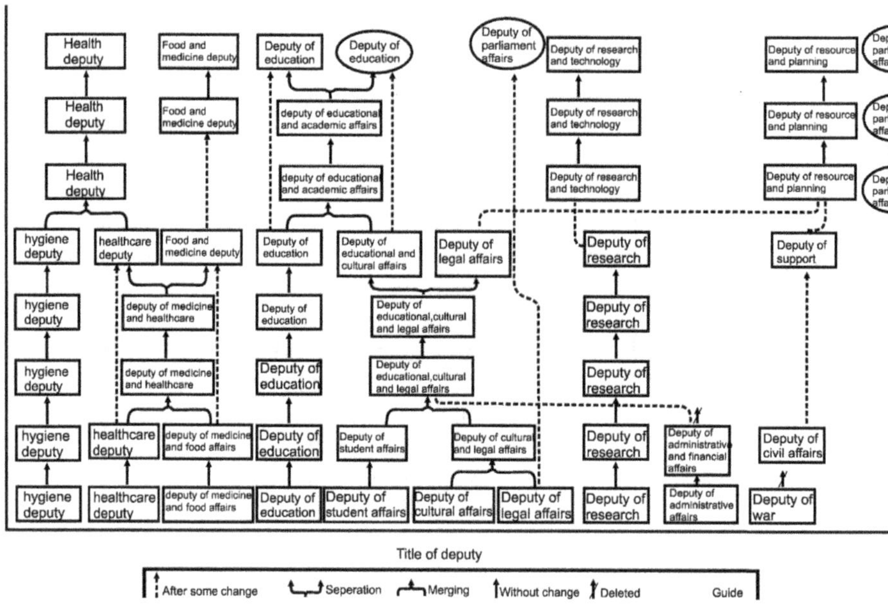

- Performing the analysis necessary to determine the roles of the Ministry in various mission areas.
- Developing and describing detailed mission of Ministry of Health and Medical education.

Based on developed detailed mission, in designing the structure of Ministry there were efforts to:

- All mission items duties of the units included in the chart.
- While there is no gap, overlap and ambiguity in the duties, the duties of the units to the lowest level of duty centers has been written.
- Strategic management roles have been delegated to headquarter and operation management tasks and operations have been delegated to universities and networks.
- The structure of departments is designed according to the following two factors:
    - The range and variety of missions of each unit (Scope).
    - The volume of missions per unit (Scale).

5. Comparative Studies

In these studies, it was necessary to study and analyze health care system and the structure of health Ministry in some countries. To this end, studies have been done considering the following steps:

- Selecting countries based on following criteria:
    - Successful implementation of structural changes in the health system.
    - Variation in concentration in health systems (being public and private in provision of services).
    - High rank on the major health characters in WHO.
- Doing studies in relation to benchmarking (comparative studies) on the subject of the structure of ministries of health (its all components) and issues of medical education in four countries, including Mexico, England, Norway and Singapore.
- About particular issues, there were conducted further studies given the importance and sensitivity of the topics . For example:
    - Checking the status of field of Food and Drugs (in regards to how to manage these areas) in 130 countries and also the exact study of the Food and Drug Administration of American (FDA).

Through the results of analysis, the main principles and policies of the benchmarking studied health systems that were used in design of different areas such as hospitals, universities and headquarters of Ministry have been extracted. In the following, the applied principals will be mentioned briefly:

1. The main principals has been observed in in all studied countries is in relation to the increase of decentralization and strengthening the role of custodianship of Ministry of Health and this will lead to an improvement of comprehensive management of the health system in various levels and dimensions.
2. Enhancing the ability of decision-making at lower levels (provincial)of Health Ministry with creating the potential of policy making and maximum delegation of authority and executive tasks to this level is another important principle.
3. Eliminating or merging organizations or sectors that have overlap and creating various organizations in the areas that need more attention or did not have at the possibility of fulfilling the duties assigned, showed the high importance in benchmarking studies. (moving towards institutional balance).
4. Necessity to develop and strengthen the use of information technology in nearly all studied cases has been emphasized t in different ways, and is one of the presuppositions used in the design of the structure (including start-up

of the information comprehensive systems, reporting systems, the electronic health, electronic health records, etc.)

5. Separation of ownership from the control sector has been observed in the studied countries and due to the separation of these two areas would further validate the efficiency of health care institutions, and other levels of health system.
6. Special attention to the health of different target groups, intellectuals and active labors in the country in offices and.... is also of those main principals.
7. Necessity of attention to establish national and professional centers in order to improve the quality of care, prevention and management of health
8. Attention to the issue of organizational excellence at all levels of the health system through creating infrastructure (including information technology), creating a system (such as knowledge management), human resources development and ....
9. Necessity to isolate the area of food and medicine (as an independent organization) were observed in these studies.
10. The need for vertical integration of the main functions of the health system, including trustee, finance, creating resources and providing services

6. Strategic Studies (Goals and Strategies)

Strategic studies conducted to evaluate the objectives, strategies and prospects facing the country's health system and the challenges they face now and in the future, have been considered in the headings and the following steps:

- Collection, review and analysis of all the existing documents about the visions, goals, strategies, policies and programs of the Ministry of Health (both strategic and operational), including:
    - 20-year-old visions of the Islamic Republic of Iran in 2025.
    - Fourth Economic, Social and Cultural Development Plan of Islamic Republic of Iran.
    - Document of Article 44 of the constitution of the Islamic Republic of Iran.
    - Document of the overall policies of fourth Economic, Social and Cultural Development Plan of Islamic Republic of Iran.
    - Document of the overall policies of fifth Economic, Social and Cultural Development Plan of Islamic Republic of Iran.
    - Documentation of Operational Planning, Ministry of Health and Medical Education.

- The National unlimited Development Plan Document for food and nutrition security on fourth Economic, Social and Cultural development plan of Islamic Republic of Iran.
- National Health Sector Development Plan Document on fourth Economic, Social and Cultural development plan of Islamic Republic of Iran.
- The draft of comprehensive scientific map in the health field.
- The plan of minister in 9th cabinet.
- The plan of minister in 10th cabinet.
- Review of Prospects and challenges facing the health system in the external environment, in three parts:
- International political environment.
- Social and cultural environment.
- Economic environment.
- Evaluation of perspectives and orientations in an indoor health system, including:
- Macro Perspectives and Directions.
- Prospects and orientation of the health care area.
- Prospects and orientation of the field of food, medicine and medical equipment.
- Perspectives and orientations of Education, Research and Technology area.
- Student perspectives and orientations, and cultural spheres.
- Perspectives and orientations of development and resource management area.

7. Strategy Structure (Conceptual Structure Studies)

According to surveys and modeling conducted, Natural model of Pine Tree -adapted from the model developed by Richard Daft (2012) -has been considered as basic model of methodology. In this model using various inputs including:

- Visions, Strategies and Directions.
- Content and structure variables.
- The distribution of organizational power.
- Integration of organizational elements.
- Strategic management and organization.
- Problems and bottlenecks of size and organizational elements.

Figure 7. Conceptual strategies of structure design in order to create status for Ministry of Health

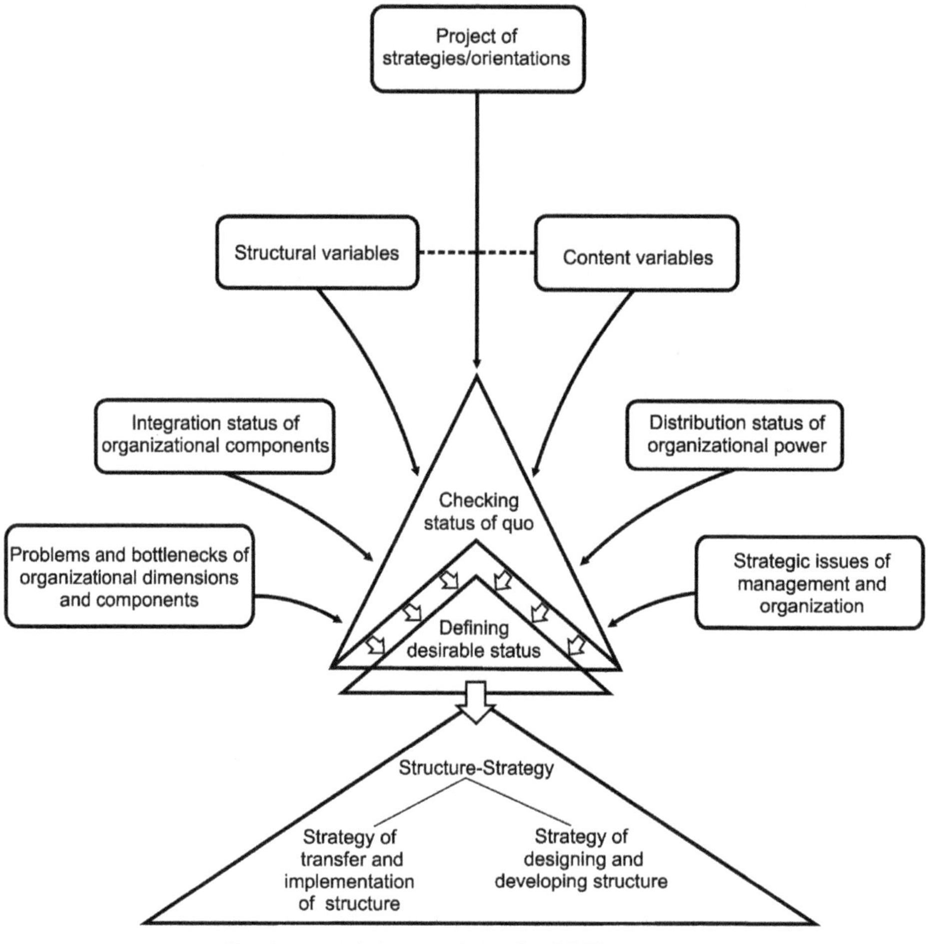

Status quo has been examined and target state has been determined. At last, conceptual strategies of structure design have been specified to create desirable status for Ministry of Health, Treatment and Medical Education. The model has been presented in Figure 7.

The conceptual structure studies in this project have been carried out in the following steps in order to developing structure strategy:

- Design of Package II includes two separate booklets for each main department, special booklet for managing director, a booklet for deputies and head of offices/groups/departments and experts (total of 68 booklets for headquarter of Ministry).

- The package design is done in three main parts:
    - **The First Part:** Analysis of the content variables (objective and strategy / environment / technology).
    - **The Second Part:** Analysis of the structural variables (concentration / recognition / complexity / standardization).
    - **The Third Part:** The design principles and policies (including variables of structural architecture based on investigating organizational power and its distribution among different units, integration of organizational elements, strategic issues such as strategic management, human resource management, information technology, management systems and processes, and knowledge management.... problems and bottlenecks of management and organization).
- Sending packages and following them to be completed.
- Analysis of 450 completed and collected booklets.
- The design of software system (using Excel) in order to enter the information of questionnaire of package II of various departments to in this system and summation and their statistical analysis.
- By analyzing the content variables, structural variables in the optimum condition were determined.

In the area of purpose and strategy, the attention to internal and external parts and the severity of control, in the area of environment the quality of complexity and environmental changes, and in the area of technology the amount of repeatability and degradation of applied technologies in every organizational areas of Ministry have been studied and due to these issues, it has been tried to consider them in designs, organic and mechanic structures.

Some of the most important results of the study of architectural variables are as follows:

- On the distribution of power between deputies, in this study, the deputy of development, health, food and medicine are ranked first to third respectively.
- Survey shows that now there is the lack of integrity in the system existing rules and upper-hand documents, objectives and strategies and programs, and management styles in headquarter of Ministry and should move towards addressing this lack of cohesion and integration.
- In the area of strategic issues, results show that in all key and strategic issues at least %77 and on average %96 and in some issues up to %131 should improve the status and necessary modification should be done. In designs have been done including designing the chart and developing duties of organizational departments this has been considered thoroughly.

- To identify organizational problems and bottlenecks two direct measurement methods and component measurement were used.

In the direct method, the average opinion suggests that financial problems are in the first place. This means when asking managers and experts in Ministry to choose between their seven problems the most important one, they all mostly refer to financial problems and resource limitation as the first problem; while in combination method this classification has been done through component measurement and human resource problems have got the first place.

Also in both methods, leadership and management problem have been in sixth place. And it seems the existence of a kind of mistake led to this result because if there is an efficient and effective management in each organization then its task is to resolve problems according to limited resources and reach targeted purposes. [1]

At the end, according to the minimal difference of "issue volume index" for each organizational problems and bottlenecks, it can be concluded that the Ministry should have a comprehensive plan to resolve these problems and structural changes cannot overcome these problems by their own. However, structural changes can be seen as "driving force" in the centerpiece of this program.

Stage II: Processing and Analysis

At this point, three main activities should to be performed simultaneously. These three activities are:

1. Developing principles and policies that govern the design.
2. Specifying the procedures and the basic views in designing structure.
3. Determining models and influencing dimensions on the design including:
    a. Organizational standards.
    b. Architecture of structure f Ministry.
    c. Models and framework of key and determining systems.
    d. A model to determine the independent agencies under supervision of the Ministry.

1. The Principles and Policies that Govern the Design

According to studies, principles and policies governing the design were divided into two categories of content and structure. In the following the more important of these principles have been provided.

Content Principles and Policies

1. To strengthen and to enhance the strategic value of integrating medical education in healthcare services and community-centered medical education
    - Consolidated integration of both medical education and health services in schools.
    - Developing duties of health, education and research units should be provided as a basis for follow-up promotion of integration at different levels of services (such as universities, hospitals and health networks).
2. Preparing context in order to improve and promote integration in the three levels of planning of health services and policy making based on:
    - Continuous monitoring of diseases and their results (remission, mortality, morbidity) and calculation of the burden of diseases.
    - Determining priorities and health needs and different target groups and policy making of interventions (with respect to resources, capabilities, and limitations...).
    - Extraction and preparation of a new comprehensive intervention plan for different target groups.
    - Integration of new intervention strategies in previous programs and integration of intervention programs in relation to different target groups or sections of society.
    - Developing models and mechanisms required (included) for the implementation of interventions in relation to different target groups or sections of society.
3. Providing infrastructures necessary to improve quality of health care and hospital management and management of health institutions
    - Strengthening the monitoring field of activities
    - Separation of audit and accreditation systems of hospitals and health care institutions from the structure of management and supervision of their operation (Accreditation, Certification and Rating hospitals and other health institutions needed done by an authority other than the trustee, the owner of their mother organization)
    - Creating mechanisms and required structures for software and managerial development and providing managerial packs for hospitals as concentrated ones(such as packs of organizational excellence system, quality systems, human resource systems and …) with the aim of:
        - Standardization.
        - Providing central services to the hospital due to low capacity of hospitals in these areas at the status quo.
        - Economic benefits.

- Creating mechanisms and required structures for the development of standards and local health care protocols, and providing health care services and hospital administration and supervision of the implementation of these standards and protocols in the country.
- Creating structures and mechanisms for developing regulation and creating related markets to health care service and management of hospitals and other health institutions, supervision and regulation of the markets, markets including
    - Market of contractors and private sector providing various services to hospitals and other health institutions by outsourcing such as clinical services. Professional services and even public services provided in hospitals must comply with the rules, and professional considerations specifically.
    - Market of providing required human resources for hospitals and health care institutions in positions that are funded by the company human resources. Occupations such as practical nurse, service personnel, etc.
    - Other issues due to different changes in different areas of treatment and management of hospitals and medical centers / educational centers and other health institutions, both public and private sector.
- Development of new approaches to medical management in health centers / educational centers.
- Strengthening the private sector (NGOs) to provide health care and increase the effective monitoring of the sector.

4. Creating contexts necessary for full implementation of the referral system and the family physicians in the country.
5. Priorities of health and education development and health promotion and creating related culture among the people towards the therapeutic_development.
6. Strengthening management and program planning and policy making, and creating required mechanisms for the development of fields below:
    - Health Economics
    - Futures Studies and Strategic Studies in the field of health and community health needs
    - Strategic value of health (integration, equity, quality, access, stability)
    - E-Health
    - Health Tourism
7. Removing the duties and functions related to health service operating in the provincial capital city from tasks and the mission of university headquarters through the creation of a network management in center of that province.

8. Creating and strengthening the foundation for required structural and institutional integration in the field of health policy and programs in the country and in different areas of the Ministry of Health and Medical Education.
9. Creating necessary contexts and structures to develop management and training of managers and improving abilities and their managerial and organizational knowledge as one of the main bottlenecks in health system and Ministry and mainly in most macro systems of country.
10. Strengthening the program of planning and organization and instructional design based on needs assessment and macro-architecture approach to training and education to strengthen the strategic values such as quality education, training responsible graduates of medical education and community-centered medical training.
11. Decentralization and delegation of maximum authority in a field of student affairs to universities.
12. Creating necessary contexts to develop and improve professional ethics among students and graduates of medical area (including doctors, paramedics, and nurses...).
13. Strengthening and enhancing mechanisms for increasing the quality and quantity of research activities and technology (especially in bio-technology and Nano).
    - Agile architecture of management structure of research and technology.
    - Creating and increasing flexibility of structure and self-organization of the structure in the field of research management.
    - Decentralization of the research and technology activities.
    - Focus on management of research, technology activities and strengthening required structures for macroeconomic policy in this area in order to:
        - The decentralized management activities based on a comprehensive map of the research and medical technology, and directing the micro/macro research activities.
        - Meeting the real needs of the mission areas of Ministry.
        - Avoiding scattered and unhelpful actions.
        - Strengthening knowledge management in order to have the synergies for technology and research activities in different parts of the country.
    - Creating and strengthening the network of researchers and research institutions in order to integrate and organize and direct all research activities.
    - Creating required platforms for recruiting and directing funding for research and technology.
    - Emphasis on the applicability of research results.

Structural Principles and Policies

In order to rationalize and resolve bottlenecks and structural strengthening of development and moving forward of health systems, the following structural principals in designing has been considered:

1. Restructuring of health area:
    - Reducing the area and increasing the effectiveness of monitoring relevant Deputy.
    - Strengthening integration of the three levels of planning and policy making and health services (as described in the description of the design process and will be described later).
2. Merger of health and treatment area in universities and establishing health deputy in order to improve mergers and also creating coordination and integration between headquarter of Ministry and head quarter of university on one hand and between head quarter of university and networks on the other hand and creating logical governing hierarchy.
3. Rationalization and standardization the organizational structure of the University of Medical Sciences and Health Services.
4. Creating "The Food and Drug Administration" (trustee of food, medicine Medical equipment area).
5. Creating a "National Centre for Standardization and Accreditation of Health Organizations."
6. Creating "the engineering and management organization of physical infrastructure," with macro missions:
    - Development of construction projects of Ministries in compliance with effective technical and economic competence.
    - Development of innovative approaches to maintain the physical infrastructure in order to increase the efficiency and lifetime of physical resources.
    - Strengthening and related issues with passive defense in physical infrastructure of health systems (especially hospitals) as part of the vital infrastructure of country.
7. Creating a "management Education and development Institute of Health Care " with aims to overcome a bottleneck for the development of the health sector as a corporate university.
8. Rationalization of education deputy structure of headquarter of Ministry; the integration of all activities of the university (academic and student) and renaming deputy to the "Deputy of Academic Affairs" or "Vice Chancellor for Academic Affairs" with regard to the following:

- Reducing the scope and increasing the effectiveness of monitoring by relevant Deputy.
- Process-centered structure of deputy and its various areas.
- Architecture approach and macro-organization of education (in terms of content and form).
- Decentralization and delegation of maximal executive activities and managing to universities.

9. Reform of the structure of resource and management development deputy:
    - The integration of system and process management and organizational architecture with IT in order to reach a logical view and real development requirements of these two areas.
    - Creating a key responsibility center that implements policy making from the beginning of "strategic studies" to "performance evaluation" integrated and based on Sigma model[2](OECD,1996) Obviously this center is responsible for integration of system policies in various areas and as a methodologist manages the planning and policy making procedures and content production of policies is the responsibility of professional and expert areas.
    - Creating approaches and new structures in the area of human capital management (HCM).
10. Reducing the scope of supervision of Minister.

2. Clarification of the Fundamental Approach to the Design of the Structure

In order to design the structure, two main approaches can be considered.

First Approach: Process

In this approach, management processes, including planning, implementation and control are considered as pillars of organizational activities and the missions of organization are organized as subsidiaries of each stage of the process. Currently, the Ministry of Health and according to historical trend of its structure, which has been organized based on the mission and operational approach; creating process approach and organization based on it leads to fundamental changes in headquarter of Ministry and main bottleneck will be reform and change management in Ministry and facing challenges should be recognized and sufficient strategies should be applied.

Second Approach: Mission

In this part, missions of organization are considered as main activities and stages of process management are organized as subsidiaries of each mission areas (figure 8).

Figure 8. Mission approach

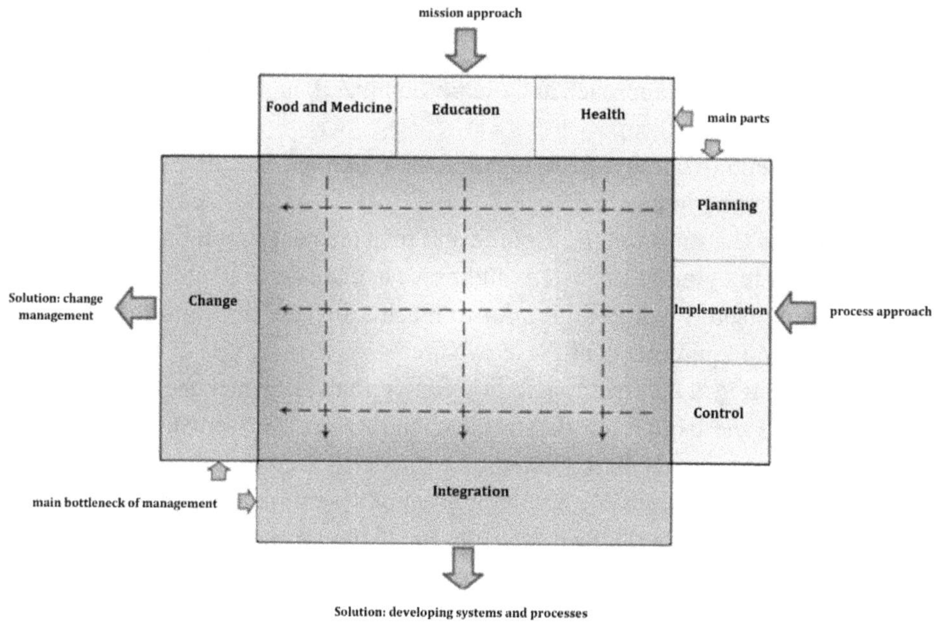

In this Ministry this approach requires the integration between health, education, food, medicine.

This type of intersection between the mission area of an organization with the process management (planning, implementation, monitoring) can be more accurately examined in order to classify tasks and organizational roles and evaluating bottleneck in organization and designing basic macro-structure. For this purpose, look at table 1. If both primary areas of mission in Health Ministry are considered as "health" and "education", each of these areas has its own content and form to achieve their goals . Content, technical topics and form contain organizing in order to reach goals and missions. On the other hand, each component of management (planning, implementation and control) has the strategic and operational dimensions. From the intersection of mission and managerial dimensions in a matrix we can categorize organizational roles and responsibilities and main bottlenecks in the design of macro- structure. Each of internal cells of matrix is an example of studied issues in organizing Ministry of Health and medical education.

For example, the "health policy making "is in the strategic planning of health content and that "the level structure of hospital care" is strategic planning in providing health care services to society.. So the "architecture of education and content of education" and "policy making of education" is strategic planning in content of education and "architecture of educational centers" is the strategic planning in form

Table 1. Categorizing tasks and organizational roles/ key bottlenecks in the design of macro structures

Solution	Main concern	Main trustee	Education		Health			
			Form(organizing)	Content(Technical)	Form(organizing)	Content(Technical)		
Organizational architecture /system and process management/integrating Processes(through centers in charge of ensuring integrating)	Form and content integration	Headquarter	Architecture of educational center	Educational architecture and content of education policy making	Structure of categorizing healthcare service	Health policy making	strategic	Planning
		Headquarter/ universities	Organizing educational groups/designing education process / evaluation	Developing cariculums/educational planning	Required structure and resources / implementation planning	Technical and content plan of fighting disease/operational plan inorder to implement policies	operational	
		Headquarter	Designing university structure/developing system of research management	Test and measurement/educational macro service	Architecture od health system/architecture of network	Implementation mechanism/developing service packages	strategic	Implementation
		Universities/ Networks	Implementation of structure/systems/making change in faculties and educational groups	Education by faculties and professors	Implementing structures/creation and management of organizational change	Providing health service	operational	
		Headquarter	Checking the compatibility of university structure with architecture and educational policies/accreditation	Control of consequences and macro indexes of medical education /accreditation	Checking the compatibility of structure with mission and health policies/accreditation	Control of consequences and macro indexes of health/accreditation	strategic	Control
		Universities/ Networks	Checking efficiency of systems/executive affairs	Checking educational service provided by professors	Checking efficiency of operational processes/administrative controls	Supervision and control of providing services	operational	
			Form Coordination	content coordination	Form Coordination	content coordination	Main concern	
			Organizational architecture and exact separation of roles and tasks	Systems and processes management (through vertical connection in cluster structure)	Organizational architecture and exact separation of roles and tasks	System and processes management (through vertical connection in cluster structure)	Solution	

area of medical education. In the field of strategic planning, headquarter of Ministry is responsible to do these activities. Operational planning are done with the cooperation of head quarter of Ministry and mainly headquarters of universities. Strategic implementation is mainly duty of Ministry and operational implementation is done with the cooperation of headquarters of universities and networks. Headquarter of Ministry is responsible for strategic control and headquarters of universities and networks are responsible for operational control.

If the mission of Ministry and health and education approach are taken into account; the main concern of managers will be content and form compatibility in strategic planning, operational planning, strategic implementation, operational implementation, strategic control and operational control. In this case, the systems and processes should be managed by using vertical connections in the cluster structure. Also both organizational architecture and the strict separation of roles and responsibilities in organizing can create form coordination in different components of management. On the other hand, if management process is taken into account, then the primary concern of managers will be the integration between health and education content and also integration in organizing health care service provision and medical education. In this regard, the content and form integration between various mission areas should be managed by creating responsible centers for integration of systems and processes and defining integrating processes and the activity of "management of organizational architecture" can be done efficiently.

3. Designing Models and Determining Dimensions Influencing the Design

3.1 Organizational Standards

One of the concerns that organizations and large companies with heavy structures having various departments or geographic dispersion or independent commercial units face due to standardization of activities, particularly in the areas of management and support is standardization and coordination and integrity of the structure design and setting of various similar units .

Designing and developing criteria and standards by which the organizational structures and the detailed structure are designed or redesigned:

- By adjusting the volume of activities and the number of employees between departments and different levels establish structural integration between them.
- Necessary contexts are created for a coordinated system of payment and incentives.
- Infrastructure necessary to create organizational justice and setting the alignment table are provided on reasonable basis.
- The specific rules for the change and dynamics of organizational structures are provided to various units and scattering is minimized.

Organizational standards try to describe any kinds of structural and organizational entities in the organization, as well as those governing the dos and don'ts by setting charts and regulations. In order to avoid the bargaining process of headquarters and provisional departments in relation to the organizational structure, occupations and positions, the coding structure has been standardized. This code completes laws and regulations in this area and it is designed flexible and comprehensive that can be provided to legislation authorities in order to use in all executive systems.

3.2 Models and Determining and Key System Framework

From the collection of models and frameworks that are designed for key systems of Ministry and are considered as a basic of macro-structure designing, here we mention three models and frameworks briefly and merely graphically.

Figure 9. Process model designed to provide health services

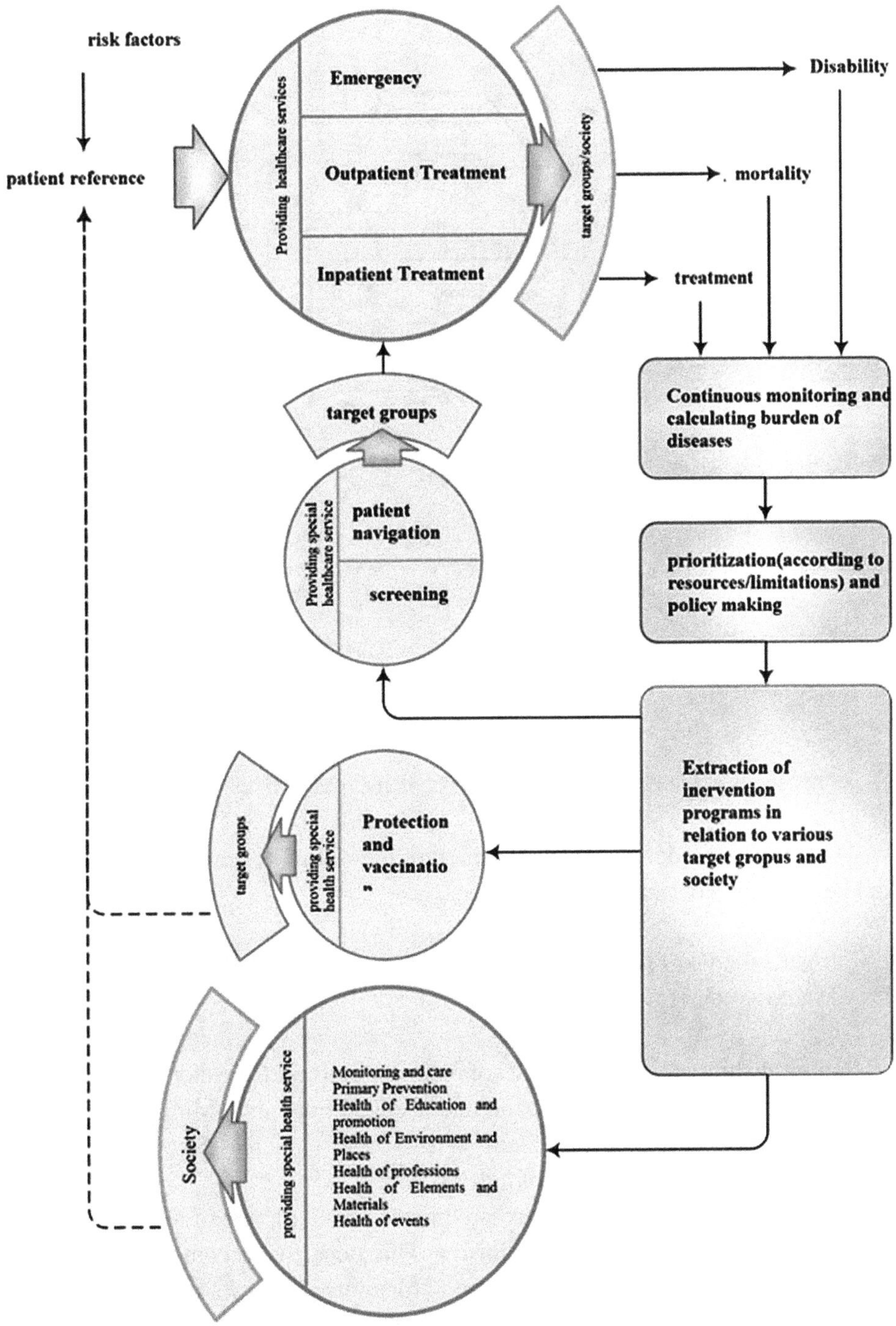

Figure 10. Macro-model of role separation in main structural levels

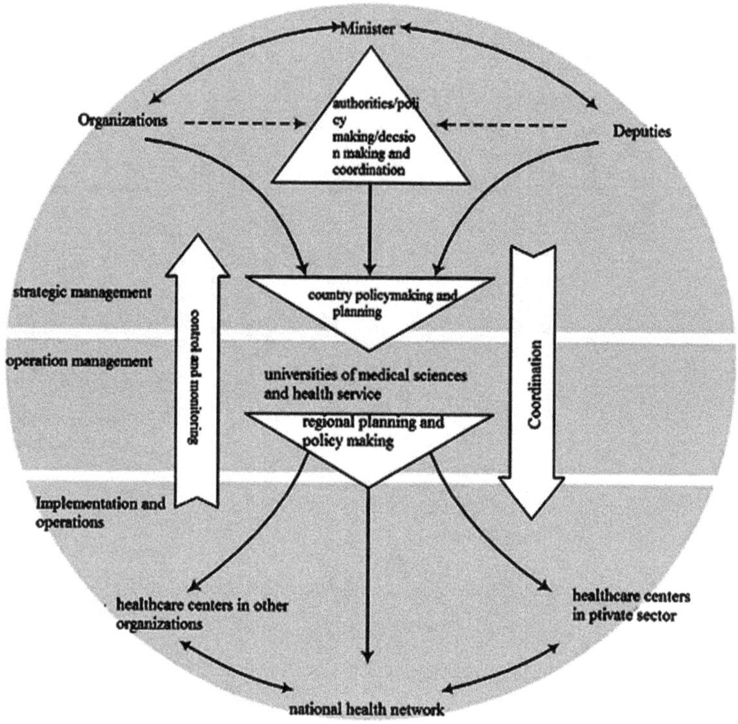

1. Designed process model to provide health care services (Levels I, II and III).

This process model is a basic of structure designing in health area of Ministry and headquarters of universities (figure 9).

2. Macro-model of role separation in main structural levels (figure 10).
3. Macro-system of planning and control.

Figure 11 shows the macro-model of planning and control system of implementing programs at three levels of Health and Medical Education Ministry.

3.3 Structure Architecture of Ministry

Figure 12 shows the designed macro-architecture for structure of Ministry. At first level, there is headquartering of Ministry. This department contains three deputies of "health"," educational affairs" and "planning and development" and some independent affiliated institutions help headquarter in reaching goals. At second level that is the provisional structure of Ministry, you can find university of medical

Figure 11. Macro-system of planning and control

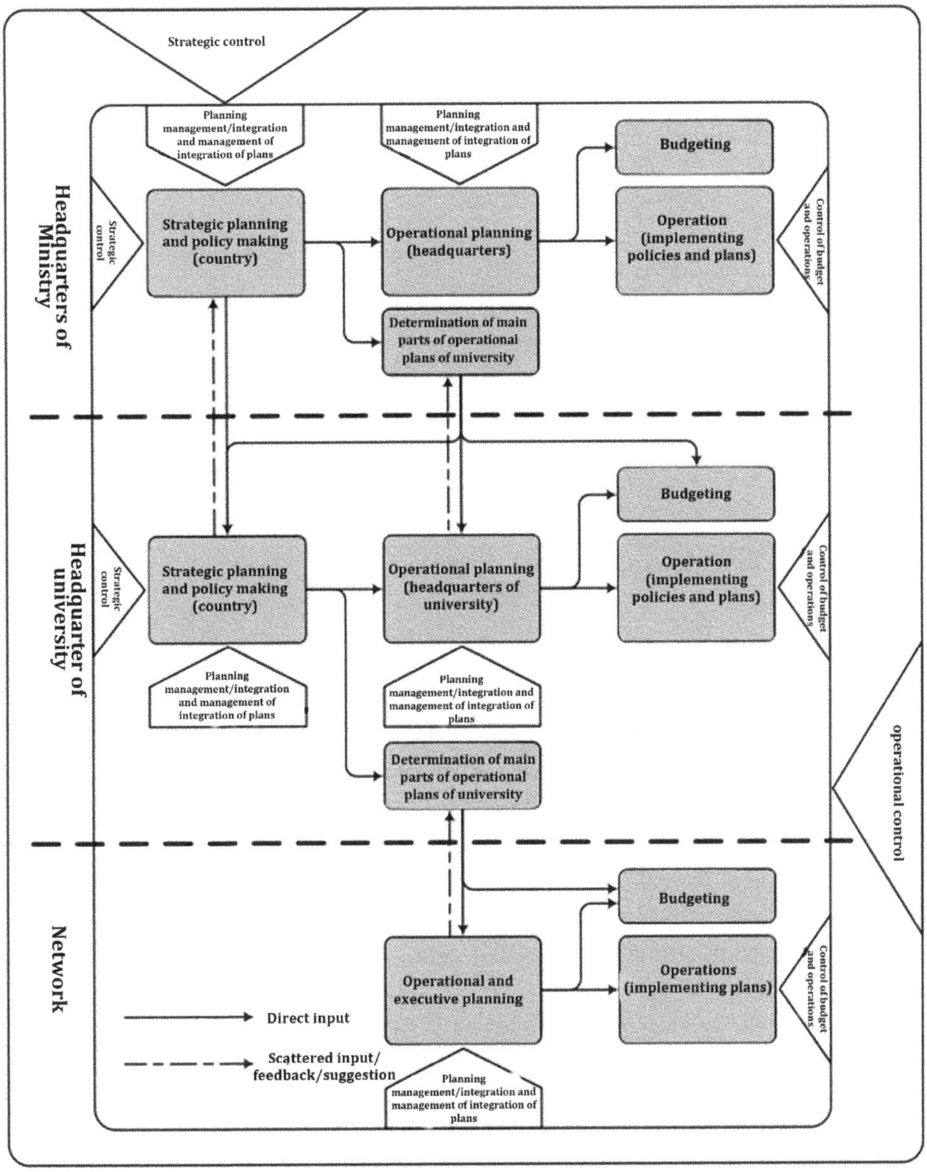

sciences and health care services that in most universities contains three deputies of "Academic affairs", "resource and management development" and "health". The deputy of health in university is a head of health in the province. In big universities two deputies of "research and technology" and "cultural and student affairs "will be added to above deputies. Affiliated organizations at provisional level have an of-

Figure 12. The designed macro-architecture for structure of Ministry

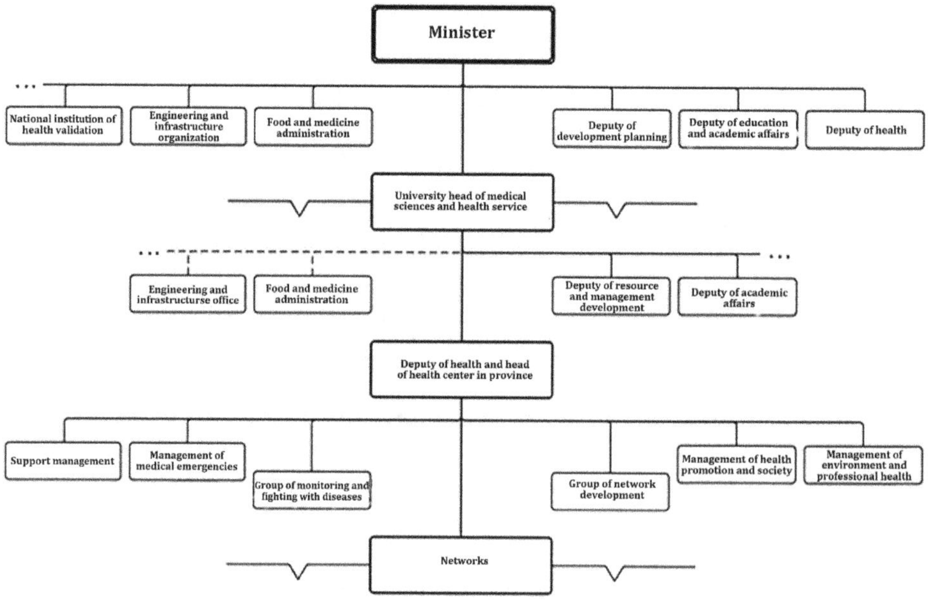

fice that is in connection with head of university and develop their regional policies with the help of university and head of university is responsible for coordinating the organizations and related departments with Ministry in target province.

Affiliated departments of health deputy in university do regional planning due to macro policy making in health area and all executive activities in province are done by networks. In order to determine the role of planning and monitoring for university and removing executive duties from missions of headquarter of university, it has been recommended that the center of that province has the separate management network.

A Model to Determine the Independent Agencies of Ministry: What is important here and before presenting scenarios, is the reasons and requirements of establishing organizations and independent institutions governing by Ministry. All these reasons and requirements can be divided into two categories:

- Reasons / requirements related to content and structural dimensions.
- Managerial reasons / requirements.

In fact, reasons and requirements of establishing an organization and institution can be investigated by this categorizing and providing sufficient indexes in each category. In new recommended scenarios, 6 new organizations and institutions have been introduced. In table 2 and table 3, rating has been done based on the severity of impact of each reason or requirement for every recommended institution (Expert Group method). Based on this analysis, prioritization of establishing recommended organizations are as follows:

1. **National Institute of Standards and accreditation of health institutions (38 points);** (National Centre for standards).
2. **Engineering and management of physical infrastructure organization (36 points);** (the engineering organization).
3. **The Food and Drugs and Medical Devices Administration (35 points);** (Food and Drug Administration).
4. **Management Development and education Institute in Health Care system (28 points);** (Institute of Management Development).
5. **National Center for Medical Technology and Research Management (23 points);** (National Research Center).
6. **Disaster Management and Medical Emergency organization (15 points);** (Disaster Management organization).

Table 2. Reasons and requirements of formation the organizations and entities affiliated to Ministry (reasons/requirements related to content and structural dimensions)

Recommended organizations and institutions						(5 points)reason/requirement with high effect ● (3 points) reason/requirement with average effect ◒ (1 points) reason/requirement with low effect ○	
Management organization	The engineering organization	National center for standards	National research center	Institute of management development	Food and drug administration	Content of reason /requirements of establishing independent Organization(governed by Ministry)	
◒			◒			Quick respond to environment	Reasons/requirement related to content and structural dimension
		◒	●	○		Higher flexibility technologic changes	
○					◒	More connections with legal and political environment	
○	◒	○	○	○	○	More connection/less complexity	
	●	●			●	Higher standardization	
						Culture / special subculture Smaller size	
	◒		◒	●	◒	Life cycle placing in growth or death stage	
5	11	9	12	7	12	Total Point	

Table 3. Reasons and requirements of formation the organizations and entities affiliated to Ministry (managerial reasons / requirements)

Recommended organizations and institutions						(5 points)reason/requirement with high effect ● (3 points) reason/requirement with average effect ◒ (1 points) reason/requirement with low effect ○	
Management organization	The engineering organization	National center for standards	National research center	Institute of management development	Food and drug administration	Content of reason /requirements of establishing independent Organization(governed by Ministry)	
	○	◒		●		Covering a bottleneck /problem /threat / special opportunities	Managerial reason/requirement
	◒	◒	◒	◒	◒	Agility of specific area to governance structure	
	◒	●			●	Connection with the market and its actors / relation with the competitive environment	
		●				Creating independency in order to monitoring public position	
◒	●	●	◒		●	Separate and distinct mission having given borders with other areas	
◒	◒	○	○		◒	Agility of strategic and macro-policy making institution	
						Preparing required context for delegation to private sector	
○	○	○			◒	Reduction of main cluster with creating side clusters	
	◒	●	◒	●	◒	Creating independency with the aim of increasing the quality of activities	
◒	○	○	○	●	○	Creating independency with the aim of preparing for fast and graphic growth	
	●			◒		Creating independency with the aim of economic and financial benefits for this system	
10	25	29	11	21	23	Total points of this part	
15	36	38	23	28	35	Total Point	

Stage III: Output

Designed Structural Scenarios

The First Approach: Fundamental Change (the Process Approach)

This approach has been developed based on the process approach previously described. In this diagram (figure 13) all operational activities in the health systems in independent organizations governing by Ministry are done. In headquarter of Ministry only policy making, planning, support and strategic monitoring are considered and consequently the deputies of " developing organization and IT", " policy making and strategic monitoring" and " support and parliament affairs" are considered for this scenario. In this case, headquarter of Ministry decreased from 3000 employees to 300 people that should be of experts in health and medical education system.According to the designers understanding of the current state of Ministry and existence of some legal, environmental, political obstacles, it seems to be difficult to implement this scenario. For this purpose the designing team did not work on detailed designing. In this scenario, the activities related to operations (including the compilation of content of operations, operational planning, and operations management) are done in affiliated organizations and the content policy making, strategic monitoring and development of large systems and related processes are done in headquarter of Ministry.

Figure 13. Fundamental change (process perspective)

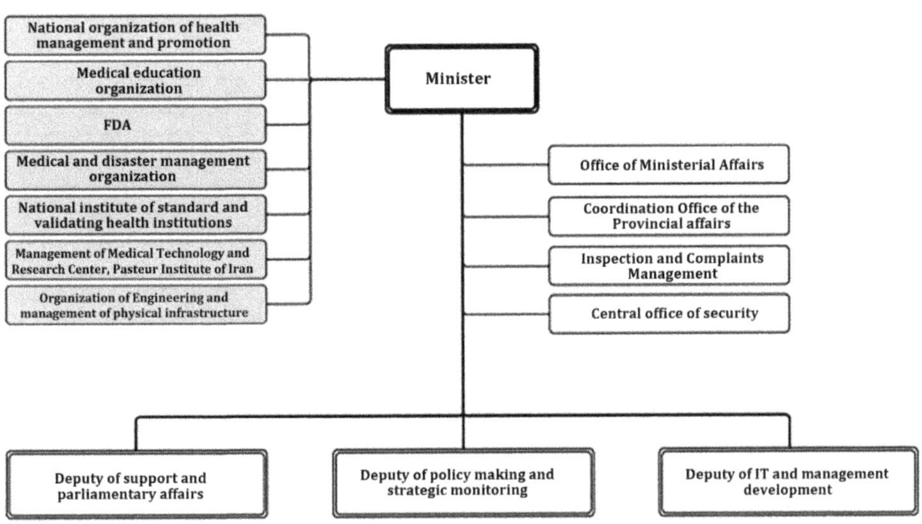

The Second Approach: Fundamental Reform (the Mission Approach)

In this approach, the primary mission and duty view of the structure (the current governing approach) has been maintained but it has been tried to design agile structures (Dove,2001) for Ministry. In this approach, two main scenarios of 3 deputies and 5 deputies have been designed.

1. Scenario 1: 3-Deputy Structure.

In this scenario, headquarter of Ministry will have three deputies of "health", "educational and Academic affairs" and "planning and development". The former "Food and Drug Department" and "Bureau of Medical Equipment" in the form of "The Food and Drugs and Medical Devices department" will be established. Meanwhile, the deputy of "technology and research" will become "center of medical research and technology management" and will be included in the deputy of "educational and Academic affairs". It should be noted that this structural change will be observed in other scenarios. This is not resulted from the lack of attention to research and

Figure 14a. Deputy structure

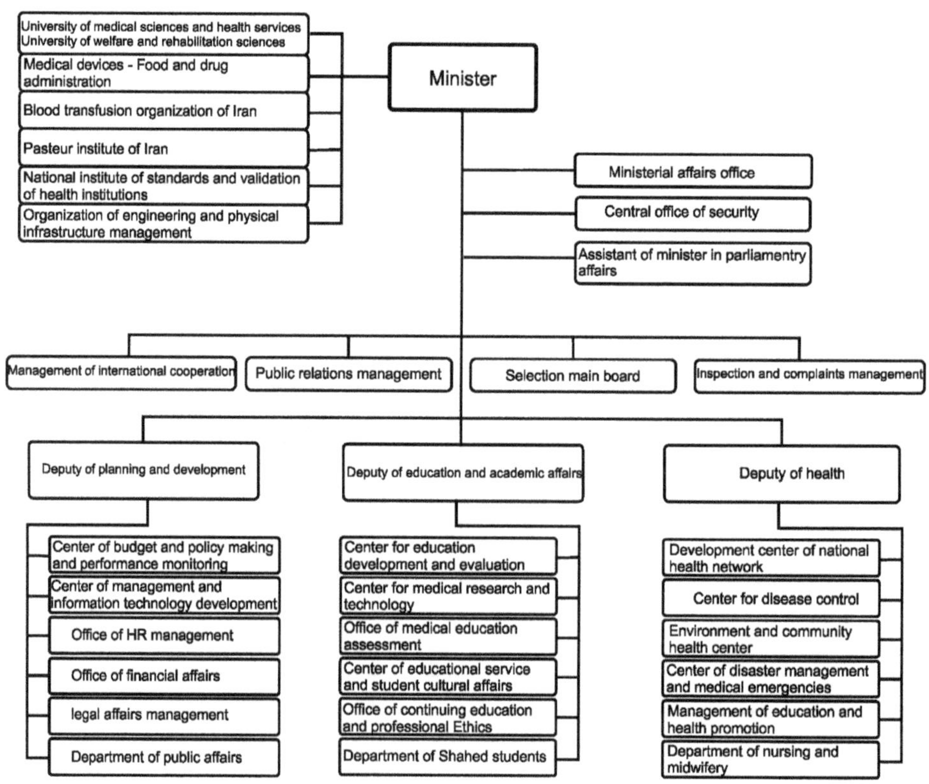

technology but the desired and detailed structure has been designed for this center more efficiently and integrated well. In fact, the load of tasks and human resource required for managing medical research and technology in Ministry has not been at the level of a deputy due to existing standards.Topics related to standardization and accreditation of health institutions are seen in an independent organization.

Also, the "management of Physical Resources" in Ministry in a form of "engineering and management of physical infrastructures organization" is included and is responsible for all issues of planning and technical and executive supervision of construction, maintenance and strengthening of physical infrastructure.Of the current organizations affiliated to the Ministry, "blood transfusion center" and "Refining and Research Company" will be merged, and "Pasteur Institute of Iran," will be responsible for "health reference laboratory" in addition to the current activities of operational issues. Topics related to standardization of hygiene medical diagnosis laboratories have been reviewed in the development center of national health network.

Figure 14b. Deputy structure continued

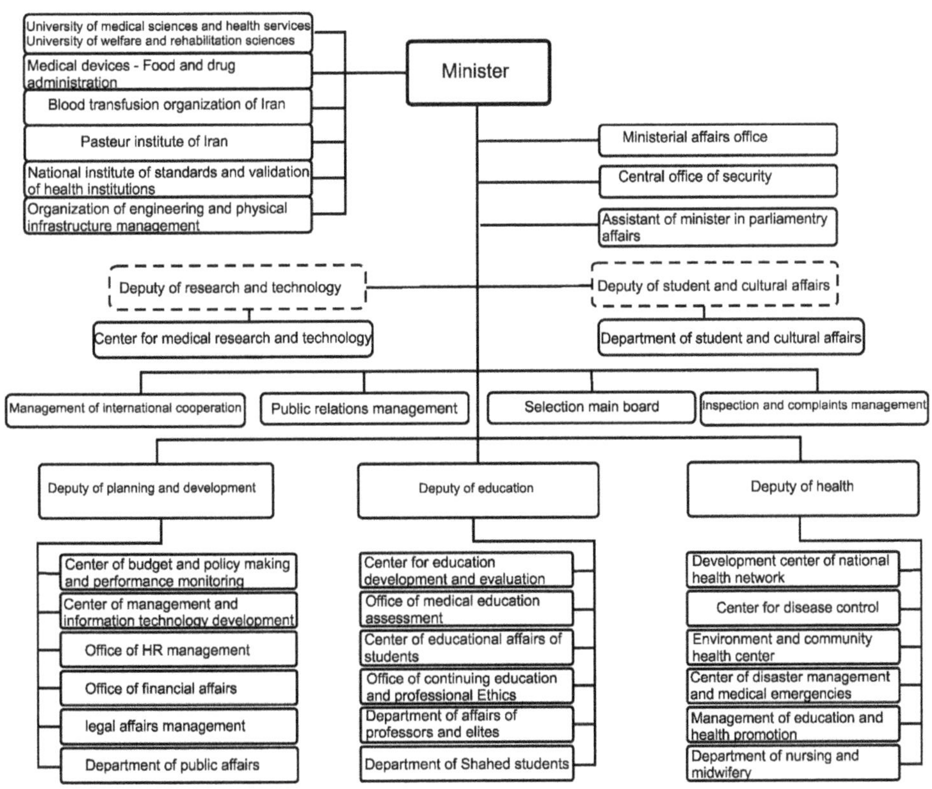

2. Scenario 2: 5-Deputy Structure.

In this scenario, "Medical Research Management Centre" has been considered as "research and technology deputy". In meantime, "Student and Cultural affairs" has been considered as separate managerial department and affiliated of "student and cultural deputy" (figure 14).

CONCLUSION

One of the concerns that organizations and large companies with heavy structures having various departments or geographic dispersion or independent commercial units face due to standardization of activities, particularly in the areas of management and support is standardization and coordination and integrity of the structure design and setting of various similar units. Health sector is facing such complications as it has to deal with aforementioned organizations to achieve its missions and visions efficiently and effectively. According to this case study, redesigning the structure of the Ministry could prove how a re-design in organizational structure followed by policy coherence can maximize the output in healthcare sector.

REFERENCES

Aldrich, H. E., & Ruef, M. (2006). Organizations evolving (2nd ed.). Sage Publishing House.

Daft, R. (2012). *Organization theory and design* (11th ed.). South-Western College Pub.

Dove, R. (2001). *Response Ability: The Language, Structure, and Culture of the Agile Enterprise*. Wiley.

Galbraith, J. (1977). *Organization design*. Addison Wesley Publishing Company.

OECD. (1996). *Budgeting and Policy Decision-Making*. SIGMA Paper No. 8, OCDE/GD(96)110. OECD.

Scott, W. R. (2005). Organizations: Rational, Natural and open systems (5th ed.). Prentice Hall.

Scott, W. R., & Davis, G. F. (2015). Organizations and organizing: Rational, Natural and open systems perspectives. Routledge.

Thurow, C. L. (1999). Building Wealth: The New Rules for Individuals, Companies, and Nations in a Knowledge-Based Economy. Harper Business.

KEY TERMS AND DEFINITIONS

Agile Enterprise: Fast moving, flexible and robust firm capable of rapid response to unexpected challenges, events, and opportunities. Built on policies and processes that facilitate speed and change, it aims to achieve continuous competitive advantage in serving its customers.

Effectiveness: The degree to which objectives are achieved and the extent to which targeted problems are solved.

Efficiency: The state or quality of being efficient, or able to accomplish something with the least waste of time and effort; competency in performance.

Natural Systems: Using a natural system perspective, Scott defines organizations as collectivities whose participants share a common interest in the survival of the system and who engage in collective activities, informally structured, to secure this end.

Organizational Change: Is about reviewing and modifying management structures and business processes.

Organizational Structure: The division of duties and coordination between personnel of the organization and it shows the framework of relationships governing occupations, systems and organizational processes and human resource (including individuals and groups) that try to achieve the specified goals.

Policy Coherence: Policy Coherence is defined by the OECD as the systematic promotion of mutually reinforcing policy actions across government departments and agencies creating synergies towards achieving the agreed objectives. Within national governments, policy coherence issues arise between different types of public policies, between different levels of government, between different stakeholders and even at an international level.

ENDNOTES

1 As an instance, during a managerial course for some of heads and managers of hospitals, in order to prioritize problems, they placed financial problems in the first rank and managerial ones in the last one. Same people at the end of the course, however, classified the managerial problems in the first and financial ones in the last rank.

2 This model with connecting the planning and policy making process to budgeting and then mission control and performance evaluation, the implementation of written policies ensures proper functioning in the context of a process presented.

Compilation of References

2001 Notices of EMS Fatalities. (2001). National EMS Memorial Service. Retrieved from http://nemsms.org/notices01.htm

29-2041 Emergency Medical Technicians and Paramedics. (n.d.). U.S. Bureau of Labor Statistics. Retrieved from http://www.bls.gov/oes/current/oes292041.htm#(1)

A Brief History of Emergency Medical Services. (n.d.). Retrieved from http://wvde.state.wv.us/abe/Public Service Personnel/HistoryofEMS.html

Aaron, H. J. (1991). *Serious and Unstable condition: Financing America's Healthcare*. Washington, DC: Brooking Institutions.

Abdollahi, M. (2007). Developing social issues in Iran: goals and requirements. Letter of Sociology Association, 3, 12.

Adedeji, A. (1999). Comprehending African Conflicts: Sub-Sahara Africa, a violent continent. In A. Adedeji (Ed.), *Comprehending and Mastering African Conflicts: The Search for Sustainable Peace and Good Governance* (pp. 3–21). London: Zed.

Advisory Commission on Intergovernmental Relations. (1980). *The Federal Role in the Federal System: The Dynamics of Growth—Public Assistance: The Growth of a Federal Function*. Washington, DC: U.S. Government Printing Office.

Affordable Care Act. (2010). Retrieved October 14, 2014, from http://hhs.gov/healthcare/rights/law/index.html

African Development Bank. (2007). *Africa's Natural Resources: The paradox of plenty*. Retrieved from http://www.afdb.org/fileadmin/uploads/afdb/Documents/Publications/(E)%20AfricanBank%202007%20Ch4.pdf

Ajaegbu, O. O. (2012). Rising youth unemployment and violent crime in Nigeria. *American Journal of Social Issues and Humanities*, *2*(5), 315–321.

Akinsola, H. A. (2007). *The Principles of Health Services Administration and Management: Perspectives from Clinical and Public Health Practices*. Ibadan: College Press and Publishers Ltd.

Aldrich, H. E., & Ruef, M. (2006). Organizations evolving (2nd ed.). Sage Publishing House.

Alesani, D., & Ancona, F. (2005). *L'innovazione nei modelli di controllo delle aziende sanitarie: evidenze dall'applicazione del modello di controllo per LEA*. Mecosan, n°53.

Alvani, M. (1992). Public issues in management. *Quarterly of Management Studies, 2*, 29-30.

Alvani, M., & Ghasemi, A. R. (1998). *Management and social responsibilities of organization*. Education Center of State Management.

American Medical Association. (1961). *House of Delegates Proceedings, Clinical Session*. Washington, DC: American Medical Association.

Aminuzzaman, S. (2002). Public Policy Making in Bangladesh: An Overview. *Public Money and Management, 2*, 1–7.

Anderson, G., & Sotir, H. (2006). Influencing government policy. In D. Pencheon, C. Guest, D. Melzer, & J. A. Gray (Eds.), *Oxford Handbook of Public Health*. Oxford University Press.

Anonymous. (2011). The doctor is in – at your workplace. *Canadian Medical Association Journal, 183*(13), E983.

Arab Uprising: Country by Country-Tunisia. (2013, December). *BBC News*. Retrieved from http://www.bbc.co.uk/news/world-12482315

Arduini, R. (2010). *Economia e gestione delle aziende sanitarie*. Milan, Italy: F. Angeli.

Auty, R. M. (1993). *Sustaining Development in Mineral Economies: The Resource Curse* (Thesis). London: Routledge.

Balestri, S., & Maggioni, M. A. (2014). Blood diamonds, dirty gold and spatial spill-overs measuring conflict dynamics in West Africa. *Peace Economics, Peace Science & Public Policy, 20*, 551–564.

Balona, D.-M. (2009). Health-care clinics for government workers may save time, money. *Orlando Sentinel*. Retrieved from http://www.orlandosentinel.com/news/orl-loc-lid-clincs031509,0,7551669.story

Bardach, E. (1977). *The implementation game: what happens after a bill comes law*. Cambridge, UK: Cambridge University Press.

Barro, J. (2011). *Cadillac coverage: the high cost of public employee health benefits*. Civic Report No. 65. Center for State and Local Leadership. Manhattan Institute. Retrieved from manhattan-institute.org/csll

Baumgartner, F. R., & Jones, B. D. (1993). *Agendas and instability in American politics*. Chicago: The University of Chicago Press.

Baumgartner, F. R., & Jones, B. D. (2008). *Agendas and Instability in American Politics*. Chicago: University of Chicago Press.

Bausch, D. G., & Schwarz, L. (2014). Outbreak of Ebola virus disease in Guinea: where ecology meets economy. *PLoS Neglected Tropical Diseases, 8*(7), e3056. Retrieved from http://journals.plos.org/plosntds/article?id=10.1371/journal.pntd.0003056

BDHS. (2007). *National Institute of Population Research and Training (NIPORT), Mitra and Associates, and Macro International. 2009. Bangladesh Demographic and Health Survey 2007.* Dhaka, Bangladesh: National Institute of Population Research and Training, Mitra and Associates, and Macro International.

Berenson, R. (2008). Health Affairs. *Medicare Advantage Plans at a Crossroads- Yet Again.* Retrieved October 14, 2014, from http://content.healthaffairs.org/content/28/1/w29.full

Berk, M. L., & Schur, C. L. (1998). Access to care how much difference does medicaid make. *Health Affairs, 17*(3), 169–180. doi:10.1377/hlthaff.17.3.169 PMID:9637973

BHW. (2007). *The Sate of Health in Bangladesh 2006: Challenges of Achieving Equity in Health, Bangladesh Health Watch (BHW).* Dhaka: BRAC University School of Public Health.

BHW. (2008). *Bangladesh Health Watch Report 2007: How Healthy is Health Sector Governance, Bangladesh Health Watch (BHW).* Dhaka: BRAC University School of Public Health.

BHW. (2009). *The Sate of Health in Bangladesh 2010: Health Workforce in Bangladesh, Bangladesh Health Watch (BHW).* Dhaka: BRAC University School of Public Health.

Biocca, M. (2010). *Bilancio di missione. Aziende sanitarie responsabili si raccontano.* Rome, Italy: Il Pensiero Scientifico Editore.

Blendon, R. (2001). The public versus the world health organization. *Health Affairs,* 18. PMID:11585157

Bossert, T. (1998). Analyzing the decentralization of health systems in developing countries: Decision space, innovation and performance. *Social Science & Medicine, 47*(10), 1513–1527. doi:10.1016/S0277-9536(98)00234-2 PMID:9823047

Bosso, C. J. (1994). The Practice and Study of Policy Formation. Northeastern University.

Brady, H. E., & Collier, D. (2004). *Rethinking social inquiry: diverse tools, shared standards.* Lanham, MD: Rowman and Littlefield Publishers, Inc.

Bretton Woods Project. (2005). *What are the Bretton Woods Institutions?* Retrieved from http://www.brettonwoodsproject.org/2005/08/art-320747/

Brewer, G., & de Leon, P. (1983). *The foundations of policy analysis.* Monterey, CA: Brooks/Cole.

Brouhard, R. (2015, March 31). *What's an Ambulance Driver.* About Health Blog.

Browne, R. S. (1987). The IMF in Africa: A case of inappropriate technology in the political morality of the International Monetary Fund. In R. J. Myers (Ed.), Ethics and Foreign Policy Series (Vol. 3, pp. 65–80). Transaction: New Jersey.

Broyles, R. W., Lutchmie, N., & Brandt, E. N. Jr. (2002). The temporarily and chronically uninsured: Does their use of primary care differ? *Journal of Health Care for the Poor and Underserved, 13*(1), 95–111. doi:10.1353/hpu.2010.0159 PMID:11836917

Brugha, R. (2005). *Global Fund Tracking Study: a cross-country comparative analysis.* Final Report. Retrieved from http://www.theglobalfund.org/en/files/links_resources/library/studies/IE13_full.pdf

Brugha, R., Donoghue, M., Starling, M., Ndubani, P., Ssengooba, F., Fernandes, B., & Walt, G. (2004). The Global Fund: Managing great expectations. *Lancet, 364*(9428), 95–100. doi:10.1016/S0140-6736(04)16595-1 PMID:15234862

Brugha, R., Starling, M., & Walt, G. (2002). GAVI, the first steps: Lessons for the Global Fund. *Lancet, 359*(9304), 435–438. doi:10.1016/S0140-6736(02)07607-9 PMID:11844535

Bruni, G., Di Lazzaro, F., & Gatti, G. (2001). *Il reporting della performance aziendale.* Milan, Italy: F. Angeli.

Buchholz, R. A., Evans, W. D., & Wagley, R. A. (1985). *Management Response Public Issues.* Prentice Hall.

Buchnolz, R. A., & Rosenthan, S. B. (2004). Stakeholder Theory and Public Policy: How Government Matters. *Journal of Business Ethics*, 51.

BUHS. (2006). *National Institute of Population Research and Training (NIPORT), MEASURE Evaluation, International Centre for Diarrhoeal Disease Research, Bangladesh (ICDDR,B), and Associates for Community and Population Research (ACPR). 2006 Bangladesh Urban Health Survey.* Dhaka, Bangladesh: NIPORT, MEASURE Evaluation, ICDDR,B, and ACPR.

Burundi. (n.d.). *The New York Times.* Retrieved from http://topics.nytimes.com/top/news/international/countriesandterritories/burundi/index.html

Buse, K. (1999). Keeping a Tight Grip in the Reins: Donor Control over Aid Coordination and. Management in Bangladesh. *Health Policy and Planning, 14*(3), 219–228. doi:10.1093/heapol/14.3.219 PMID:10621239

Buse, K., Mays, N., & Walt, G. (2005). *Making health policy.* Milton Keynes, UK: Open University Press.

Buse, K., Mays, N., & Watts, G. (2005). *Making Health Policy: Understanding Public Health Series.* Open University Press.

Byrne, R. (2009). *Worksite health clinics put new focus on employee health.* HealthLeaders InterStudy's Ohio, Kentucky, and Indiana Health Plan Analysis 10:1, 1-5. Retrieved from: http://www.noviacareclinics.com/assets/uploads /IKO_WorksiteHealth_09.pdf

Caccioppoli, L. (2014). Cultural competency and the rollout of the affordable care act. *PA Times Online.* Retrieved October 14, 2014, from: http://patimes.org/cultural-competency-rollout-affordable-care-act/

Camussone, P. F. (1998). *Il sistema informativo aziendale*. Milan, Italy: Etas libri.

CDC SARS Response Timeline, SARS: Key Events. (2013). Retrieved from http://www.cdc.gov/about/history/sars/timeline.htm

CDC. (2015). *Outbreaks chronology; Ebola virus disease*. Retrieved from http://www.cdc.gov/vhf/ebola/outbreaks/history/chronology.html

Cecchella, A. (1971). *Microeconomia*. Pisa, Italy: ETS.

Census. (2004). *Health Insurance*. Retrieved October 14, 2014, from http://www.census.gov/hhes/www/hlthins/hlthins.html

Census. (2013). *47° Rapporto annuale sulla situazione sociale del Paese*. Retrieved from www.censis.it

Centers for Disease Control and Prevention. (2009). *The power of prevention: chronic disease . . . the public health challenge of the 21st century*. National Center for Chronic Disease and Health Promotion. Retrieved from: http://www.cdc.gov/chronicdisease/pdf/2009-power-of-prevention.pdf

Cepiku, D. (2006). L'esternalizzazione nelle amministrazioni pubbliche. Teorie, politiche ed esperienze a livello internazionale. Rome, Italy: Aracne, Roma.

Cesare, M. D., Marmot, M. G., Blakely, T., Asaria, P., Khang, Y., & Ezzati, M. (2013). Inequalities in non-communicable diseases and effective responses. *Lancet*, *381*(9866), 585–597. doi:10.1016/S0140-6736(12)61851-0 PMID:23410608

Chase, D. (2011). Employers solving healthcare crisis one on-site clinic at a time. *Insurance Thought Leadership*. Retrieved from http://www.insurancethoughtleadership.com/index.php/site/healthcare/employers-solving-healthcare-crisis-one-onsite-clinic-at-a-time/#axzz1x1a44iPx

Chase, D. (2012). Marcus Welby is dead – long live Marcus Welby. *Insurance Thought Leadership*. Retrieved from http://www.insurancethoughtleadership.com/index.php/site/authors/69#axzz1x1a44iPx

Chaudhury, N., & Hammer, J. S. (2004). Ghost Doctors: Absenteeism in Rural Bangladeshi Health Facilities. *The World Bank Economic Review*, *18*(3), 423–441. doi:10.1093/wber/lhh047

Chenoweth, D. H., & Garrett, J. (2006). Cost-effectiveness analysis of a worksite clinic. *AAOHN Journal*, *54*(2), 84–89. PMID:16509183

Childrens Defense Fund. (2012). *Uninsured children*. Retrieved October 14, 2014, from http://www.childrensdefense.org/policy-priorities/children-health/uninsured-children/

Chordas, Lori. (2009). On-the-spot care. *Best's Review*, (May), 74-75.

Cifalà, S. S. (2008). Il sistema di reporting in sanità. Rome, Italy: Aracne.

Claxton, G., Rae, M., Panchal, N., Damico, A., Lundy, J., Bostick, N., . . . Whitmore, H. (2012). *Employee health benefits 2012 annual survey*. Kaiser Family Foundation, Health Research & Educational Trust, and NORC. Retrieved from http://ehbs.kff.org/pdf/2012/8345.pdf

Cochran, C. L., & Malone, E. F. (2005). Public Policy Perspective and Choices (3rd ed.). Academic Press.

Cochran, C. E., Mayer, L. C., Carr, T. R., & Cayer, N. J. (1986). *American Public Policy: An introduction* (2nd ed.). New York: St Martins Press.

Cohen, B. C. (1963). *The Press and Foreign Policy*. Princeton, NJ: Princeton University Press.

Collins, S. R., Davids, K., Doty, M., & Ho, A. (2004). *Wages, benefits, and workers' health*. New York: The Commonwealth Fund. Congressional Budget Office. Cost estimates for health care legislation. Congressional Budget Office. Retrieved October 14, 2014 from http://www.cbo.gov/publications/collections

Collins, S. R., Robertson, R., Garber, T., & Doty, M. M. (2013). *Insuring the Future: Current Trends in Health Coverage and the Effects of Implementing the Affordable Care Act*. New York: The Commonwealth Fund.

Comite, U. (2004). *La comunicazione sanitaria: i rapporti tra personale, paziente e struttura organizzativa*, working paper n°1, Dipartimento di Organizzazione aziendale e amministrazione pubblica, Facoltà di Economia, Università della Calabria, Italy.

Comite, U. (2013). *Accountability e bilancio sociali nei tribunali*. Padova, Italy: Cedam.

Commission on Nonprofit Health and Human Services. (2011). *State of Connecticut*. Retrieved October 14, 2014, from http://ct.gov/opm/lib/opm/finance/hhs_commission/final_report_comission_on_nonprofit_health_and_human_services.pdf

Committee on the Consequences of Uninsurance. (2002). *Institute of Medicine. Care Without Coverage: Too Little, Too Late*. Washington, DC: National Academy Press.

Community H. S. I. (CHSI). (n.d.). Retrieved 22 April 2010 from: http://www.communityhealth.hhs.gov/homepage.aspx?j=1

Congressional Quarterly Almanac. (1960). 36(76-77), 148-164. Washington, DC: Congressional Quarterly.

Congressional Quarterly Weekly Report. (1960). 18(1), 6-8, 18(29), 1236-1250. Washington, DC: Congressional Quarterly.

Corson, J. J. (1939). Wage reports for workers covered by federal old-age insurance in 1937. *Social Security Bulletin*, *2*(3), 3–9.

Cox, W. (2011). Out of sync: Government and private employee compensation in Illinois. Illinois Policy Institute.

Crutchfield, L. R., & Grant, H. M. (2008). *Forces For Good: the six practices of high-impact nonprofits*. San Francisco: Jossey-Bass.

CSG. (2008). *State Policy Guide: Using Research in Public Health Policymaking*. Retrieved from http://stacks.cdc.gov/view/cdc/5233

Cuccurullo, C. (2003). *Il management strategico nelle aziende sanitarie pubbliche*. Milan, Italy: Mc Graw-Hill.

Daft, R. (2012). *Organization theory and design* (11th ed.). South-Western College Pub.

Davis, K., Schoen, C., Schoenbaum, S. C., & Doty, M. M. (2007, May). *Mirror, Mirror on the Wall: An International Update on the Comparative Performance of American Health Care, The Commonwealth Fund*. Retrieved from http://www.commonwealthfund.org/

de Tocqueville, A. (1945). *Democracy in America* (Vol. 2). (H. Reeve, Trans.). New York: Random House. (orig. publ. 1835)

Dearing, J. W., & Rogers, E. M. (1996). *Agenda-setting*. Thousand Oaks, CA: Sage.

Del Bene, L. (2000). *Criteri e strumenti gestionali nelle aziende sanitarie*. Milan, Italy: Giuffrè.

Dery, D. (2000). Agenda Setting and Problem Definition. *Policy Studies*, *21*(1), 37–47.

Devins, N. (2012). Party polarization and judicial review: Lessons learned from the affordable care act. *Northwestern University Law Review*, *106*(4), 1821–1848. Retrieved from http://www.law.northwestern.edu/depts/legalpub/lawreview/v106/n4/1821/LR106n4Devins.pdf

Dove, R. (2001). *Response Ability: The Language, Structure, and Culture of the Agile Enterprise*. Wiley.

Dray-Spira, R., Gueguen, A., Persoz, A., Deveau, C., Lert, F., Delfraissy, J.-F., & Meyer, L. (2005). Temporary employment, absence of stable partnership, and risk of hospitalization or death during the course of HIV infection. *Journal of Acquired Immune Deficiency Syndromes*, *40*(2), 190–197. doi:10.1097/01.qai.0000165908.12333.4e

Dunn, W. (2007). *Public policy analysis: An introduction*. Englewood Cliffs, NJ: Prentice-Hall.

Dye, T. R. (1997). Understanding Public Policy. Prentice Hall.

Dye, T., & Thomas, R. (2001). *Understanding public policy*. Prentice Hall.

Dye, T. (2001). *Top down policy making*. New York: Chatham House.

Edgell, S., Hetherington, K., & Warde, A. (Eds.). (1996). *Consumption matters*. Oxford, UK: Blackwell Publishers.

Egypt under Sisi. (n.d.). *BBC News*. Retrieved from http://www.bbc.co.uk/news/world-middle-east-12315833

Elmore, R. (1979). Backward mapping. *Political Science Quarterly*, *94*(4), 601–616. doi:10.2307/2149628

Elmore, R. (1985). Forward and backward mapping. In K. Hanf & T. Toonen (Eds.), *Policy Implementation in Federal and Unitary Systems* (pp. 33–70). Dordrecht: Martinus Nijhoff. doi:10.1007/978-94-009-5089-4_4

Engel, J. (2006). *Poor People's Medicine: Medicaid and American Charity Care since 1965*. Durham, NC: Duke University Press. doi:10.1215/9780822387633

Ensor, T., & Cooper, S. (2002). *Resource Allocation and Purchasing: Influencing the demand side*. York: Centre for Health Economics, University of York. Prepared for the World Bank, Resource Allocation and Purchasing Project.

Enthoven, A. (2003). Employment-based health insurance is failing: Now what? *Health Affairs*. doi:10.1377/hlthaff.w3.237 PMID:14527258

Eurodad. (2006). *World Bank and IMF Conditionality; A development injustice*. Retrieved from http://www.eurodad.org/uploadedfiles/whats_new/reports/eurodad_world_bank_and_imf_conditionality_report.pdf

Exworthy, M. (2007). *Policy to tackle the social determinants of health: Using conceptual frameworks to understand the policy process*. Paper presented to a Workshop on Health Policy Analysis, London, UK.

Fairbrother, G., Gusmano, M. K., Park, H. L., & Scheinmann, R. (2003). Care for the uninsured in general internists' private offices. *Health Affairs*, *22*(6), 217–264. doi:10.1377/hlthaff.22.6.217 PMID:14649449

Falk, J. (2012). *Comparing the compensation of federal and private-sector employees*. Congressional Budget Office.

Fassin, D., & Schneider, H. (2003). The politics of AIDS in South Africa: Beyond the controversies (Education and Debate). *British Medical Journal*, *326*(7387), 495–497. doi:10.1136/bmj.326.7387.495 PMID:12609950

Feagin, J., Orum, A., & Sjoberg, G. (Eds.). (1991). *A Case for Case study*. Chapel Hill, NC: University of North Carolina Press.

Ferrara, G., & Pozzoli, S. (2006). *Sistemi sanitari regionali tra razionalizzazione degli acquisti e qualità*. Torino, Italy: Giappichelli.

Field, H. H. (1973). Environmental Design Implications of a Changing Health Care System. In Environment and Cognition (pp. 127-157). New York: Seminar Press.

Firestone, W. (1989). Educational policy as ecology of games. *Educational Researcher*, *18*(7), 18–24. doi:10.2307/1177165

Fontana, F., & Lorenzoni, G. (2000). *L'architettura strategica delle aziende ospedaliere: un'analisi empirica*. Milan, Italy: F. Angeli.

Freeman, R. E. (1984). *Strategic management: a stakeholder approach*. Boston: Pitman.

Frenk, J., & Donabedian, A. (1987). State intervention in medical care: types, trends and variables. *Health Policy and Planning*, *2*(1), 17–31. doi:10.1093/heapol/2.1.17 PMID:10282125

Fullan, M. (2000). The three stories of education reform. *Phi Delta Kappan*, 581–584.

Fullan, M. (2007). *The new meaning of educational change*. New York: Teacher's College Press.

Fullan, M. (2009). Large-scale reform comes of age. *Journal of Educational Change*, *10*(2-3), 101–113. doi:10.1007/s10833-009-9108-z

Funkhouser, G. R. (n.d.). The Issues of the Sixties: An Exploratory Study in the Dynamics of Public Opinion. *Public Opinion Quarterly*, *62*.

Galbraith, J. (1977). *Organization design*. Addison Wesley Publishing Company.

Galewitz, P. (n.d.). *Most states to rely on federal website for2015enrollment*. Kaiser Health News. Retrieved October 14, 2014, from http://www.kaiserhealthnews.org/stories/2014/april/24/two-states-likely-to-set-up-own-exchange-for-2015.aspx

George, A. L., & Bennett, A. (2004). *Case studies and theory development in the social sciences*. Cambridge, MA: MIT Press.

Gholipour, R. (2008). *Organizational decision making and public policy making*. Samt Publication.

Gholipour, R., &Faghihi, M. (2014). *Policy making and public policy analysis*. Mahkame Publication.

Giarelli, G., & Venneri, E. (2009). *Sociologia della salute e della medicina*. Milan, Italy: F. Angeli.

Gilman, J. D. (1998). *Medicaid and the Costs of Federalism, 1984-1992*. New York, NY: Garland Publishing, Inc.

Gilson, L., & Raphaely, N. (2007). The terrain of health policy analysis in low and middle income countries: a review of the literature 1994–2005. Paper presented to a Workshop on Health Policy Analysis, London, UK.

Givarian, H., &Rabiei, M. R. (2005). *Decision making and state policy making* (2nd ed.). Yekan Publication.

Global Health Observatory, Life Expectancy Situation. (n.d.). *WHO*. Retrieved from http://www.who.int/gho/mortality_burden_disease/life_tables/situation_trends_text/en/

Gorman, K., & Miller, R. (2011). Managing the risks of on-site health centers. *AAOHN Journal*, *59*(11), 483–490. doi:10.3928/08910162-20111017-02 PMID:22017191

Gornick, M. E., Eggers, P. W., Reilly, T. W., Mentnech, R. M., Fitterman, L. K., Kucken, L. E., & Vladeck, B. C. (1996). Effects of race and income on mortality and use of services among medicare. *The New England Journal of Medicine*, *335*(11), 791–799. doi:10.1056/NEJM199609123351106 PMID:8703185

Gornitzka, A., Kyvik, S., & Stensaker, B. (2005). Implementation analysis in higher education. In A. Gornitzka, M. Kogan, & A. Amaral (Eds.), *Reform and change in higher education: analyzing policy implementation* (pp. 35–56). Dordrecht: Springer. doi:10.1007/1-4020-3411-3_3

Greene, M. (2013). 2013 JEMS Salary and Workplace Survey. *A Journal of Emergency Medical Services*, (Oct), 8.

Greene, M. (2014). 2014 JEMS Salary and Workplace Survey. *A Journal of Emergency Medical Services*, (Oct), 6. PMID:25630146

Grieve, H. R. (1995). Health for All by 2000: Some issues of Health and Health Care in Bangladesh. In Bangladesh Strategy for Development. Dhaka: University Press Limited.

Grindle, M., & Thomas, J. (1991). *Public choice and policy change*. Baltimore, MD: Johns Hopkins University Press.

Gross, L., Huh, K., Sylvester, A., & Zahradnik, R. (2012). *The local squeeze: falling revenues and growing demand for services challenge cities, counties, and school districts*. The Pew Charitable Trust. Retrieved from: http://www.pewstates.org/uploadedFiles/PCS_Assets/2012/Pew_Local_Squeeze(1).pdf

Grossman, M. (2000). The human capital model. In Handbook of Health economics. Amsterdam: North-Holland.

Haas, P. (1992). Introduction: Epistemic communities and international policy coordination. *International Organization*, *46*(01), 1–18. doi:10.1017/S0020818300001442

Hajer, M. A., & Wagenaar, H. (Eds.). (2003). *Deliberative policy analysis*. Cambridge, UK: Cambridge University Press. doi:10.1017/CBO9780511490934

Hall, P., & Taylor, R. (1996). Political science and the three new institutionalisms. *Political Studies*, *64*(5), 936–957. doi:10.1111/j.1467-9248.1996.tb00343.x

Hanf, K., Hjern, B., & Porter, D. (1978). Local networks of manpower training in the Federal Republic of Germany and Sweden. In K. Hanf & F. Scharpf (Eds.), *Interorganisational Policy Making: Limits to Coordination and Central Control* (pp. 303–344). London: Sage.

Haque, M. S. (2002). The Changing Balance of Power between the Government and NGOs in Bangladesh. *International Political Science Review*, *23*(4), 411–435. doi:10.1177/0192512102023004006

Hardey, M. (2001). E-health: The internet and the transformation of patients into consumers and producers of health knowledge. *Information Communication and Society*, 4.

Hasan. (2008). *Challenges of governmental management in Iran*. Samt Publication.

Health Insurance Association of America. (1993). *Source Book on Health Insurance*. Washington, D.C.: The Association.

HealthCare.gov. (2014). Fees you pay if you don't have health insurance coverage. *HealthCare.gov*. Retrieved October 12, 2014, from http://www.healthcare.gov/fees-exemptions/fee-for-not-being-covered/

Hegel, G. W. F. R., & Wood, A. W. (1991). *Hegel: Elements of the Philosophy of Right*. Cambridge University Press.

Hewitt Associates. (2008). *Wellness and beyond: employees examine ways to improve employee health and productivity and reduce costs*. Retrieved from: http://www.aon.com/attachments/thought-leadership/Wellness_and_Beyond.pdf

Hill, M. J., & Hupe, P. L. (2002). *Implementing public policy: governance in theory and practice*. London: Sage.

Hirsch, B. T., Macpherson, D. A., & Vroman, W. G. (2001). Estimates of union density by State. *Monthly Labor Review*, (July): 51–55.

Hirschmann, A. O. (1970). *Exit, Voice and Loyalty: Responses to decline in firms, organizations and states*. Cambridge, MA: Harvard University Press.

Hjern, B., & Hull, C. (1982). Implementation research as empirical constitutionalism. *European Journal of Political Research*, *10*(2), 105–116. doi:10.1111/j.1475-6765.1982.tb00011.x

Hjern, B., & Porter, D. O. (1981). Implementation structures: A new unit of administrative analysis. *Organization Studies*, *2*, 211–227.

Hoffman, C., Carbaugh, A., & Cook, A. (2004). *Health insurance coverage in america: 2003 data update*. Washington, DC: Kaiser Commission on Medicaid and the Uninsured.

Hoffman, C., Schoen, C., Rowland, D., & Davis, K. (2001). Gaps in health coverage among worker-age americans and the consequences. *Journal of Health Care for the Poor and Underserved*, *12*(3), 272–289. doi:10.1353/hpu.2010.0739 PMID:11475546

Hofstede, G. (1980). *Culture's Consequences: International Differences in Work-Related Values*. Beverly Hills, CA: Sage Publications.

Hogwood, G., & Gunn, L. (1984). *Policy analysis for the real world*. Oxford, UK: Oxford University Press.

Hollingsworth, J. R., Hage, J., & Hanneman, R. (1990). *State intervention in medical care: consequences for Britain, France, Sweden, and the United States, 1890-1970*. Chicago: Cornell Univ Press.

How Long are African Presidents Staying in Power?. (2015, May). *BBC News*. Retrieved from http://www.bbc.com/news/world-africa-32624979

Howlett, M., & Ramesh, M. (2003). *Studying Public Policy*. Oxford University Press.

Howlett, M., & Romesh, M. (1995). *Studying Public Policy-Policy Cycles and Policy Subsystems*. New York: Oxford University Press.

Hsiao, W. (1998). *Health care financing in developing nations*. Paper prepared for the World Bank Institute Flagship Course on Integrated Health Care Financing Approaches.

Hsiao, W. C. (2003). *What is a health system? Why should we care*. Harvard School of Public Health, working paper, 33.

Hunter, D. J. (2003). Evidence-based policy and practice: Riding for a fall? *Journal of the Royal Society of Medicine*, *96*(4), 194–196. doi:10.1258/jrsm.96.4.194 PMID:12668712

IDA. (2015). *What is IDA?* Retrieved from http://www.worldbank.org/ida/what-is-ida.html

IDMC. (2015). *The Norwegian Refugee Council's Internal Displacement Monitoring Center Global Overview; People internally displaced by conflict and violence*. Retrieved from http://www.internal-displacement.org/assets/library/Media/201505-Global-Overview-2015/20150506-global-overview-2015-en.pdf

ILO. (2010). *ILO Global Employment Trends*. Retrieved from http://www.ilo.org/wcmsp5/groups/public/---ed_emp/---emp_elm/---trends/documents/publication/wcms_120471.pdf

ILO. (2013). *ILO Global employment Trends 2013*. Retrieved from http://www.ilo.org/wcmsp5/groups/public/---dgreports/---dcomm/---publ/documents/publication/wcms_202326.pdf

IMF. (2015a). *About the IMF*. Retrieved from http://www.imf.org/external/about.htm

IMF. (2015b). *IMF Executive directors and voting powers*. Retrieved from http://www.imf.org/external/np/sec/memdir/eds.aspx

IMF. (2015c). *IMF Executive Directors and Voting Powers*. Available from: http://www.imf.org/external/np/sec/memdir/eds.aspx

IMF. (2015c). *IMF Lending*. Retrieved from http://www.imf.org/external/np/exr/facts/howlend.htm

Infoplease. (2014). *Population Distribution by Age, Race, and Nativity, 1860-2010*. Retrieved July 2014, from http://www.infoplease.com/ipa/A0110384.html

Ingram, H., Schneider, A. L., & De Leon, P. (2007). Social construction and policy design. In Theories of the policy process. Boulder, CO: Westview Press.

Ingram, H., & Schneider, A. (1990). Improving implementation through framing smarter statutes. *Journal of Public Policy*, *10*(1), 67–88. doi:10.1017/S0143814X00004682

International City-County Management Association. (2011). *Local government employee Insurance Program*. Accessed at: https://icma.org/Documents/Document/Document/303133.Washington

IRS.gov. (2014). Exemption requirements – 501(c)3 organizations. *IRS.gov*. Retrieved October 14, 2014, from http://www.irs.gov/charities-&-non-profits/charitabale-organizations/exemption-requirements-section-501%28c%29%283%29-Organizations

Jahan, R., & Salehin, M. (2006). Health Care for Rural People of Bangladesh: Overview of Some Governance Issues. In Governance and Development: Bangladesh and Regional Experiences. Dhaka: Shrabon Prokashoni.

Jahan, R. (2003). Restructuring the Health System: Experiences of Advocates for Gender Equity in Bangladesh. *Reproductive Health Matters*, *11*(21), 183–191. doi:10.1016/S0968-8080(03)02173-6 PMID:12800715

Jecker, N. (1993). Can an employer-based health insurance system be just? *Journal of Health Care Politics. Policy and Law*, *18*(3), 657–673.

Jenkin, R. A., Frommer, M. S., & Rubin, G. L. (2006). Translating indicators and targets into public health action. In D. Pencheon, C. Guest, D. Melzer, & J. A. Muir Gray (Eds.), *Oxford Handbook of Public Health*. Oxford University Press.

John, P. (2003). Is there a life after policy streams, advocacy coalitions and punctuations: Using evolutionary theory to explain policy change? *Policy Studies Journal: the Journal of the Policy Studies Organization*, *31*(4), 481–498. doi:10.1111/1541-0072.00039

Johnson, L. B. (1971). *The Vantage Point: Perspectives of the Presidency, 1963-1969*. Chicago, IL: Holt, Rinehart & Winston.

Jordan, M. M. (2003). Punctuations and Agendas: A New Look at Local Government Budget Expenditures. *Journal of Policy Analysis and Management*, *22*(3), 345–360. doi:10.1002/pam.10136

Kaiser Family Foundation. (2012). *Premiums, cost-sharing and coverage at public, private and non-profit employers: a view from the 2012 employer health benefit survey*. Retrieved from: http://www.kff.org/insurance/ snapshot/chcm112012oth.cfm

Kaler, A., & Watkins, S. C. (2001). Disobedient distributors: street-level bureaucrats and would-be patrons in community-based family planning programs in rural Kenya. *Studies in Family Planning, 32*, 254-69.

Kamuzora, P., & Gilson, L. (2007). Factors influencing implementation of the Community Health Fund in Tanzania. *Health Policy and Planning*, *22*(2), 95–102. doi:10.1093/heapol/czm001 PMID:17299023

Kavanaugh, S. (2011). *Containing health care costs: proven strategies for success in the public sector*. Government Finance Officers Association and Colonial Life.

Keck, M. E., & Sikkink, K. (1998). *Activists beyond borders*. Ithaca, NY: Cornell University Press.

Kiewiet, D., & McCubbins, M. (1991). *The logic of delegation*. Chicago: University of Chicago Press.

Kingdon, J. W. (1995). Agendas, Alternatives, and Public Policies (Second Ed.). New York, NY: Harper Collins.

Kingdon, J. W. (1984). *Agendas, alternatives and public policies*. Boston, MA: Little, Brown and Company.

Kingdon, J. W. (1995). *Agendas, Alternatives, and Public Policies*. New York: HarperCollins College Publishers.

Kiser, E. (1999). Comparing varieties of agency theory in economics, political science and sociology: An illustration from state policy implementation. *Sociological Theory, 17*(2), 146-170.

Kleczkowski, B. M., Roemer, M. I., & Werff, A. V. D. (1984). *National health systems and their reorientation towards health for all: guidelines for policy-making*. Academic Press.

Kolodrubetz, W. W. (1972). Two decades of employee-benefit plans, 1950-70: A review. *Social Security Bulletin, 35*(4), 10–22.

Koremenos, B., & Lynn, L. (1996). Leadership of a state agency. In D. Kettl & H. Brinton Milward (Eds.), The State of Public Management. Baltimore, MD: Johns Hopkins University Press.

Kraft, M. E., & Furlong, S. R. (2012). Public policy: Politics, Analysis, and alternatives (4th ed.). CQ Press.

Krause, E. A. (1977). *Power and illness: the political sociology of health and medical care*. New York: Elsevier.

Lambert, J. (2013, December 10). *NPQ. Infographic: what is driving nonprofit sector's growth?* Retrieved October 13, 2014, from https://nonprofitquarterly.org/policysocial-context/23359-infographic-what-is-driving-nonprofit-sectors-growth.html

LaPenna, A. M. (2010). Workplace Clinics and employer managed healthcare: a catalyst for cost savings and improved productivity. Boca Raton, FL: CRC Press.

Laraway, A. S., & Jennings, C. P. (2002). Health Insurance Flexibility and Accountability Demonstration Initiative (HIFA): A Policy Analysis Using Kingdon's Policy Streams Model. *Policy, Politics & Nursing Practice, 3*(4), 358–366. doi:10.1177/152715402237970

Lasswell, H. (1956). *The decision process*. College Park, MD: University of Maryland Press.

Lasswell, H. D. (1971). *A Pre-view of Policy Sciences*. New York: American Elsevier Publishing Co.

Laurent Gbagbo. (n.d.). *The New York Times*. Retrieved from http://topics.nytimes.com/top/reference/timestopics/people/g/laurent_gbagbo/index.html

Le Guenno, B., Formentry, P., Wyers, M., Gounon, P., Walker, F., & Boesch, C. (1995). Isolation and partial characterization of a new strain of Ebola virus. *Lancet, 345*(8960), 1271–1274. doi:10.1016/S0140-6736(95)90925-7

Lee, K., Fustukian, S., & Buse, K. (2002). *Health policy in a globalizing world*. Cambridge, UK: Cambridge University Press.

Lee, K., Lush, L., Walt, G., & Cleland, J. (1998). Family planning policies and programmes in eight low-income countries: A comparative policy analysis. *Social Science & Medicine*, *47*(7), 949–959. doi:10.1016/S0277-9536(98)00168-3 PMID:9722114

Lee, S. Y., Chun, C. B., Lee, Y. G., & Seo, N. K. (2008). The National Health Insurance system as one type of new typology: The case of South Korea and Taiwan. *Health Policy (Amsterdam)*, *85*(1), 105–113.

Libya Country Profile-Overview. (2015, June). *BBC News*. Retrieved from http://www.bbc.co.uk/news/world-africa-13754897

Liddick, Betty. (2005). Sick over health care costs, companies get some relief with on-site medical centers. *Workforce Management, 84*(5), 82.

Liedtke, M. (2009, August 9). Small Is Beautiful (and Successful) for Newspapers. *Palestine (Texas) Herald.*

Lincoln, Y. (1995). Emerging criteria for quality in qualitative and interpretive research. *Qualitative Inquiry*, *1*(3), 275–289. doi:10.1177/107780049500100301

Lindblom, C. E. (2002). *The Market System: What it Is, how it Works, and what to Make of it.* Yale University Press.

Lipsky, M. (1980). *Street-level bureaucracy: dilemmas of the individual in public services.* New York: Russell Sage Foundation.

Londoño, J. L., & Frenk, J. (1997). Structured pluralism: Towards an innovative model for health system reform in Latin America. *Health Policy (Amsterdam)*, *41*(1), 1–36. doi:10.1016/S0168-8510(97)00010-9 PMID:10169060

Long, S. K. (2003). *Hardship among the uninsured: choosing among food, housing and health insurance. New Federalism.* Washington, DC: The Urban Institute.

LowsPa, D. (2004). *New approach in social issue analysis.* Tehran: Amirkabir Publication.

Mahmud, S. (2007). Spaces for Participation in Health Systems in Rural Bangladesh: The Experience of Stakeholder Community Groups. In Spaces for Change? The Politics of Citizen Participation in New Democratic Arenas. London: Zed Books.

Malaria. (2015, April). *The World Bank.* Retrieved from http://www.worldbank.org/en/topic/health/brief/malaria

Marinò, L. (2008). *La ricerca dell'economicità nelle aziende sanitarie locali. Concetti, modelli, decisioni.* Torino, Italy: Giappichelli.

Marsh, D. (Ed.). (1998). *Comparing policy networks.* Buckingham, UK: Open University Press.

Marsh, D., & Rhodes, R. A. W. (1992). *Policy networks in British Government.* Buckingham, UK: Open University Press. doi:10.1093/acprof:oso/9780198278528.001.0001

Marx, K. (2011). *Capital: volume one, A critique of political economy*. Dover Publications.

Matland, R. (1995). Synthesising the implementation literature: The ambiguity-conflict model of policy implementation. *Journal of Public Administration: Research and Theory*, *5*(2), 145–174.

Mazmanian, D., & Sabatier, P. (1983). *Implementation and Public Policy*. Glenview: Scott, Foresman.

McCallion, T. (2013). Feds Make Sweeping Changes to HIPAA Privacy and Security Rules. *A Journal of Emergency Medical Services*.

McCarthy, D., & Klein, S. (2010). *QuadMed: transforming employer-Sponsored health care through workplace primary care and wellness programs*. The Commonwealth Fund. Retrieved from: http://www.commonwealthfund.org/~/media/Files/Publications/Casepercent20Study/2010/Jul/Triplepercent20Aimpercent20v2/1424_McCarthy_QuadMed_triple_aim_case_study_v2.pdf

McCombs, M., & Valenzuela, S. (2014). *Agenda-Setting Theory: The Frontier Research Questions*. Retrieved from http://www.academia.edu/8239537/Agenda-Setting_Theory_The_Frontier_Research_Questions

McCombs, M. E. (2004). *Setting the Agenda: The Mass Media and Public Opinion*. Malden, MA: Blackwell Publishing.

McCombs, M. E., & Shaw, D. L. (1972). The Agenda-Setting Function of Mass Media. *Public Opinion Quarterly*, *36*(2), 176–187. doi:10.1086/267990

McKeown, T. J. (2004). Case studies and the limits of the quantitative worldview. In H. E. Brady & D. Collier (Eds.), *Rethinking social inquiry: diverse tools, shared standards* (pp. 139–168). Lanham, MD: Rowman and Littlefield Publishers, Inc.

McLaughlin, M. W. (1987). Learning from experience: Lessons from policy implementation. *Educational Evaluation and Policy Analysis*, *9*(2), 171–178. doi:10.3102/01623737009002171

MDG 6. Combat HIV/AIDS, Malaria and Other Diseases. (2014, December). *WHO*. Retrieved from http://www.who.int/topics/millennium_development_goals/diseases/en/

Merriam, S. B., Johnson-Bailey, J., Lee, M. Y., Kee, Y., Ntseane, G., & Muhamad, M. (2001). Power and positionality: Negotiating insider/outsider status within and across cultures. *International Journal of Lifelong Education*, *20*(5), 405–416. doi:10.1080/02601370120490

MIC. (2006). *Multi-indicator Cluster Survey, 2006, BBS, UNICEF*. Dhaka: GOB.

MICS. (2009). *Multi-indicator Cluster Survey, 2009, BBS, UNICEF*. Dhaka: GOB.

Mills, C. (2013, July 8). EMS Run by Idiots. *WRDW*.

Mills, A. J., & Ranson, M. K. (2001). *The design of health systems. International Public Health*. Gaithersburg, MD: Aspen Publishers.

MoHFW. (2010). Final Draft of Health Policy. Dhaka: Ministry of Health and Family Welfare (MoHFW).

Mooradian, D. (2008). Jobsite health clinics open doors to savings. *HealthLeaders InterStudy – Tennessee Health Plan Analysis, 20*(4), 1-4.

Moore, A. V. (2011). The doctor is in – at the workplace. *Benefits Magazine,* (December), 14-19.

Mortensen, P. B., & Serritzlew, S. (2006). Newspapers and Budgeting: The Effects of Media Coverage on Local Expenditure Decisions. *Scandinavian Political Studies, 29*(3), 236–260. doi:10.1111/j.1467-9477.2006.00151.x

Muller, P. (1999). *Les politiques publiques*. Montchrestien.

Murray, S. F. (2007). *Illuminating unintended consequences: a case study using retrospective policy analysis linking the macro, meso, and micro*. Paper presented to a Workshop on Health Policy Analysis, London, UK.

Myott, S. (2010). 2009 *County Long-Term Care Gaps Analysis Survey*. Department of Human Services Continuing Care Administration. Retrieved October 14, 2014, from http://dhs.state.mn.us/main/groups/aging/documents/pub/dhs16_153750.pdf

Narayan, T. (2007). *Policy Processes underlying Health and Equity Initiatives in a rapidly globalizing context – a case study from Bangalore, Karnataka, India*. Paper presented to a Workshop on Health Policy Analysis, London, UK.

Nash, J. L. (2005). *Making the business case for integrated health and wellness*. Academic Press.

National Center for Health Statistics. (2004). *Health United States 2004*. Hyattsville, MD: Centers for Disease Control and Prevention, U.S. Department of Health and Human Services.

National Multiple Sclerosis Society. (2014). *Home*. Retrieved October 12, 2014, from http://www.nationalmssociety.org/

Navarro, V. (1989). Why some countries have national health insurance, others have national health services, and the US has neither. *Social Science & Medicine, 28*(9), 887–898. doi:10.1016/0277-9536(89)90313-4 PMID:2652327

Navarro, V. (2004). *A critique of social capital. In Political and Economic Determinants of Population Health and well-being*. Amityville, NY: Baywood.

Nazneen, K. (2001). *Governance of the Healthcare Sector in Bangladesh*. Dhaka: University Press Limited.

Negredo, A., Palacios, G., Vázquez-Morón, S., González, F., Dopazo, H., Molero, F., & Tenorio, A. et al. (2011). Discovery of an Ebolavirus-like filovirus in Europe. *PLoS Pathogens, 7*(10), e1002304.

Ng, S., Basta, N. E., & Cowling, B. J. (2014). Association between temperature, humidity and ebolavirus disease outbreaks in Africa, 1976 to 2014. *Eurosurveillance*, *19*(35), 20892. doi:10.2807/1560-7917.ES2014.19.35.20892

Njoku, A. C., & Ihugba, O. A. (2011). Unemployment and Nigerian Economic Growth (1985-2009). *Mediterranean Journal of Social Sciences*, *2*(6), 23–32.

O'Toole, L. (1995). Rational choice and policy implementation: Implications for interorganisational network management. *American Review of Public Administration*, *25*(1), 43–57. doi:10.1177/027507409502500103

Oberlander, J. (2003). *The Politics Of Health Reform: Why Do Bad Things Happen To Good Plans?* Health Affairs Web Exclusive. Retrieved 27 August 2009 from: http://content.healthaffairs.org/cgi/reprint/hlthaff.w3.391v1?maxtoshow=&hits=10&RESULTFORMAT=&fulltext=The+Politics+Of+Health+Reform%3A&searchid=1&FIRSTINDEX=0&resourcetype=HWCIT

Obilade, T. T. (2015a). Ebola virus disease stigmatization: The role of societal attributes. *International Archives of Medicine*, *8*(14), 1-19. Retrieved from http://imed.pub/ojs/index.php/iam/article/view/1007/674

Obilade, T. T. (2015b). The political economy and stigmatization of HIV/AIDS in patients attending a clinic in Lagos, Nigeria. *The International Archives of Medicine*, *8*(26), 1-11. Retrieved from http://imed.pub/ojs/index.php/iam/article/view/997/687

OECD. (1987). *The Reform of Health Care: A Comparative Analysis of Seven OECD Countries*. OECD.

OECD. (1992). *The Reform of Health Care: A Comparative Analysis of Seven OECD Countries*. OECD.

OECD. (1996). *Budgeting and Policy Decision-Making*. SIGMA Paper No. 8, OCDE/GD(96)110. OECD.

OECD. (2004). The Reform of Health Care: A Comparative Analysis of Seven OECD Countries. Paris: Organisation for Economic Co-operation and Development.

OECD. (2013). *Health at a Glance 2013*. Retrieved October 14, 2014 from http://oecd.org/els/health-systems/health-at-a-glance-2013.pdf

Office of Management and Budget. (2015). *Historical Tables*. Retrieved July 2014, from https://www.whitehouse.gov/omb/budget/Historicals

Office of the National Coordinator for Health Information Technology. (n.d.). *Benefits of EHRs: improved diagnostics and patient outcomes*. Retrieved from http://www.healthit.gov/providers-professionals/improved-diagnostics-patient-outcomes

Ogden, J., Walt, G., & Lush, L. (2003). The politics of 'branding' in policy transfer: The case of DOTS for tuberculosis control. *Social Science & Medicine*, *57*(1), 179–188. doi:10.1016/S0277-9536(02)00373-8 PMID:12753826

Oleszek, W. J. (2014). *Congressional Procedures and the Policy Process*. Washington: Congressional Quarterly Press.

Oliphant, L. T., & Murray, C. C. (2012). Fit for an on-site clinic. *HRMagazine*, *57*, 1, 61, 63, 65.

Oliver, T. R., & Dowell, E. B. (1994). Interest groups and health reform: Lessons from California, *Health Affairs. Supplement*, *13*(2), 123–141.

Olson, L. K. (2010). *The Politics of Medicaid*. New York, NY: Columbia University Press.

Omar al-Bashir wins Sudan Elections by a Landslide. (2015, April). *BBC News*. Retrieved from http://www.bbc.com/news/world-africa-32481013

Onida, P. (1961). Economicità, socialità ed efficienza nell'amministrazione d'impresa. *Stato sociale*, 3.

Osman, F. A. (2004). *Policy Making in Bangladesh: A Study of the Health Policy Process*. Dhaka: A H Development Publishing House.

Osman, F. A. (2005). Implementation Constrained by a Lack of Policy Ownership: Evidence from Bangladesh. *The Asia Pacific Journal of Public Administration*, *27*(1), 19–36. doi:10.1080/23276665.2005.10779297

Osman, F. A. (2008). Health Policy, Programs and System in Bangladesh: Achievement and Challenges. *South Asian Survey*, *15*(2), 23–288. doi:10.1177/097152310801500206

Ostrom, E. (2007). Institutional rational choice: an assessment of the institutional analysis and development framework. In P. A. Sabatier (Ed.), *Theories of the policy process* (2nd ed.; pp. 21–64). Boulder, CO: Westview Press.

Pachman, J. S., Stempien, D., Milles, S. S., & O'Neill, F. N. (1996). The hidden savings of a corporate on-site medical center. *Journal of Occupational and Environmental Medicine*, *83*(10), 1047–1048. PMID:8899583

Paessler, S., & Walker, D. H. (2013). Pathogenesis of the viral hemorrhagic fevers. *Annual Review of Pathology*, *8*(1), 411–440. doi:10.1146/annurev-pathol-020712-164041

Page, B. I., & Shapiro, R. Y. (1992). *The Rational Public Fifty Years of Trends in Americans' Policy Preferences*. Chicago: University of Chicago Press. doi:10.7208/chicago/9780226644806.001.0001

Panday, P. K. (2008). Women's Political Participation in Bangladesh: Institutional Reforms, Actors and Outcomes. (Unpublished PhD thesis). City University of Hong Kong. Retrieved from http://dspace.cityu.edu.hk/handle/2031/5426

Panday, P. K. (2001). The Role of Bureaucratic Elite in the Policy Making Process in Bangladesh., *Socialist Perspective: A Quarterly. Journal of Social Sciences*, *29*(1-2), 47–60.

Pang, T., Sadana, R., Hanney, S., Bhutta, Z. A., Hyder, A. A., & Simon, J. (2003). Knowledge for better health - a conceptual framework and foundation for health research systems. *Bulletin of the World Health Organization*, *81*, 777–854. PMID:14758408

Parkhurst, J. O. (2002). The Ugandan success story? Evidence and claims of HIV-1 Prevention. *Lancet, 360*(9326), 78–80. doi:10.1016/S0140-6736(02)09340-6 PMID:12114061

Patel, K., & Rushefsky, M. (2006). *Health Care Politics and Policy in America* (3rd ed.). Armonk, NY: M. E. Sharpe.

Payne, C. (2008). *So much reform, so little change: the persistence of failure in urban schools.* Cambridge, MA: Harvard Education Press.

Pelone, F., & Ricciardi, W. (2013). Il public reporting in sanità: Riflessioni e proposte di un nuovo strumento operative. *Quaderni dell'Italian. Journal of Public Health, 2*(10).

Perry, A. (2010, June 28). Brief History: The Resource Curse. *Time Magazine.* Retrieved from http://content.time.com/time/magazine/article/0,9171,1997460,00.html

Perry, H. B. (1999). *Quest for a Healthy Bangladesh: A Vision for the Twenty-First Century.* Dhaka: University Press.

Perry, H. B. (2000). *Health for All in Bangladesh.* Dhaka: University Press.

Peteromode, V. F., & Peretomode, O. (2005). *Human Resource Management.* Lagos: Onoosomegbwho Ogbinaka Publishers.

Peters, R. A. (2004). The Social Security Amendments of 1960: Completing the foundation for Medicare and Medicaid. *Journal of Health and Human Services Administration, 26*(4), 438–469. PMID:15704642

Peter, T. (Ed.). (1988). *Inequalities in Health: The Black Report.* London: Penguin.

Pew Research Center. (2013). *Partisan polarization in congress and among public is greater than ever.* Retrieved October 14, 2014, from http://www.pewresearch.org/fact-tank/2013/07/17/partisan-polarization-in-congress-and-among-public-is-greater-than-ever/

Pippin, J. (2014, August 8). Richlands EMS Suspended from Medical Calls. *The Daily News.* Retrieved from: http://www.jdnews.com/news/local/richlands-ems-suspended-from-medical-calls-1.356331

Politico. (2014). *Protecting the sick? Not so easy.* Retrieved October 14, 2014, from http://www.politico.com/story/2014/08/insurance-discrimination-obamacare-110095.html

Population Reference Bureau. (2011). *The World's Women's and Girls' 2011 Data Sheet.* Retrieved from http://www.prb.org/pdf11/world-women-girls-2011-data-sheet.pdf

Population Reference Bureau. (2014). *Population Reference Bureau 2014 World Population Data Sheet.* Retrieved from http://www. prb.org/pdf14/2014-world-population-data-sheet_eng.pdf

Porter, E. (2013). Health care and profits, a poor mix. *The New York Times.* Retrieved October 14, 2014, from http://www.nytimes.com/2013/01/09/business/health-care-and-pursuit-of-profit-make-a-poor-mix.html?pagewanted=all&_r=0

Pozzoli, S. (2001). *Il controllo direzionale negli enti locali.* Milan, Italy: F. Angeli.

Pressman, J., & Wildavsky, A. (1984). *Implementation* (3rd ed.). Berkeley, CA: University of California Press.

Putnam, R. (2000). *Bowling Alone: The collapse and Revival of American community.* New York: Simon and Schuster. doi:10.1145/358916.361990

Quality Assurance Project TASC 2, Eritrea. (2003). *Quality Assurance Core Course.* Associate Student Nurses State of Eritrea, Ministry of Health.

Rabbani, G. (2009). Non-Governmental Actors are Coming Forward as Policy Actors: Example from Operational Framework for Pre-Primary Education. *Social Change, 3*(2), 7–20.

Ragin, C., & Becker, H. S. (1992). *What is a case? Exploring the foundations of social enquiry.* New York: Cambridge University Press.

Rahman, R. M. (2006). Human rights, health and the state in Bangladesh. *BMC International Health and Human Rights, 6*(4). Retrieved 22 May 2990 from http://www.biomedcentral.com/1472-698X/6/4

Rashid, S. F., Hadin, A., Afsana, K., & Begum, S. A. (2001). Acute respiratory infections in rural Bangladesh: Cultural understanding, practices and the role of mothers and community health volunteers. *Tropical Medicine & International Health, 6*(4), 249–255. doi:10.1046/j.1365-3156.2001.00702.x PMID:11348514

Reich, M. R., & Cooper, D. (1996). *Policy Maker* [Software tool]. Available from http://www.hsph.harvard.edu

Reich, M. R. (1995). The politics of agenda setting in international health: Child health versus adult health in developing countries. *Journal of International Development, 7*(3), 489–502. doi:10.1002/jid.3380070310 PMID:12290763

Reich, M. R. (1995). The Politics of Health Sector Reform in Developing Countries: Three Cases of Pharmaceutical Policy. *Health Policy (Amsterdam), 32*(3), 47–77.

Reich, M. R., & Govindaraj, R. (1998). Dilemmas in drug development for tropical diseases. Experiences with praziquantel. *Health Policy (Amsterdam), 44*(1), 1–18. doi:10.1016/S0168-8510(98)00002-5 PMID:10180198

Reid, T. R. (2010). *The Healing of America: a global quest for better, cheaper, fairer health care.* New York: Penguin Press.

Reporter's Guide to Medical Privacy Law. (2007). Reporters Committee for Freedom of the Press.

Rhodes, R. A. W. (1997). *Understanding Governance: Policy Networks, Governance, Flexibility and Accountability.* Buckingham, UK: Open University Press.

Robinson, S. E., & Eller, W. S. (2010). Participation in Policy Streams: Testing the Separation of Problems and Solutions in Subnational Policy Systems. *Policy Studies Journal: the Journal of the Policy Studies Organization, 38*(2), 199–216. doi:10.1111/j.1541-0072.2010.00358.x

Roemer, M. I. (1956). *Medical Care in Relation to Public Health: A Study of Relationships Between Preventive and Curative Health Services Throughout the World.* World Health Organization.

Roemer, M. I. (1991). Health care costs and financing in world perspective. *The Yale Journal of Biology and Medicine, 64*(5), 435. PMID:1814057

Roemer, M. I., & Axelrod, S. J. (1977). A National Health Service and Social Security. *American Journal of Public Health, 67*(5), 462–465. doi:10.2105/AJPH.67.5.462 PMID:324295

Rogers, E. M., Dearing, J. W., & Bregman, D. (1993). The Anatomy of Agenda-Setting Research. *Journal of Communication, 43*(2), 68–84. doi:10.1111/j.1460-2466.1993.tb01263.x

Roper, W. L. (2007). Here We Go Again-Lessons On Health Reform Advances in science and clinical practice, not the political process, will continue to drive the pace of reform. *Health Affairs, 26*(6), 1551–1552. doi:10.1377/hlthaff.26.6.1551 PMID:17978372

Rose, G. (1997). Situating knowledges: Positionality, reflexivity and other tactics. *Progress in Human Geography, 21*(3), 305–320. doi:10.1191/030913297673302122

Rosenbaum, W.A. (1985). *Environmental Politics and Policy*. Washington, DC: CQ Press.

Ross, W. (2008, August 6). Guinea Turmoil Threatens Mine Deal. *BBC News*. Retrieved from http://news.bbc.co.uk/2/hi/africa/7544046.stm

Sabatier, P. (2005). From policy implementation to policy change: a personal odyssey. In A. Gornitzka, M. Kogan, & A. Amaral (Eds.), *Reform and change in higher education: analyzing policy implementation* (pp. 17–34). Dordrecht: Springer. doi:10.1007/1-4020-3411-3_2

Sabatier, P. A. (Ed.). (1999). *Theories of the policy process*. Boulder, CO: Westview Press.

Sabatier, P., & Jenkins-Smith, H. (1999). The advocacy coalition framework: an assessment. In P. Sabatier (Ed.), *Theories of the Policy Process* (pp. 117–168). Boulder, CO: Westview Press.

Sachs, J. D., & Warner, A. M. (1999). The big push, natural resource booms and growth. *Journal of Development Economics, 59*(1), 43–76. doi:10.1016/S0304-3878(99)00005-X

Saetren, H. (2005). Facts and myths about research on public policy implementation: Out-of-fashion, allegedly dead, but still very much alive and relevant. *Policy Studies Journal: the Journal of the Policy Studies Organization, 33*(4), 559–582. doi:10.1111/j.1541-0072.2005.00133.x

Saita, M. (2007). Governance ed economicità nelle aziende sanitarie. Il Sole 24 Ore, Milano.

Sandy, L. G., Bodenheimer, T., Pawlson, L. G., & Starfield, B. (2009). The political economy of U.S. primary care. *Health Affairs, 28*(4), 1136–1144. doi:10.1377/hlthaff.28.4.1136 PMID:19597213

Santi, M. (1998). *I sistemi informativi per il controllo di gestione nelle aziende sanitarie. In Sanità pubblica* (p. 3). Rimini: Maggioli.

Sargeant, A., & Shang, J. (2010). *Fundraising Principles and Practice*. San Francisco: Jossey-Bass.

Savely, S., Hamilton, W., Degani, F., Weinberg, A., & Muraca, P. (2011). A survey of environmental safety at 20 medical clinics. *Journal of Environmental Health*, *73*(6), 86–94. PMID:21306100

Scheiffer, B. (2014, September 7). Remembering 9/11, when Americans Came Together. *Face the Nation*.

Schlager, E. (2007). A comparison of frameworks, theories, and models of policy processes. In P. A. Sabatier (Ed.), *Theories of the policy process*. Boulder, CO: Westview Press.

Schneider, A., & Ingram, H. (1993). Social Construction of target populations: Implications for politics and policy. *The American Political Science Review*, *87*(2), 334–347. doi:10.2307/2939044

Schneider, H., Gilson, L., Ogden, J., Lush, L., & Walt, G. (2006). Health systems and the implementation of disease programmes: Case studies from South Africa. *Global Public Health: An International Journal for Research, Policy and Practice*, *1*(1), 49–64. doi:10.1080/17441690500361083 PMID:19153894

Schottland, C. I. (1956). Social Security Amendments of 1956: A Summary and Legislative History. *Social Security Bulletin*, (September), 1956.

Schramm, W. (1963). *The Science of Human Communication; New Directions and New Findings in Communication Research*. New York: Basic Books.

Schurmann, A. T., & Mahmud, S. (2009). Civil society, health, and social exclusion in Bangladesh. *Journal of Health, Population, and Nutrition*, *27*, 536–544. PMID:19761087

Scott, W. R. (2005). Organizations: Rational, Natural and open systems (5th ed.). Prentice Hall.

Scott, W. R., & Davis, G. F. (2015). Organizations and organizing: Rational, Natural and open systems perspectives. Routledge.

Sherman, B. W., & Fabius, R. J. (2012). Quantifying the value of worksite clinic nonoccupational health care services. *Journal of Occupational and Environmental Medicine*, *54*(4), 394–403. doi:10.1097/JOM.0b013e31824b2157 PMID:22418274

Sherman, B. W., Frazee, S. G., Fabius, R. J., Broome, R., Manfred, J. R., & Davis, J. (2009). Impact of workplace health services on adherence to chronic medications. *The American Journal of Managed Care*, *15*(7), 53–59. PMID:19589007

Shiffman, J. (2007). Generating political priority for maternal mortality reduction in 5 developing countries. *American Journal of Public Health*, *97*(5), 796–803. doi:10.2105/AJPH.2006.095455 PMID:17395848

Shiffman, J., Beer, T., & Wu, Y. H. (2002). The emergence of global disease control priorities. *Health Policy and Planning*, *17*(3), 225–234. doi:10.1093/heapol/17.3.225 PMID:12135988

Shiffman, J., & Wu, Y. (2003, November). Norms in tension: Democracy and efficiency in Bangladeshi health and population sector reform. *Social Science & Medicine*, *57*(9), 1547–1557. doi:10.1016/S0277-9536(02)00547-6 PMID:12948566

Shi, L. (1995). Balancing primary versus specialty care. *Journal of the Royal Society of Medicine*, *88*, 428–432. PMID:7562823

Slomin, H. (1942). State and Regional Differences in Covered Employment and Taxable Wages, 1939. *Social Security Bulletin*, *5*(1), 35–44.

Smedley, B. D., Stith, A. Y., & Nelson, A. R. (2003). *Racial and Ethnic Disparities in Healthcare: a Background and History. In Unequal Treatment: Confronting Racial and Ethnic Disparities in Health Care* (pp. 455–527). Washington, DC: National Academy Press.

Smedley, B. D., Stith, A. Y., & Nelson, A. R. (2003). *Unequal Treatment Confronting Racial and Ethnic Disparities in Health Care*. Washington, DC: National Academies Press.

Smith, D. G., & Moore, J. D. (2009). *Medicaid Politics and Policy: 1965-2007*. New Brunswick, NJ: Transaction Publishers.

Social Security Act Amendments of 1950, Pub. L. No. 81-734, sections 6, 323, 1006, and 1405, 64 Stat 477–561 (1950).

Social Security Act Amendments of 1956, Pub. L. No. 84-880, sections 301-304, 70 Stat. 846-848 (1956).

Social Security Act of 1935, Pub. L. No. 74-271, sections 3, 403, and 1002, 49 Stat. 620-648 (1935).

Social Security Administration. (1951). *Social Security Bulletin. Annual Statistical Supplement*, *14*(9).

Social Security Administration. (1951-1964). *Social Security Bulletin*, *14*(12)-*27*(12).

South Sudan Profile- Overview. (2015, August). *BBC News*. Retrieved from http://www.bbc.com/news/world-africa-14069082

Staeheli, L. A., & Lawson, V. A. (1995). Feminism, praxis and human geography. *Geographical Analysis*, *27*(4), 321–328. doi:10.1111/j.1538-4632.1995.tb00914.x

Starfield, B., Shi, L., Grover, A., & Macinko, J. (2005). The effects of specialist supply on populations' health: Assessing the evidence. *Health Affairs*. Retrieved from http://content.healthaffairs.org/content/early/2005/03/15/hlthaff.w5.97.full.pdf

Starfield, B., Shi, L., & Macinko, J. (2005). Contribution of primary care to health systems and health. *The Milbank Quarterly*, *83*(3), 457–502. doi:10.1111/j.1468-0009.2005.00409.x PMID:16202000

Stoddard, J., St. Peter, R., & Newacheck, P. (1994). Health insurance status and ambulatory care for children. *The New England Journal of Medicine*, *330*(20), 1421–1425. doi:10.1056/NEJM199405193302006 PMID:8159197

Stone, R. W. (2004). The political economy of IMF lending in Africa. *The American Political Science Review*, *98*(04), 577–591. doi:10.1017/S000305540404136X

Stout, K. E., & Stevens, B. (2000). The Case of the Failed Diversity Rule: A Multiple Streams Analysis. *Educational Evaluation and Policy Analysis*, *22*(4), 341–355. doi:10.3102/01623737022004341

Suggett, D. (2011). *The implementation challenge: strategy is only as good as its execution.* State Services Authority Occasional Paper No. 15.

Sundewall, J., Forsberg, B. C., & Tomson, G. (2006). Theory and practice—a case study of coordination and ownership in the Bangladesh health SWAp. *Health Research Policy and Systems*, *4*(5), 1–8. PMID:16704726

Sundquist, J. L. (1968). *Politics and Policy: The Eisenhower, Kennedy, and Johnson Years.* Washington, DC: The Brookings Institution.

Talukder, M. N., Rob, U., & Mahabub, U A M. (2007). Lessons learned from health sector reform: A four-country comparison. *International Quarterly of Community Health Education*, *28*(2), 153–164. doi:10.2190/IQ.28.2.e PMID:19131306

Tandon, A., Murray, C. J. L., & Evans, D. (2000). *Measuring overall health system performance for 191 countries*. World Health Organization.

Tanner, M. (2008). The grass is not always greener: A look at national health care systems around the world. *Cato Policy Analysis Paper,* (613).

Taylor, K. (2009). Paternalism, participation and partnership. The evolution of patient centeredness in the consultation. *Patient Education and Counseling*, 74. PMID:18930624

Terris, M., Cornely, P. B., Daniels, H. C., & Kerr, L. E. (1977). The case for a national health service. *American Journal of Public Health*, *67*(12), 1183–1185. doi:10.2105/AJPH.67.12.1183 PMID:596502

Thatcher, M. (1998). The development of policy network analyses. *Journal of Theoretical Politics*, *10*(4), 389–416. doi:10.1177/0951692898010004002

The African Leaders Who Chose Power above the People. (2015, January). *BBC News*. Retrieved from http://www.bbc.com/news/world-africa-30886067

The Daily Star. (05June2010).

The Daily Star. (10January, 2009).

The Daily Star. (10March2010).

The Daily Star. (13September, 2008).

The Daily Star. (16September, 2009).

The Daily Star. (1November, 2009).

The Daily Star. (23September, 2008).

The Daily Star. (26July2008).

The Daily Star. (29April, 2004).

The History of EMS at NHTSA. (n.d.). NHTSA EMS. Retrieved from http://www.ems.gov/history.htm

The World Bank Group & International Monetary Fund. (2015). *Global Monitoring Report 2014/2015; Ending Poverty and Sharing Prosperity*. Retrieved from http://www.worldbank.org/content/dam/Worldbank/gmr/gmr2014/GMR_2014_Full_Report.pdf

The World Bank. (2014). *Country and Lending Groups; Sub-Saharan Africa*. Retrieved from http://data.worldbank.org/about/country-and-lending-groups#Sub_Saharan_Africa

The World Bank. (2015). *The International Bank for Reconstruction and Development*. Retrieved from http://www.worldbank.org/en/about/what-we-do/brief/ibrd

Thurow, C. L. (1999). Building Wealth: The New Rules for Individuals, Companies, and Nations in a Knowledge-Based Economy. Harper Business.

Togo Profile Leaders-Togo. (2015, May). *BBC News*. Retrieved from http://www.bbc.com/news/world-africa-14106787

Togo's Faure Gnassingbe Wins Third Term as President. (2015, April). *BBC News*. Retrieved from http://www.bbc.com/news/world-africa-32512615

Top Ten Causes of Death: How Has the Situation Changed in the Past Decade?. (n.d.). *WHO*. Retrieved from http://www.who.int/mediacentre/factsheets/fs310/en/index2.html

Towers-Watson. (2012). *2012 Onsite health center survey report*. Retrieved from: http://www.towerswatson.com/assets/pdf/7705/Realizing-the-Potential-of-Onsite-Health-Centers.pdf

Trafton, G. H., & Feinroth, L. H. (1944). State differences in insurance status under Old-Age and Survivors Insurance. *Social Security Bulletin*, *7*(8), 6–11.

Triassi, M. (2011). *Il management in sanità*. Rome, Italy: Società Editrice Universo.

Tu, H. T., Boukus, E., & Cohen, G. (2010). *Workplace clinics: a sign of Growing employer interest in wellness*. Center for Studying Health System Change Research Brief.

U.S. Census Bureau. (1968). *Current Population Reports, Population Estimates, Series P-25, No. 384*. Retrieved July 2014, from https://www.census.gov/prod/1/pop/p25-384.pdf

U.S. Census Bureau. (2014). *Median family income by State: 1959, 1969, 1979, 1989, and 1999*. Retrieved July 2014, from https://www.census.gov/hhes/www/income/data/historical/state/state2.html

U.S. Department of Health and Human Services. (1991). *Health Status of Minorities and Low Income Groups* (3rd ed.). Washington, DC: U.S. Government Printing Office.

U.S. House. (1949). Congressional Record. 95(August 15), Part 9.

U.S. Senate (1950). Congressional Record. 96(June 13), Part 6.

U.S. Senate (1956). Congressional Record. 102(July 17), Part 10.

Ugolini, C. (1999). *Libertà di scelta in sanità*. Bologna, Italy: Il Mulino.

UHS. (2006). *Urban Health Survey 2006*. Bangladesh: BBS.

UNAIDS. (2013). *Global Report: UNAIDS report on the global AIDS epidemic 2013*. Retrieved from http://www.unaids.org/sites/default/files/en/media/unaids/contentassets/documents/epidemiology/2013/gr2013/UNAIDS_Global_Report_2013_en.pdf

UNDP Human Development Reports. (n.d.). *Table 1: Human Development Index and Its Components*. Available from: http://hdr.undp.org/en/content/table-1-human-development-index-and-its-components

UNDP Human Development Reports. (n.d.). *Table 1: Human Development Index and its components*. Retrieved from http://hdr.undp.org/en/content/table-1-human-development-index-and-its-components

United Nations, UN List of Least Developed Countries. (2015). Retrieved from http://www.un.org/en/development/desa/policy/cdp/ldc/ldc_list.pdf

United Nations. (2015). *We can end poverty; Millennium Development Goals*. Retrieved from http://www.un.org/millenniumgoals/

United Nations. (n.d.). *UN List of Least Developed Countries*. Available from: http://www.un.org/en/development/desa/policy/cdp/ldc/ldc_list.pdf

USAID. (2009). *Sustaining health gains –Building systems*. Washington, DC: United States Agency for International Development.

Varvasovszky, Z., & Brugha, R. (2000). How to do a stakeholder analysis. *Health Policy and Planning*, *15*(3), 338–345. doi:10.1093/heapol/15.3.338 PMID:11012410

Vasselli, S., Filippetti, G., & Spizzichino, L. (2005). *Misurare la performance di un sistema sanitario*. Rome, Italy: Il Pensiero Scientifico.

Vendramini, E. (2004). *Il sistema di budget per le aziende sanitarie pubbliche*. Milan, Italy: McGraw-Hill.

Verschuere, B. (2009). The role of public agencies in the policy making process: Rhetoric versus reality. *Public Policy and Administration*, *24*(1), 22–46. doi:10.1177/0952076708097907

Walt, G., & Gilson, L. (1994). Reforming the health sector in developing countries: the central role of policy analysis. *Health Policy and Planning, 9*(4).

Walt, G., & Gilson, L. (1994). Reforming the health sector in developing countries: The central role of policy analysis. *Health Policy and Planning*, *9*(4), 353–370. doi:10.1093/heapol/9.4.353 PMID:10139469

Walt, G., Pavignani, E., Gilson, L., & Buse, K. (1999). Health sector development: From aid coordination to resource management. *Health Policy and Planning*, *14*(3), 207–218. doi:10.1093/heapol/14.3.207 PMID:10621238

Ward, B. (2014, September 1). *Journalists Are Losing Access, but the Public Still Expects the Story*. Academic Press.

Watson, S. (1994). Minority access and health reform: A civil right to health care. *The Journal of Law, Medicine & Ethics*, *22*(2), 127–137. doi:10.1111/j.1748-720X.1994.tb01285.x PMID:7921079

WB. (2005). *The Economics and Governance of Non Governmental Organizations (NGOs) in Bangladesh*. Poverty Reduction and Economic Management Sector Unit South Asia Region.

Weaver, D., McCombs, M., & Spellman, C. (1975). Watergate and the Media: A Case Study of Agenda-Setting. *American Politics Research*, *3*(4), 458–472. doi:10.1177/1532673X7500300407

Weber, M. (1994). *Political Writings*. University of Cambridge Press.

Weingast, B., & Moran, M. (1983). Bureaucratic discretion or congressional control? Regulatory policy-making by the Federal Trade Commission. *Journal of Political Economy*, *91*(5), 765–800. doi:10.1086/261181

Weiss, C. H. (1997). *Evaluation* (2nd ed.). Prentice Hall.

Whiteford, L. M., & Szelag. (2000). Access and Utility as reflections of culture construction of pregnancv. *Primary Care Update*, *7*, 98-104.

WHO. (1978a). Report of a WHO/International Study Team. (1978). Ebola Haemorrhagic Fever in Sudan, 1976. *Bulletin of the World Health Organization*, *56*, 247–270.

WHO. (1978b). Report of an International Commission. (1978). Ebola Haemorrhagic Fever in Zaire, 1976. *Bulletin of the World Health Organization*, *56*, 271–293.

WHO. (2000). *The World Health Report*. Geneva: WHO.

WHO. (2000). *World Health Report 2000 – Health systems: improving performance*. Geneva: WHO Press.

WHO. (2007). *Everybody's business. Strengthening health systems to improve health outcomes: WHO's framework for action*. WHO.

WHO. (2014a). *The health of the people-what works: The African regional health report*. Retrieved from http://apps.who.int/iris/bitstream/10665/137377/4/9789290232612.pdf?ua=1

WHO. (2014b). *The 10 leading causes of death in the world 2000 and 2012*. Retrieved from http://www.who.int/mediacentre/factsheets/fs310/en/

WHO/UNICEF/UNFPA. (1999). *Women-friendly health services Experiences in maternal care, Report of a WHO/UNICEF/UNFPA Workshop, Mexico City, 26-28 January*. Retrieved from http://www.unicef.org/health/files/womenfriendlyhealthservices.pdf

Wilson, B. (2012). *The Impact of Media Agenda Setting on Local Governments*. (Dissertation). North Carolina State University, Raleigh, NC. Retrieved from http://repository.lib.ncsu.edu/ir/bitstream/1840.16/7870/1/etd.pdf

Winter, S. (2003). Implementation perspectives: status and reconsideration. In G. Peters & J. Pierre (Eds.), *Handbook of Public Administration* (pp. 212–222). London: Sage. doi:10.4135/9781848608214.n17

Wolff, M. J. (2013). Failure of the International Monetary Fund and World Bank to Achieve Integral Development: A Critical Historical Assessment of Bretton Woods Institutions Policies, Structures & Governance. *Syracuse Journal of International Law & Commerce*, *41*, 71–144.

World Bank. (2007). *Healthy development: the World Bank strategy for health, nutrition and population results*. Washington, DC: The World Bank.

Yin, R. (1994). *Case study research: design and methods* (2nd ed.). Thousand Oaks, CA: Sage Publications.

Yin, R. (2004). *The case study anthology*. Thousand Oaks, CA: Sage Publications.

Yurk, M. J., Christensen, K., & Wright, E. (2008). *Overuse of specialty care increases costs in Indiana*. Center for Health Policy.

About the Contributors

Khadijeh Rouzbehani is a distinguished researcher in university of Tehran who has been running her consulting firm for roughly a decade. She has been consulting and running workshops in Iran .Her expertise is Policy analysis, policy evaluation, Health policy, organizational behavior and leadership, ethics and KM.

* * *

Laura Caccioppoli has a Masters in Political Science and certificate in Nonprofit Management from Villanova University.

Ubaldo Comite was born in Cosenza, Italy, June 14 1971. He has a degree in Law (1994) and Economics (1996) at the University of Messina (Italy), and earned his Ph.D. in Public Administration at the University of Calabria, Rende (Cs) Italy, in 2005. Currently he is a professor of Budget and Business Organization at the Faculty of Economy, Department of Business Sciences, University of Calabria. Furthermore he is a professor of Business Administration at the Faculty of Economy, University Giustino Fortunato (Benevento – Italy). His Research interests are: Private and Public Management, Non profit Organizations and Accounting.

Minerva Cruz joined Western Michigan University in Fall 2014. She holds a Ph.D. in Political Science with a specialization in Public Administration and Public Policy from Purdue University. She also specializes in Political Economy, Quantitative Methods, Organizational Behavior and Human Resources, and has a M.A. in Public Administration from the University of Puerto Rico. Her teaching regimen includes Health Care policies and courses in Public Administration and Public Policy. Her most recent publication can be found in the book The Theories of Decentralization and Local Government: Implementation, Implications, and Realities. A Global Perspective, 2013, entitled "Medicaid: The Decentralization of Health Policies in the United States and Puerto Rico." Dr. Cruz has varied research interests, including Public Health Care Administration, Public Policy Implementation, Comparative Studies, and Culture, among others. A particular area of interest is social policy regarding the elderly population in the United States and Puerto Rico. Dr. Cruz has earned various awards, including the Frank Wilson Award given by the Purdue University Political Science Department, the Rosa E. Axtmayer Fellowship from the University of Puerto Rico, the Public Employees Fellowship from the Association of Employees of Puerto Rico, and the Rector's Honor Role at the University of Puerto Rico.

Zohreh Karimmian took her master in Industrial Engineering from Tehran Polytechnic. She is working as Advisor to some Iranian public organizations and after passing some experiences in strategic planning and public policy-making, she is now a PhD candidate in"Science & Technology Policy-making" at university of Tehran.

Titilola Obilade is a medical doctor and a senior education specialist. She earned her Ph.D. in Learning Sciences and Technologies from Virginia Polytechnic Institute and State University. She is also an alumnus of University of Lagos, Nigeria where she earned her MBBS in Medicine and Surgery. She has authored and coauthored more than 20 refereed articles, book chapters and a textbook in areas of instructional design and technology, human computer interaction, health education and infectious diseases. Her most recent work is a textbook on visual literacy.

Robert Peters is a professor in the School of Public Affairs and Administration at Western Michigan University. He teaches courses in government and health care finance, intergovernmental relations, health care policy, and statistics. His research focuses on the politics of public budgeting, intergovernmental relations, and pedagogy.

Virginia Sizemore is a healthcare administration professional with over 26 years of experience in the field. She has served in a variety of roles, including regulatory compliance, internal audit, training and development, financial planning, revenue cycle, data analytics and cost accounting. Ms. Sizemore is currently a doctoral candidate pursuing a Doctor of Public Administration degree with a concentration in Healthcare Policy from Valdosta State University. She holds certifications in Healthcare Compliance (CHC) and is a Certified Internal Auditor (CIA).

Mary Eleanor Wickersham has a B.A. from Emory University, the M.A. in Public Affairs from Georgia College and State University, and a Doctorate in Public Administration from Valdosta State University. She is an Assistant Professor of Public Affairs at the College of Coastal Georgia.

Bradley Wilson, Ph.D., is an assistant professor at Midwestern State University. He is the editor of the national magazine of the Journalism Education Association — Communication: Journalism Education Today and co-managing editor of College Media Review, the magazine and research journal of the College Media Association. In 2014, the National Press Photographers Association named him the Robin F. Garland Educator of the Year and the College Media Association named him a Four-Year Newspaper Honor Roll Adviser. He worked for more than two decades in pre-hospital healthcare in three states as an EMT-I.

Mostafa Zamanian has been working as Advisor to many Iranian public organizations since 2002. Particularly in 2004, he was Advisor in the Ministry of Health and Medical Education were he gained excellent experiences in Public Health. He took his master in Industrial Engineering and after several years of advising in various fields, especially public policy and strategic planning, he is PhD in public administration & policy making.

Index

I

L

M

N

O

P

www.ingramcontent.com/pod-product-compliance
Lightning Source LLC
LaVergne TN
LVHW061549290926
849162LV00004B/958